Geriatric Psychiatry: Advances and Directions

Guest Editors

GEORGE S. ALEXOPOULOS, MD
DIMITRIS N. KIOSSES, PhD

PSYCHIATRIC CLINICS OF NORTH AMERICA

www.psych.theclinics.com

June 2011 • Volume 34 • Number 2

SAUNDERS an imprint of ELSEVIER, Inc.

MT

W.B. SAUNDERS COMPANY
A Division of Elsevier Inc.

1600 John F. Kennedy Boulevard • Suite 1800 • Philadelphia, PA 19103-2899

http://www.theclinics.com

PSYCHIATRIC CLINICS OF NORTH AMERICA Volume 34, Number 2
June 2011 ISSN 0193-953X, ISBN-13: 978-1-4557-0499-6

Editor: Sarah E. Barth
Developmental Editor: Jessica Demetriou

Psychiatric Clinics of North America (ISSN 0193-953X) is published quarterly by Elsevier Inc., 360 Park Avenue South, New York, NY 10010-1710. Months of issue are March, June, September, and December. Business and Editorial Offices: 1600 John F. Kennedy Blvd., Suite 1800, Philadelphia, PA 19103-2899. Periodicals postage paid at New York, NY and additional mailing offices. Subscription prices are $265.00 per year (US individuals), $473.00 per year (US institutions), $131.00 per year (US students/residents), $321.00 per year (Canadian individuals), $589.00 per year (Canadian Institutions), $399.00 per year (foreign individuals), $589.00 per year (foreign institutions), and $194.00 per year (international & Canadian students/residents). Foreign air speed delivery is included in all *Clinics'* subscription prices. All prices are subject to change without notice. **POSTMASTER:** Send address changes to *Psychiatric Clinics of North America*, Elsevier Health Sciences Division, Subscription Customer Service, 3251 Riverport Lane, Maryland Heights, MO 63043. Customer Service: 1-800-654-2452 (US). From outside the United States, call 1-314-447-8871. Fax: 1-314-447-8029. E-mail: journalscustomerservice-usa@elsevier.com (for print support) and journalsonlinesupport-usa@elsevier.com (for online support).

Reprints. For copies of 100 or more, of articles in this publication, please contact the Commercial Reprints Department, Elsevier Inc., 360 Park Avenue South, New York, New York 10010-1710. Tel.: (212) 633-3813, Fax: (212) 462-1935, E-mail: reprints@elsevier.com.

Psychiatric Clinics of North America is covered in *MEDLINE/PubMed (Index Medicus)*, *Current Contents/Social and Behavioral Sciences*, *Social Science Citation Index*, *Embase/Excerpta Medica,* and PsycINFO.

Printed in the United States of America.

10/17/11

Contributors

GUEST EDITORS

GEORGE S. ALEXOPOULOS, MD
SP Tobin and AM Cooper Professor; Director, Weill-Cornell Institute of Geriatric Psychiatry, White Plains, New York

DIMITRIS N. KIOSSES, PhD
Associate Professor of Psychology in Clinical Psychiatry, Weill-Cornell Institute of Geriatric Psychiatry, White Plains, New York

AUTHORS

GEORGE S. ALEXOPOULOS, MD
SP Tobin and AM Cooper Professor; Director, Weill-Cornell Institute of Geriatric Psychiatry, White Plains, New York

CARMEN ANDREESCU, MD
Department of Psychiatry, Western Psychiatric Institute and Clinic, University of Pittsburgh, Pittsburgh, Pennsylvania

PATRICIA A. AREÁN, PhD
Professor, Department of Psychiatry, University of California, San Francisco, San Francisco, California

SOPHIYA BENJAMIN, MD
Geriatric Psychiatry Fellow, Department of Psychiatry, Duke University Medical Center, DHSP, Durham, North Carolina

ERIC D. CAINE, MD
Professor and John Romano Chair, Department of Psychiatry, University of Rochester Medical Center, Rochester, New York

PEIJUN CHEN, MD, PhD, MPH
Assistant Professor of Psychiatry, Geriatric Psychiatry, Department of Psychiatry, Louis Stokes Cleveland Veterans Affairs Medical Center, Case Western Reserve University School of Medicine, Brecksville, Ohio

YEATES CONWELL, MD
Professor of Psychiatry, Department of Psychiatry, University of Rochester Medical Center, Rochester, New York

FAITH M. GUNNING, PhD
Associate Professor of Psychology, Weill-Cornell Institute of Geriatric Psychiatry, White Plains, New York

ALANA IGLEWICZ, MD
Geriatric Psychiatry Research Fellow, Department of Psychiatry, University of California, San Diego, San Diego, California

DILIP V. JESTE, MD
Estelle and Edgar Levi Chair in Aging; Distinguished Professor of Psychiatry and
Neurosciences; Director, Sam and Rose Stein Institute for Research on Aging,
University of California, San Diego, San Diego, California

DIMITRIS N. KIOSSES, PhD
Associate Professor of Psychology in Clinical Psychiatry, Weill-Cornell Institute
of Geriatric Psychiatry, White Plains, New York

ANDREW C. LEON, PhD
DeWitt Wallace Senior Scholar; Professor of Biostatistics in Psychiatry; Professor of
Public Health; Weill-Cornell Institute of Geriatric Psychiatry, New York, New York

FRANCIS E. LOTRICH, MD, PhD
Assistant Professor of Psychiatry, Western Psychiatric Institute and Clinics,
University of Pittsburgh Medical Center, Pittsburgh, Pennsylvania

CONSTANTINE G. LYKETSOS, MD, MHS
Elizabeth Plank Althouse Professor and Chairman, Department of Psychiatry,
Johns Hopkins Bayview Medical Center, Baltimore, Maryland

THOMAS W. MEEKS, MD
Assistant Professor of Psychiatry, Department of Psychiatry, University of California,
San Diego, San Diego, California

SARAH SHIZUKO MORIMOTO, PsyD
Research Fellow, Weill-Cornell Institute of Geriatric Psychiatry, White Plains,
New York

MILAP A. NOWRANGI, MD, MBe
Postdoctoral Fellow, Department of Psychiatry and Behavioral Sciences,
Johns Hopkins University School of Medicine; Department of Psychiatry,
Johns Hopkins Bayview Medical Center, Baltimore, Maryland

MIJUNG PARK, RN, PhD
Post-doctoral Fellow, University of Washington, Seattle, Washington

VANI RAO, MD
Associate Professor, Department of Psychiatry, Johns Hopkins Bayview
Medical Center, Baltimore, Maryland

PATRICK J. RAUE, PhD
Associate Professor of Psychology in Psychiatry, Weill-Cornell Institute of Geriatric
Psychiatry, White Plains, New York

CHARLES F. REYNOLDS III, MD
Department of Psychiatry, Western Psychiatric Institute and Clinic,
University of Pittsburgh, Pittsburgh, Pennsylvania

MARTHA SAJATOVIC, MD
Professor of Psychiatry; Director of Geriatric Psychiatry, Department of Psychiatry;
Director, Neurological Outcomes Center, Neurological Institute, University
Hospitals of Cleveland, Case Western Reserve University School of Medicine,
Cleveland, Ohio

JO ANNE SIREY, PhD
Associate Professor of Psychology in Psychiatry, Weill-Cornell Institute of Geriatric Psychiatry, White Plains, New York

GWENN S. SMITH, PhD
Professor, Department of Psychiatry and Behavioral Sciences, Johns Hopkins Bayview Medical Center, Baltimore, Maryland

DAVID C. STEFFENS, MD, MHS
Professor and Head, Division of Geriatric Psychiatry, Department of Psychiatry and Behavioral Sciences, Duke University Medical Center, DHSP, Durham, North Carolina

JÜRGEN UNÜTZER, MD, MPH, MA
Professor and Vice Chair, Psychiatry and Behavioral Sciences; Chief of Psychiatry, University of Washington Medical Center; Director, UW AIMS Center; Director, IMPACT Implementation Program, University of Washington, Seattle, Washington

KIMBERLY VAN ORDEN, PhD
Instructor, Department of Psychiatry, University of Rochester Medical Center, Rochester, New York

Contents

> The risk of developing dementia is associated with increasing age, life-style, and cardiovascular health. Alzheimer dementia is characterized by progressive cognitive deficits and decline in functional ability. Using history, examination, and laboratory testing, the clinician can evaluate the patient with dementia. Specific to these conditions are assessments of cognition, neuropsychiatric symptoms, and level of functioning. Managing neuropsychiatric symptoms is challenging and requires a team approach in which nonpharmacological strategies are preferred before medications are considered. Various diagnostic methods are being developed to discriminate disease from nondisease and track progression. Drug discovery is identifying novel molecules that target underlying disease mechanisms.

> Psychosis is common in late-life and exacts enormous costs to society, affected individuals, and their caregivers. A multitude of etiologies for late-life psychosis exist, the two most prototypical being schizophrenia and psychosis of Alzheimer disease (AD). As such, this article focuses on the nonaffective, neuropsychiatric causes of chronic psychosis in the elderly, specifically schizophrenia, delusional disorder, and the psychosis of AD and other dementias.

> Because the elderly are the fastest growing segment of the population, the number of older adults with bipolar disorder is increasing. Geriatric bipolar disorder is relatively rare, with an estimated lifetime prevalence of 0.5% to 1%, although approximately 4% to 17% of older patients in clinical psychiatric settings have bipolar disorder. Bipolar elders are disproportionately affected by medical burden. Given the complex nature of this disorder, comorbidity, and behavioral disturbances, various interventions may be indicated, including pharmacotherapies, electroconvulsive therapy, psychotherapies, and integrated care models. Additional research is needed to better understand the epidemiology, phenomenology, and treatment of geriatric bipolar disorder.

> As the population ages, successive cohorts of older adults will experience depressive disorders. Late-life depression (LLD) carries additional risk for

suicide, medical comorbidity, disability, and family caregiving burden. Although response and remission rates to pharmacotherapy and electro-convulsive therapy are comparable with those in midlife depression, relapse rates are higher, underscoring the challenge to achieve and maintain wellness. This article reviews the evidence base for LLD treatment options and provides an analysis of treatment options for difficult-to-treat LLD variants (eg, psychotic depression, vascular depression). Treatment algorithms are also reviewed based on predictors of response and promising novel treatment options.

In older adults, several environmental challenges can potentially trigger the onset of an episode of major depression. Vulnerability to these challenges can be influenced by genetics. There is accumulating evidence for an interaction between stress and a serotonin transporter polymorphism, though there is also heterogeneity among studies. Other relevant genes include those encoding for the neuroendocrine stress axis, growth factors, and other monoaminergic systems. Each of these may interact with either predisposing traumas in early childhood or precipitating events later in life.

This systematic review evaluates the efficacy of psychosocial interventions for the acute treatment of late-life depression and identifies predictors of treatment outcomes and moderators of treatment effects. Problem-solving therapy, cognitive behavioral therapy, and treatment initiation and participation program have supportive evidence of efficacy, pending replication. Although the data on predictors of treatment outcomes and moderators of treatment effects are preliminary, it appears that baseline anxiety and stress level, personality disorders, endogenous depression, and reduced self-rated health predict worse depression outcomes. Future research may examine the moderating effects of baseline depression severity and identify other clinical or demographic moderators.

Abnormalities in specific cerebral networks likely confer vulnerability that increases the susceptibility for development of geriatric depression and affect the course of symptoms. Functional neuroimaging enables the in vivo identification of alterations in cerebral function that characterize disease vulnerability and contribute to variability in depressive symptoms and antidepressant response. Judicious use of functional neuroimaging tools can advance pathophysiologic models of geriatric depression. Furthermore, geriatric depression provides a logical context within which to study the role of specific functional abnormalities in both antidepressant response and key behavioral and cognitive abnormalities of mood disorders.

of engaging and supporting family caregivers of depressed older adults and the 3 strategic areas to improve the treatment of geriatric depression in primary care are also discussed.

Designing Personalized Treatment Engagement Interventions for Depressed Older Adults

Patrick J. Raue and Jo Anne Sirey

Despite the benefits of treatment for late-life depression, underutilization of mental health services by older adults and nonadherence to offered interventions exist. This article describes psychosocial and interactional barriers and facilitators of treatment engagement among depressed older adults served by community health care settings. The authors describe the need to engage older adults in treatment using interventions that: (1) target psychological barriers such as stigma and other negative beliefs about depression and its treatment; and (2) increase individuals' involvement in the treatment decision-making process. Personalized treatment engagement interventions designed by the authors' group for various community settings are presented.

RELATED INTEREST

Clinics in Geriatric Medicine, February 2010 (Vol. 26, No. 1)
**Healthy Brain Aging: Evidence Based Methods to Preserve Brain
Function and Prevent Dementia**
Abhilash K. Desai, MD, *Guest Editor*

THE CLINICS ARE NOW AVAILABLE ONLINE!
Access your subscription at:
www.theclinics.com

Preface

Geriatric Psychiatry: Advances and Directions

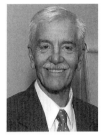 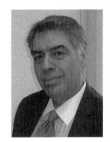

George S. Alexopoulos, MD   Dimitris N. Kiosses, PhD
Guest Editors

As the population of older adults is expected to rise in the next two decades, a significant number of older adults will be in need of treatment for mental disorders. The demographic imperative mandates awareness of safe and reliable facts about geriatric mental disorders and of cutting edge findings on their management. Written by distinguished investigators and thinkers in our field, this issue offers an up-to-date summary of where our field is now and where we hope to go in the near future. We are grateful to our contributors, whose pioneering work has made Geriatric Psychiatry what it is today. Their thoughtful writing conveys these achievements with clarity and reflects their research creativity and clinical experience and judgment. We greatly appreciate the help of Sarah Barth, Peg Ennis, and the rest of the Elsevier staff, whose help was critical in producing this issue.

Old age is associated with cognitive impairment and poses a risk for dementing disorders. Dementia contributes to increased morbidity and mortality and exorbitant costs for patients, families, and society. Nowrangi and coworkers provide a clear review on the epidemiology, assessment, and treatment of dementia and highlight promising diagnostic methods and novel biological discoveries that may help improve the lives of patients with dementia and their families.

Although severe mental illnesses shorten the sufferers' life span, many survive into old age and new cases are added. Iglewicz and colleagues offer a review of late-life psychosis covering early-onset and late-onset schizophrenia, delusional disorder, and psychoses of patients with dementing disorders. They focus on the neuropsychiatric causes of psychoses in the elderly, the existing pharmacological and psychosocial treatments, as well as directions for future research. Sajatovic and Chen present an overview of the epidemiology, phenomenology, assessment, and diagnosis of geriatric bipolar disorder and underline the complexities of pharmacological treatment, electroconvulsive therapy, and psychosocial interventions. Because of the dearth of research on late-life bipolar disorder, many findings are a thoughtful extrapolation

Psychiatr Clin N Am 34 (2011) xiii–xv
doi:10.1016/j.psc.2011.03.002
psych.theclinics.com

from studies of mixed-aged and young adults. The authors point out areas in which findings on young adults may offer inadequate guidance, highlight the need for prospective studies on geriatric bipolar disorder, and outline a research agenda for future studies.

Andreescu and Reynolds, in a well-targeted review of evidence-based treatments for late-life depression, highlight the difficulties of achieving and maintaining remission with the available pharmacotherapy and psychosocial treatments. They also discuss novel treatments, such as transcranial magnetic stimulation, deep brain stimulation, vagus nerve stimulation, and magnetic seizure therapy. Finally, they propose future research directions including genetic studies to develop individualized treatments. Lotrich follows with an exceptional review of the methodologies and results of genetic studies and discusses the potential interaction of genes with environmental factors.

Fewer than 50% of older adults on antidepressants achieve remission of late-life major depression. As a result, psychosocial interventions addressing the clinical complexity and the interplay of depressive symptoms with the cognitive impairment and disability remain critical. The review by Kiosses and colleagues summarizes the psychosocial interventions with evidence of efficacy in late-life major depression and proposes recommendations for future research including application of interventions in nontraditional settings and expansion of research to include more racially and ethnically diverse populations.

Many of the brain structures implicated in late-life depression are preferentially affected by aging. For this reason, geriatric depression provides the context for studying functional abnormalities due to age-related vulnerability of brain systems. Gunning and Smith present a comprehensive review of functional neuroimaging studies and point out strategies for identifying dysfunctions of networks contributing to late-life depression and interfering with treatment response.

The developments of advanced structural neuroimaging techniques enable us to see aspects of the brain microstructure that could not be seen or measured earlier. Benjamin and Steffens provide an in-depth review of structural neuroimaging findings in geriatric depression derived from studies of magnetic resonance morphometry, diffusion tensor imaging, and magnetic resonance spectroscopy. Beyond outlining where the field is, they offer guidance for future research neuroanatomic markers in geriatric depression.

Increased inflammatory responses occur during aging, during exposure to stress, and in medical and neurological illnesses often comorbid with late-life depression. Brain areas related to mood processing have increased inflammatory responses, and connectivity among mood-regulating structures may be modulated by inflammatory responses. Geriatric depression exacerbates comorbid medical and neurological disorders, raising the question whether depression-related inflammatory changes mediate the worsening of their outcomes. Morimoto and Alexopoulos present theoretical arguments for the "inflammatory hypothesis" in late-life depression and a research agenda that may further clarify the role of inflammation and contribute to novel therapeutics.

Late-life mental disorders pose the highest risk for suicide. Conwell and coworkers argue that "suicide is a developmental process to which risk and protective factors contribute in defining a trajectory to suicide over time." They describe the risk and protective factors of late-life suicide and present three levels of preventive interventions: indicated (targeting individuals with detectable symptoms and other proximal risk factors), selective (targeting asymptomatic or presymptomatic individuals or groups with more distal risk factors), and universal (targeting an entire population).

Most patients with late-life depression are treated in the primary care sector, and despite efforts to improve diagnosis and treatment, many cases remain underdiagnosed and incorrectly treated. Park and Unützer offer a thoughtful review of depression seen in primary care settings, identify barriers to treatment, and explore treatment strategies, including stepped-care and collaborative care, to improve the effectiveness of depression treatment. Important areas of intervention include engagement of patients and families, providers' training, and organizational changes to facilitate the implementation of evidence-based treatment programs. Raue and Sirey discuss psychosocial and communication barriers and facilitators of treatment engagement among older adults in community health care settings and describe personalized treatment engagement interventions in community agencies and primary care, targeting the referral process, early adherence, and participation in treatment as well as shared decision-making.

Health care needs of older adults are highlighted as a national priority by the Surgeon General and National Institutes of Health. Late-life mental disorders may have detrimental consequences for patients and their families, increasing medical morbidity, mortality, and disability, and often requiring relocation or institutionalization. We hope that this issue will serve as a guide to clinical care and add to the evolving research agenda on the biology and treatment of late-life mental disorders.

George S. Alexopoulos, MD
Dimitris N. Kiosses, PhD

Weill-Cornell Institute of Geriatric Psychiatry
21 Bloomingdale Road
White Plains, NY 10605, USA

E-mail addresses:
gsalexop@med.cornell.edu (G.S. Alexopoulos)
dkiosses@med.cornell.edu (D.N. Kiosses)

Epidemiology, Assessment, and Treatment of Dementia

Milap A. Nowrangi, MD, MBe[a,b,*], Vani Rao, MD[b],
Constantine G. Lyketsos, MD, MHS[b]

KEYWORDS

- Dementia • Alzheimer Disease • Epidemiology • Assessment
- Treatment

As our population ages, clinicians will see increasing numbers of patients who seek medical attention with memory or other cognitive complaints. The clinician is faced with the challenge of understanding these conditions to reach a diagnosis and offer treatment. This article contributes to this endeavor by synthesizing what is currently known about the epidemiology, clinical evaluation, and guidelines for treatment of the cognitive disorders, with special emphasis on Alzheimer dementia (AD), to give the clinician a sense of promising experimental diagnostic techniques and novel treatments currently in development that may soon come to practice as cutting-edge research in the field continues. It provides a basic conceptual framework on which we will build later material.

NOSOLOGY AND PHENOMENOLOGY

Criteria for the diagnosis of dementia are included in the Diagnostic and Statistics Manual fourth Text Revision (DSM-IV-TR).[1] Criteria for AD were established by the National Institute of Neurological Disorders and Stroke/Alzheimer's Disease and Related Disorders Association (NINDS/ADRDA) in 1984 and include definitions for definite, probable, possible, and unlikely AD.[2] Together, criteria for dementia, more specifically AD, identify progressive cognitive impairments in multiple domains and deficits in functioning as core features. Recently, proposals for updated criteria that would reflect the major scientific advances in the last 25 years were provided at the 2010 Alzheimer's Association International meeting, and these are discussed later in this article.

The authors have nothing to disclose.
[a] Department of Psychiatry and Behavioral Sciences, Johns Hopkins University School of Medicine, Baltimore, MD 21287, USA
[b] Department of Psychiatry, Johns Hopkins Bayview Medical Center, 5300 Alpha Commons Drive, 4th Floor, Baltimore, MD 21224, USA
* Corresponding author. Department of Psychiatry and Behavioral Sciences, Johns Hopkins University School of Medicine, Baltimore, MD.
E-mail address: mnowran1@jhmi.edu

Psychiatr Clin N Am 34 (2011) 275–294
doi:10.1016/j.psc.2011.02.004
0193-953X/11/$ – see front matter © 2011 Elsevier Inc. All rights reserved.

Because dementia is a syndrome, it is defined entirely on clinical grounds. Four key elements of this syndrome are (1) dementia affects cognition (ie, processes involved in memory, attention, perception, abstract thought, judgment, and the abilities to think, organize, learn, and execute purposeful action); (2) several areas of cognition are affected (ie, it is global); (3) the symptoms represent a decline in functioning; (4) there is an absence of delirium.[3] In addition, many patients with dementia exhibit neuropsychiatric symptoms that may include changes in mood, perceptual discrimination, agitation, wandering, and violence. Neurological symptoms such as changes in gait, continence, other focal neurological findings, and seizures may also be present. The complexity and wide range of clinical presentations reinforces the concept of syndrome rather than a discrete disease process.

Dementia is at the severe end of a continuum of cognitive effects of brain diseases. **Table 1** presents several key concepts that illustrate this continuum. Syndromal states (cognitive impairment not dementia [CIND]) are differentiated from subsyndromal states (mild cognitive impairment [MCI]). Disease, which is characterized by the presence of identifiable pathological changes, is a discrete brain process that presumably causes the observed syndrome.[4] These pathological changes are discussed briefly later.

The more common dementia causes are listed in **Table 2**. Although these seem to exist independently of each other, postmortem autopsy of those diagnosed with dementia in the community typically show mixed, rather than unitary, brain abnormalities (eg, presence of both plaques and tangles as well as microinfarcts).[5–7] Most agree that Alzheimer disease is the most prevalent cause of dementia, followed by vascular dementia (VaD), and then either frontotemporal dementia (FTD) or Lewy body disease (LBD).[5,6,8] Less common causes of dementia include normal-pressure hydrocephalus (NPH), traumatic brain injury (TBI), acquired immune deficiency syndrome (AIDS), Huntington disease (HD), prion diseases (eg, Creutzfeldt-Jakob disease), primary progressive aphasia (PPA), corticobasal degeneration (CBD), and dementia of depression (in the past referred to as pseudodementia). Although not as rare as was once believed, an extended discussion of these is beyond the scope of this article.[9]

PATHOPHYSIOLOGY

Although an in-depth review of the pathophysiology of these neurodegenerative diseases exceeds the boundaries this article, the clinician is well served to become familiar with several basic genetic and neurochemical concepts. Although the exact

Table 1 Key definitions related to dementia	
CIND	A clinical syndrome with deficits in memory or other cognitive abilities that have minimal impact on day-to-day functioning and does not meet criteria for dementia
MCI	A clinical subsyndrome of CIND. Amnestic or nonamnestic
Dementia	A clinical syndrome consisting of global cognitive decline, memory deficits plus 1 other area of cognition, and significant effect on day-to-day functioning. Not delirium
Alzheimer dementia	A dementia syndrome that has gradual onset and slow progression and is best explained as caused by Alzheimer disease
Alzheimer disease	A brain disease characterized by plaques, tangles, and neuronal loss

Abbreviations: CIND, cognitive impairment not dementia; MCI, mild cognitive impairment.

Table 2
Major types of dementia

	Hallmark Features	Estimated Prevalence Range (%)
Alzheimer disease	Brain disease characterized by plaques, tangles, and neuronal loss. Clinically manifested with slow cognitive decline and loss of functioning	60–80
Vascular dementia	Also known as multi-infarct dementia. Stepwise progression. Symptoms overlap with AD. Focal neurologic signs	20–40
Lewy body disease	Deficits of memory, judgment, behavior. Visual hallucinations and muscle rigidity (parkinsonism) are common. α-Synuclein deposits in neurons	5–20
Frontotemporal dementia	Focal atrophy of frontal and temporal lobes; knife-edge atrophy on MRI. Changes in personality and behavior. Deficits in language	5–20

Abbreviation: MRI, magnetic resonance imaging.

mechanisms remain unknown, dementia, regardless of cause, is the result of pathological processes that represent a departure from normal aging. In AD, the best-established etiologic hypothesis involves the development of proteinaceous senile plaques and neurofibrillary tangles along 2 parallel pathways. Plaques are formed by proteolytic processing of the amyloid precursor protein (APP) producing β amyloid peptide (Aβ) through APP-cleaving enzyme and γ-secretase action on the β site.[10] Aggregation of Aβ has several deleterious effects that are believed to result in neuronal death, the proximal event to symptom manifestation. Tau proteins are the major component of the neurofibrillary tangles. Tau hyperphosphorylation is a purported mechanism by which a cascade of neurochemical steps is set into motion, resulting in neuronal death.[11,12] Four major genes have been associated with AD: *APOE*, *SORL1*, *PSEN1*, and *PSEN2*.[13] An allele of apolipoprotein called ε4 (ApoE4) is associated with more than 50% of cases of AD.[14,15] The *SORL1* gene has recently been associated with late-onset AD.[16–18] The SORL1 protein may alter intracellular trafficking of APP, causing aggregated Aβ to accumulate, ultimately causing cell death.[16] Mutations in the *PSEN1* gene account for 18% to 55% of early-onset familial AD cases, whereas mutations in *PSEN2* and *APP* genes are less common.[19] These genetic loci interact through mechanisms that are currently being studied. A 2010 meta-analysis by Jun and colleagues[20] confirmed that the *APOE* and *PICALM* (encoding phosphatidylinositol-binding clathrin assembly protein) gene products interact in a pathogenic pathway with other β-amyloid–producing genes (*PSEN1*, *PSEN2*, *APP*), leading to AD.

EPIDEMIOLOGY
Prevalence

Estimates by the United Nations indicate that the world's population is aging at an accelerated rate, especially in the more developed regions **Fig. 1**. By 2050, the number of those older than 65 years is expected to grow more rapidly than any other age group and, in 2006, their numbers exceeded 700 million.[21] The greatest rates of

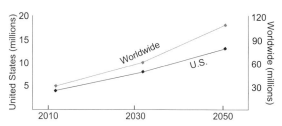

Fig. 1. Projected prevalence of dementia. (*Data from* Refs.[21–23])

increase will occur among the very old, those aged more than 90 years. Because increasing age is the major risk factor for dementia (AD in particular), the prevalence of AD and other dementias will also increase. The latest figures from the Alzheimer's Association indicate that there are an estimated 5.3 million Americans living with AD. By 2050, an estimated 11 million to 16 million people are expected to be diagnosed with AD in the United States.[22] Data from Alzheimer's Disease International (ADI) forecast that the prevalence of AD will double every 20 years, to 65.7 million by 2030 and 115.4 million by 2050, with higher proportions in developed versus undeveloped countries.[23,24]

Demographics

Studies of dementia incidence from the Aging, Demographics, and Memory Study (ADAMS) and the Cache County study suggest that women are at greater risk for developing dementia than men, especially among the very old.[25,26] Other studies of age-specific incidence and analysis of patterns of cognitive decline show no significant gender difference.[26–28] One explanation for the lack of agreement between these sets of studies is that women tend to live longer than men and would be expected, as a group, to have more cases of dementia.[22]

The presence of cognitive disorders varies by racial and ethnic group. The Alzheimer's Association estimates that African Americans are twice as likely as whites to develop AD and other dementias, whereas Hispanic Americans are 1.5 times more likely.[22,29] One reason for this is that these other ethnic and racial groups are more likely to suffer from cardiac disease, hypertension, diabetes, and cerebrovascular disease, all of which are risk factors for dementia. Moreover, despite a higher incidence of dementia, ethnic minorities are more cognitively impaired and less likely to access health care services (including treatment with medications) for their disease.[30]

Mortality

Dementia increases the risk of death. One study found that, as the severity of dementia increased, mean survival times decreased in a dose-response pattern.[31] Another study found that the presence of AD increased the risk of death by 40%, with a mean survival of 5.9 (standard deviation 3.7) years after diagnosis.[32] The most common causes of death in people with dementia are bronchopneumonia, cardiovascular disease, or neurologic causes.

Costs

The economic costs of caring for those with dementia are huge. The Alzheimer's Association estimates that total health care costs for patients with AD are expected to exceed $172 billion, including $123 billion in costs to Medicaid and Medicare.[22]

Globally, ADI estimates that current total annual costs from AD exceed $315 billion, with 70% of the costs in developed countries.[23,33] However, these estimates of direct costs are considerably smaller than the indirect costs of caring for those with dementia, which include costs to caregivers, caregiver loss of productivity, and use of long-term care facilities and hospice.

Risk

A considerable amount of effort has been put into delineating risk factors for dementia. Because it is not the focus of this article, these are summarized in **Table 3**. We have chosen to group these risk factors along 4 broad categories, as shown, but could also have grouped them according to whether or not the risk factor is modifiable. However, advancing age is the strongest risk factor.

CLINICAL EVALUATION

Careful attention to the individual components of evaluating a patient suspected of having dementia allows the clinician to form an informed differential diagnosis (**Fig. 2**) that may suggest the underlying etiopathology.

History

By definition, a diagnosis of dementia is based solely on clinical grounds. For the clinician, this requires a thorough inventory of the history of present illness. The clinician should pay special attention to the timing of onset, including the time when the patient was last well rather than when symptoms first started. The time course of the illness should be elicited (ie, whether the symptoms had a sudden onset or slowly developed in a longer period of time). Symptoms that develop insidiously for years point more to a diagnosis of AD, for example, than ones that develop in the course of days, which may point to a more rapidly developing brain disease. A special consideration is that often patients are not able to recount accurate historical information. Accordingly, a reliable informant such as a spouse or child should be present to provide information that the patient cannot.

Symptom characterization is the next step in coloring the clinical picture. We first introduce aspects of eliciting cognitive symptoms and discuss neuropsychiatric symptoms later. Cognitive symptoms can be considered in terms of cortical and subcortical subsyndromes of the illness. In general, deficits in cortical functioning involve the loss of abilities such as amnesia, apraxia, aphasia, and agnosia; the

Table 3 Risk factors associated with the development of dementia	
Sociodemographic	Age Race Education
Vascular/metabolic	Hypertension, Hyperlipidemia Diabetes
Lifestyle	Diet Obesity Smoking Head injury
Genetic	ApoE4

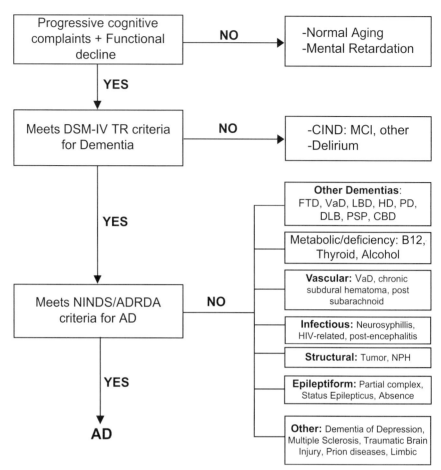

Fig. 2. Forming a diagnosis.

4 As. Subcortical deficits involve the loss of coordination of these abilities and include dysmnesia, delay, dysexecutive, and depletion; the 4 Ds.[34] This is important because a great deal of work in neuropsychology has gone into characterizing patterns of cognitive deficits and correlating them with brain structure and function. For example, the preservation of episodic learning often discriminates between AD and other dementias, which include better verbal recall in vascular dementia, better contextual verbal delayed recall in dementia with Lewy body (DLB) and better multimodal retention in FTD.[35] However, the difference between cortical and subcortical is more a heuristic separation than an anatomical one, but it is helpful in conceptualization.

Examination

The physical, neurological, and mental status examinations are a fundamental part of the evaluation but are often shortchanged. Of great importance is the general physical examination, which is most helpful in eliciting medical causes of cognitive deficits. For example, a patient who presents with cognitive complaints may also have an abnormal thyroid, which may raise suspicion for hypothyroidism, or if a patient presents with a distended abdomen, icteric skin, and spider angiomas the clinician would be well advised to consider hepatic dysfunction as a potential cause.

The purpose of a complete neurological examination is to assess for neurological conditions that may cause cognitive symptoms. Although the list is long, these conditions include stroke, seizure, tumor, Parkinson disease, and hemorrhage. In most patients with AD, the neurological examination is benign, especially in early stages of the disease, except for mild abnormalities of tone. Primitive reflexes such as the grasp, root, and suck reflexes emerge primarily in advanced stages of dementia. The clinician should be aware of gait abnormalities that may point toward a diagnosis of NPH. Parkinsonian features may suggest a diagnosis of DLB rather than AD or FTD.[9]

A careful mental status examination is critical to the overall evaluation. Appearance and behavior often lead to gross estimations of dementia severity and may raise concerns about safety and independence. Speech should be evaluated for hesitancy, word-finding difficulties, and paraphasic errors. Disturbances in mood are common in dementia syndromes. Likewise, primary disorders of mood, in particular long-standing major depression, can lower the threshold for developing dementia. Assessing risk for suicide and harm to others is a task that should not be overlooked. The presence of fluctuating cognition, visual hallucinations early on, and parkinsonism may suggest DLB, although 30% to 40% of patients with AD have these as well.[34]

Cognitive Assessment

In the office, the clinician is likely to use screening tests such as the Mini Mental State Examination (MMSE) developed by Folstein and colleagues[36] This tool, despite its brevity and ease of use, has the limitations of not being able to detect very mild dementia, especially with subcortical features, and its inability to discriminate degree of impairment in very severe dementia. The Modified Mini Mental State (3MS), developed by Teng and Chui,[37] offers a broader assessment of cognition because it assesses abstract thinking, delayed recall, and verbal fluency better than the MMSE. Cutoff scores are typically 25 on the MMSE, which roughly correlates with a 75 on the 3MS. In addition to these tests, the sophisticated clinician should incorporate other bedside assessments such as clock drawing,[38] Frontal Assessment Battery,[39] and Mental Alternation Test[40] to complete the initial cognitive evaluation.[41] More thorough assessments of cognition are typically performed by neuropsychologists who parse fine differences in a few key domains: (1) memory (verbal and nonverbal), (2) language, (3) executive functions, (4) visuospatial abilities.[35,42–45] These detailed evaluations provide valuable information that helps differentiate one type of dementia from another when uncertainties exist.

Neuropsychiatric Assessment

Neuropsychiatric symptoms are highly prevalent because nearly all patients with dementia exhibit 1 or multiple symptoms in the course of the disease.[46–48] The presence of these symptoms often portends a worse outcome because patients suffer poorer quality of life and tend to be institutionalized sooner.[49,50] Symptoms can range from mild (depression, anxiety, irritability, apathy) to severe (aberrant vocalizations, hallucinations, disinhibition).[51] Several scales have been developed to assess these symptoms. The best known is the Neuropsychiatric Inventory (NPI), which has been considered the standard assessment for neuropsychiatric symptoms for the past decade.[52] Recently, a revised version of the NPI, the Neuropsychiatric Inventory Clinician reported (NPI-C) has been developed and validated to address several shortcomings of the NPI and other rating scales and is now considered the gold standard assessment.[53] A major improvement in NPI-C was addition of a clinician rating methodology, which mitigates the reliance on caregiver provided information.

Functional Assessment

Dementia syndromes almost always affect ability to independently perform activities of daily living (ADL) such as grooming, toileting, and eating. Instrumental ADLs (IADLs) include complex activities such as meal preparation, banking, driving,[54] and decision making.[55,56] Changes in functional abilities correlate with cognitive deficits[57] and have been shown to prognosticate clinical course because it significantly affects caregiver burden and rates of institutionalization.[58] In addition to collecting information from patient and caregiver, the clinician may use a variety of functional assessment scales to quantify impairment. The Functional Activities Questionnaire (FAQ)[59] and the Assessment of Motor and Processing Skills (AMPS)[60] are 2 such tools. Occupational therapists are especially skilled at administering these and the clinician should have a low threshold for referring patients to them if there are questions about the ability of the patient to live alone or with other related level-of-care questions.

Laboratory Testing

Forming a complete differential diagnosis requires ruling out other potential causes of disease. The American Academy of Neurology recommends serum analyses that include thyroid function tests, hepatic panels, metabolic panel, complete blood count, vitamin B12 levels, and folate levels. In addition, heavy metal screens, syphilis serology, urine or serum toxicology, electrocardiogram, and chest radiograph may be considered.[61] Brain imaging may include either noncontrast head computed tomography, brain magnetic resonance imaging (MRI), and positron emission tomography (PET) (discussed later) based on clinical findings. Other biomarkers, such as cerebrospinal fluid tau, amyloid-β levels, and genetic screening for ApoE4, continue to be used in research but may soon be used in the clinical setting.

TREATMENT
General Principles

Treating dementia requires a comprehensive multidimensional approach. A thoughtful model of treatment is presented in *Practical Dementia Care*,[34] in which the 4 pillars of dementia care are considered to be (1) treating the disease, (2) treating the symptoms, (3) supporting the patient, and (4) supporting the caregiver. There is strong clinical evidence to suggest that delivering dementia care as a comprehensive package has many positive effects to both the patient and caregiver. Furthermore, a team approach that incorporates and values communication, collaboration, and has a shared therapeutic relationship with the patient is an effective way of delivering high-quality care.[62] The Prevention of Recurrent Venous Thromboembolism (PREVENT) trial in the United States used a collaborative care intervention delivered by a nurse with supervision from a specialist team. It showed that there were significant improvements in time to institutionalization, caregiver distress, and lower rates of behavioral and psychological symptoms.[63] The dementia care specialist should assemble a team of clinicians that includes occupational therapists, psychologists, and case managers working closely with the primary care physician to provide the best care.

Because there are currently no approved disease-modifying therapies for dementia, the clinician is charged with managing the cognitive and neuropsychiatric symptoms that define the syndrome while at the same time supporting the patient and caregivers. The therapies used today are either pharmacological or nonpharmacological modalities. The best treatment involves the concurrent application of both. There are several factors that should be considered when starting treatment with medication. First, the elderly have decreased renal clearance and slowed hepatic metabolism. Second, these patients likely suffer from other medical illnesses and may come with a long list of medications, so drug interactions need to be carefully evaluated before starting. Third, falls from orthostasis are common because of decreased vascular tone. The adage start low and go slow should apply to each patient as medications are considered. However, this does not mean that full doses should be avoided; they should be used if they are indicated and tolerated.

Although medications are often considered by many clinicians to be a first-line therapy, the importance of psychosocial and psychotherapeutic strategies should be emphasized. These treatments have not only shown effectiveness but they also avoid the inherent risks of pharmacotherapy: side effects, intolerability, and even death. This article discusses both strategies in the context of cognitive and neuropsychiatric symptoms.

Cognition

The US Food and Drug Administration (FDA) approves 5 medications for the treatment of cognitive symptoms in AD. The cholinesterase inhibitors tacrine, donepezil, rivastigmine, and galantamine are available in a variety of preparations including delayed-release pills and in patch form (rivastigmine only). Their effect in the brain is through the relative increase of acetylcholine, a hypothesized mechanism for improvements in cognition. Memantine is an N-methyl-D-aspartate (NMDA) antagonist that purportedly works by preventing the excitotoxic effects of glutamate in the brain. These medications typically benefit patients for a period of months and, in 10% to 15%, lead to notable, albeit temporary, symptomatic improvements. As such, these medications, also summarized in **Table 4**, provide only a modest temporary stabilization of the cognitive changes that define Alzheimer disease. Head-to-head comparative effectiveness trials have been small, open label, and have failed to show consistent differences in efficacy between medications.

Tacrine is used infrequently because it causes hepatotoxicity in some patients (transient and reversible increases in hepatic transaminase levels) and should generally be avoided. Donepezil (Aricept) has shown a modest effect in patients with AD with mild to moderate cognitive impairments. In 2 meta-analyses combining a total of 37 high-quality studies, all but 3 showed statistically significant positive effects in at least 1 measure of cognition; however, the clinical importance of this change (as defined by a >4-point increase on the Alzheimer Disease Assessment

Table 4
Cholinesterase inhibitors for the treatment of dementia

Drug	Dosing	Common Side Effects
Donepezil (Aricept)	Start 5 mg once daily then may increase to 10 mg in 4–6 weeks	Nausea, headache, diarrhea, malaise
Rivastigmine (Exelon)	Start 1.5 mg twice daily. Increase by 1.5 mg every 4 weeks to maximum dose of 6 mg twice daily	Gastrointestinal related: nausea, vomiting, diarrhea
Galantamine (Reminyl)	Start 4 mg twice daily. Increase to 8 mg twice daily after 4 weeks. May increase to 12 mg twice daily if indicated	Mild nausea, vomiting, diarrhea. Take with food. Caution in patients with renal or hepatic impairments
Tacrine (Cognex)	Start 10 mg 4 times daily. Increase by 10 mg/dose every 4 weeks to max of 40 mg doses or as tolerated	Various gastrointestinal side effects. Hepatotoxicity

Scale-Cognitive [ADAS-cog]) was inconclusive. However, higher doses of the medication produced more benefit.[64,65] A recent Cochrane Review examining the effect of donepezil in patients with MCI concluded that there was no evidence to either support the use of donepezil in patients with MCI or suggest that it delayed the conversion of MCI to AD. Furthermore, there were significantly more side effects associated with donepezil than placebo.[66] Ongoing studies are examining the effects of medications and other treatments on delaying or preventing the progression of MCI to AD.

Nine high-quality studies in a recent Cochrane Review comparing rivastigmine with placebo showed that, at high doses (6 mg to 12 mg daily), its use was associated with statistically significant benefits on several measures of cognition as assessed by the ADAS-cog. There was a 2.2-point improvement in ADLs as approximated by the Progressive Deterioration Scale. The review concluded that there appeared to be a beneficial effect for people with mild to moderate AD and that the lower-dose transdermal patch had comparable efficacy with both high-dose pills and the higher-dose patch.[67]

As stated earlier, the effect of memantine is exerted through an NMDA receptor mechanism. Studies of efficacy have shown that, compared with placebo, memantine was well tolerated and showed a small, but significant, statistical as well as clinical benefit for patients with moderate to severe, but not mild to moderate, AD.[68]

The American Association for Geriatric Psychiatry's principles of care concluded that estrogen, anti-inflammatory agents, and ginkgo biloba are not effective treatments for Alzheimer dementia.[4] High doses of the antioxidant vitamin E were shown in the only randomized controlled trial (RCT) of the drug to delay time to predetermined end points (death, institutionalization, loss of basic ADLs) over 2 years.[69] Higher quality studies are needed to establish clinical recommendations for its use. The 3-hydroxy-3-methyl-glutaryl enzyme A reductase inhibitors (statins) effectively reduce serum cholesterol concentrations. Two large, randomized, placebo-controlled trials (Heart Protection Study and Prospective Study of Pravastatin in the Elderly at Risk [PROSPER]) have examined the effects of statins on cognitive decline and dementia but neither showed any significant effect of statin therapy on cognition.[70,71] Aggressive management of cardiovascular risk factors such as blood pressure management (especially keeping systolic blood pressure <160 mm Hg), weight loss, exercise, management of diabetes, and a healthy diet all probably constitute a significant part of effective AD therapy.[72,73]

Nonpharmacological, evidence-based interventions span a broad range of modalities and include cognitive behavioral therapy (CBT), cognitive rehabilitation, reminiscence therapy, and environmental manipulation. They provide a noninvasive, holistic approach that has been shown to improve cognition and psychological well-being.[74–77] Combining cognitive strategies, such as spaced retrieval, with errorless learning, for example, is based on preserved implicit memory function and has been shown to be effective in maximizing memory function in patients with AD.[78–81] Although these techniques and others seem to provide some benefit, monitoring the patient's level of frustration, especially for the inability to recall memories, is important to prevent depression in patients and caregivers. Balancing risks with benefits continues to be an important part of choosing a treatment, especially in this case.

Neuropsychiatric Symptoms

As discussed earlier, these disturbances are common in dementia and, when present, lead to significant disability for both the patient and caregiver. A useful approach to the management of neuropsychiatric symptoms is presented in *Practical Dementia Care*[34] and defined by a mnemonic of 4 Ds: define, decode, devise, and determine. Define refers to an evaluation phase and has already been presented. Identifying contributing factors describes the decode phase. Such factors may include biological stress or delirium, identifiable psychiatric syndrome, environmental stressors, unmet needs, or medication side effects. The devise phase consists of pharmacological, behavioral, environmental, and educational approaches that target the identified causes. The determine phase involves goal setting and forming contingency plans should an intervention not produce desired results.

Because of the increased risks of using medications to treat these symptoms in patients with dementia, nonpharmacological interventions should be considered as first line. A wide range of different types of therapies have been studied. Some small studies have shown modest benefit with such strategies as aromatherapy, bright light therapy, and music therapy. Behavior therapy using antecedent-behavior-consequence (ABC) diary assessment has provided good sustained improvements in behavior.[82,83] One meta-analysis found that behavioral management techniques focused on individual patients' behavior and individually oriented psychoeducation provided longer-lasting (several months) positive effects on behavior compared with placebo.[82] Music therapy and Snoezelen were 2 other types of therapies that provided positive, but short-lived, effects. Staff education has been shown to lead to reductions in behavioral outbursts and fewer episodes of restraint use. Despite the promising results from these studies, there is little controlled evidence that they work, and they are often difficult to implement in real-world settings. These drawbacks, as well as a perceived lack of other options, have led to the increasing use of medications.

The process of selecting a medication to treat neuropsychiatric symptoms should weigh the risks and benefits of its use. A useful strategy for choosing an appropriate medication involves isolating a target symptom then choosing a medication that is known to treat it. There are several broad categories of psychotropics used in the treatment of the neuropsychiatric symptoms of dementia today: antipsychotics, anticonvulsants, antidepressants, and anxiolytics. Recent evidence has shown that the use of typical and atypical antipsychotics has been associated with increased rates of cardiovascular and cerebrovascular events, and even death, in patients with dementia.[84] However, use of antidepressants or anticonvulsants does not carry these particular concerns but has other risks to consider. There is poor evidence to suggest that cholinesterase inhibitors or memantine effectively treat neuropsychiatric symptoms, although they may delay their emergence.

Antipsychotic medications are the mainstays for the treatment of agitation and psychosis, which often are associated with aggression, shouting, wandering, and similar behaviors. In the Clinical Antipsychotic *Trial* of International Effectiveness-Alzheimer's Disease (CATIE-AD) trial, risperidone and olanzapine have shown the most benefits, although still only a modest effect of symptom reduction as assessed by various rating scales. These modest benefits must be balanced against the significant adverse effects of these medications in dementia elders, including the higher mortality risks.[85] They had no effect in other clinical outcome measures such as cognition, functioning, or quality of life.[86,87] One important consideration is that patients suspected of having dementia with Lewy bodies are known to be exquisitely sensitivity to all antipsychotics. Adverse events have ranged from acute dystonia to drug-induced parkinsonism to life-threatening neuroleptics malignant syndrome.[88] There are some data suggesting that the antiepileptic drug carbamazepine may have some positive effect, although these studies have not established information about adverse events from long-term effects.[89,90]

The patient with dementia with depressive symptoms (eg, depressed mood, apathy, loss of appetite) should be considered for treatment with antidepressant medications.

The presence of major depression places the patient at risk for several adverse outcomes, including death from suicide. The antidepressant medication should be tailored to the patient and should be based on the drug's side effect profile and the patient's general medical and psychiatric status. Selective serotonin reuptake inhibitors (SSRI) tend to be prescribed more frequently than tricyclic antidepressants (TCA) or monoamine oxidase inhibitors (MAOI), largely because of the ease of use and better side effect profiles.[91] A Cochrane Review of antidepressants in dementia concluded that the evidence was weak in terms of the effectiveness of these medications but that the results of 1 small study showed more significant differences between sertraline and placebo groups.[92] Duration of treatment is unclear, although general clinical practice patterns suggest that a minimum treatment of 6 months is indicated for most cases of major depression. The most recent study in the area, DIADS-2, did not find efficacy for sertraline compared with placebo.[93–95]

Supporting the Patient and Caregiver

Systematic provision of care to both patient and caregiver is essential to effective comprehensive dementia care. For the patient, care is typically tailored to each patient with other members of a collaborative team as discussed earlier. Areas that should be addressed in every case should include comfort and emotional support, safety at home and local environment, structure in activities and stimulation in day-to-day life, and planning with decision making. When appropriate, patients should be educated about their condition, including giving them their diagnosis and anticipated course.

Caregiver burden is a well-documented phenomenon that affects not only the caregiver but the patient as well. Increased stress, incidence of depression, and adverse effects on physical health and financial security are a few of the recognized negative outcomes of caregiving.[22,91,96,97] Ultimately, poor caregiver status leads to earlier institutionalization of the patient.[98,99] Mittelman and colleagues[77,100] showed that caregiver interventions had effect sizes as large or larger than medications in delaying out-of-home placement. Key interventions that the clinician should provide include psychoeducation, instruction in the skills of caregiving, support with problem solving, availability of an expert clinician, and instructions on obtaining respite. When applied thoughtfully, these measures help reinforce a positive caregiver-recipient relationship, which has been shown to attenuate AD decline.[101]

FUTURE DIRECTIONS
Diagnosis

At the most recent Alzheimer's Association International Conference on Alzheimer's Disease (AAICAD) in July 2010, several scientists presented arguments for refining the diagnostic criteria for Alzheimer disease. Noting that the field has advanced considerably since the original criteria were issued nearly 25 years ago, new criteria could reflect potentially 3 stages of the disease (preclinical, MCI, AD) as well as the inclusion of biomarkers in diagnosis. Dubois and colleagues[102] suggested that minor criteria include presence of temporal lobe atrophy as shown with MRI, abnormal cerebrospinal fluid (CSF) biomarkers, and functional neuroimaging changes as seen with PET. These diagnostic modalities are among several others that are currently being refined, standardized, and validated.

The use of PET has been revolutionized in the last 10 years by the discovery of several highly lipophilic compounds that bind to the amyloid plaques and neurofibrillary tangles of AD.[11] C-labeled Pittsburgh compound B (PIB) binds more specifically to amyloid than neurofibrillary tangles. ^{18}F-FDDNP is able to bind to both amyloid as well as neurofibrillary tangles and has been able to predict progression from MCI to AD.[103] Among the several other ligands currently in development, ^{18}F-BAY94-9172 and ^{18}F-AV-45 (Florbetapir) are compounds that are similar to PIB but with the advantage of having a half-life that is nearly 5 times longer.[104,105] With these ligands, PET imaging could help with establishing diagnosis as well as localizing disease burden and tracking response to treatment of future disease-modifying drugs.

MRI is perhaps the most accessible of the imaging modalities and therefore the most likely to be used clinically. Morphometric and volumetric analyses of whole brain, as well as cortical and subcortical (entorhinal cortex, hippocampus, parahippocampal gyrus) structures, have been used to discriminate subjects with and without disease. Automated methods of analysis are being refined to provide highly sensitive and specific measurements. These methods may become more important because longitudinal data, which show rates of change (calculated as slopes), tend to provide better discrimination than single time point measurements and may also be able to track and prognosticate disease progression. Diffusion tensor imaging (DTI) and related methods are being shown to discriminate between groups by measuring relative values of fractional anisotropy (FA) and mean diffusivity, values that assess the integrity of white matter tracts in the brain.[106]

There are primarily 4 established core biomarkers identified in the CSF: $A\beta_{40}$, $A\beta_{42}$, total tau, and phosphorylated tau.[107,108] These markers (with the exception of total tau) reflect the underlying disease process in AD. CSF studies showing high levels of total and phosphorylated tau together with reduced levels of $A\beta_{42}$ or reduced $A\beta_{40}/A\beta_{42}$ ratio in the CSF have been consistent findings in patients with AD. Several other candidate markers have been identified and are currently being studied. Some of these include $A\beta$ oligomers, β-site amyloid precursor protein–cleaving enzyme 1 (BACE1), secreted isoforms of APP, and $A\beta$ degradation products. Several of these markers have recently shown the ability to predict longitudinal decline in AD and, as such, have shown promise as biomarkers for disease progression.[109]

Treatment

The development of disease-modifying drugs for AD is progressing quickly. Mangialasche and colleagues[110] summarized approximately 75 compounds that are currently in FDA phase I to III testing. These candidate drugs are broadly grouped according to their mechanism of action: (1) modulators of the amyloid cascade, primarily $A\beta$ production or aggregation; (2) immunotherapy targeting $A\beta$ clearance; (3) tau modulators. Other targets have included modulators of neuroinflammation and metal ion metabolism but there are no compounds currently in clinical trials.

AD drug development has focused on the amyloid hypothesis in which most studies are designed to target $A\beta$ production, aggregation, and clearance. $A\beta$ production is regulated by β-secretase, α-secretase, and γ-secretase action. These 4 enzymes have attracted the attention of drug developers for more than a decade. γ-Secretase was the earliest target but problems with slowed cleavage of an essential substrate, Notch 1, halted further development. Eli Lilly overcome this challenge and developed a candidate drug named semagacestat (LY450139), which entered phase III clinical trials. However, in August 2010 these trials were stopped because of concerns of cognitive worsening and adverse affects.[111]

Tramiprostrate is a synthetic glycosaminoglycan that acts as a chaperone for $A\beta$, effectively disrupting the hydrophobic core sequence preventing aggregation. Tramiprostrate is currently in phase III trials but was discontinued in Europe because of discouraging findings from one large RCT and has received some skepticism in the

US after the manufacturer began marketing the compound as a nutriceutical. Scyllo-inositol (scyllo-cyclohexanehexol, AZD-103, ELND-005), is an orally administered stereoisomer of inositol, which crosses the blood-brain barrier. It is believed to bind to $A\beta$, inhibit its aggregation, and increase dissociation of aggregates.[112] In animal studies, it reduced brain concentrations of soluble and insoluble $A\beta_{1-40}$ and $A\beta_{1-42}$, plaque burden, synaptic loss, and glial inflammatory reaction, and improved spatial memory function. The drug was found to be well tolerated in healthy volunteers[113] and recently completed a phase 2 RCT in patients with mild to moderate Alzheimer disease (NCT00568776). However, high doses of the drug (1000–2000 mg) have resulted in a total of 9 deaths. Lower doses (500 mg) are currently being tested.[114] The drug is expected to move to phase III trials in 2011.

Active and passive immunization have been proposed as mechanisms in the clearance of soluble $A\beta$. Bapineuzumab and solanezumab are monoclonal antibodies that bind to soluble $A\beta$, promoting its removal from the brain through the blood. Both are currently in phase III clinical trials. Intravenous immunoglobulin (IVIg) is another form of passive immunotherapy that has already shown good tolerability and side effect profile in the treatment of various immune deficiency syndromes. IVIg has shown similar profiles along with positive effects on cognition and is currently in phase III investigation.[115]

Anti-tau compounds have targeted tau hyperphosphorylation and inhibition of tau aggregation. Currently, several other compounds, including lithium and methylthioninium chloride (methylene blue), are in phase II trials because they have shown antiaggregant effects. Results from the Alzheimer's Disease Cooperative Study (ADCS) trial showed that treatment with valproate had no effect on cognition and functional status, but reduced rates of agitation.[116] Although these results are promising, the true test will be whether these drugs can improve cognition on clinical measures.

SUMMARY

Dementia is a complex disorder. As the population of the world ages, clinicians will see many more patients who either have dementia or have cared for someone with dementia. At the same time, the clinician is charged with treating the disease, the symptoms, the patient, and the caregiver, which is a challenge that may seem overwhelming at first but, equipped with guidelines and skills that afford more accurate diagnosis and effective treatment, the clinician should be able to provide care that is informed, comprehensive, and compassionate. Although current diagnostic and treatment strategies leave much to be desired, it is exciting to see how biomedical research will provide us with the understanding and tools to help fight these diseases and care for the patients they afflict for the next 25 years.

REFERENCES

1. American Psychiatric Association, American Psychiatric Association, Task Force on DSM-IV. Diagnostic and statistical manual of mental disorders: DSM-IV. 4th edition. Washington, DC: American Psychiatric Association; 1994. p. xxvii, 886.
2. McKhann G, Drachman D, Folstein M, et al. Clinical diagnosis of Alzheimer's disease: report of the NINCDS-ADRDA Work Group under the auspices of Department of Health and Human Services Task Force on Alzheimer's Disease. Neurology 1984;34(7):939–44.
3. Lyketsos C. Dementia and milder cognitive syndromes. In: Steffens BA, editor. Textbook of geriatric psychiatry. APPI; 2009. p. 243–60.

4. Lyketsos CG, Colenda CC, Beck C, et al. Position statement of the American Association for Geriatric Psychiatry regarding principles of care for patients with dementia resulting from Alzheimer disease. Am J Geriatr Psychiatry 2006;14(7):561–72.

5. Schneider JA, Arvanitakis Z, Bang W, et al. Mixed brain pathologies account for most dementia cases in community-dwelling older persons. Neurology 2007; 69(24):2197–204.

6. White L, Petrovitch H, Ross GW, et al. Prevalence of dementia in older Japanese-American men in Hawaii: the Honolulu-Asia Aging Study. JAMA 1996;276(12):955–60.

7. Kovacs GG, Alafuzoff I, Al-Sarraj S, et al. Mixed brain pathologies in dementia: the BrainNet Europe consortium experience. Dement Geriatr Cogn Disord 2008; 26(4):343–50.

8. Kelley RE, Minagar A. Memory complaints and dementia. Med Clin North Am 2009;93(2):389–406, ix.

9. Bradley WG, editor. Neurology in clinical practice, vol. 1. 5th edition. Philadelphia: Butterworth-Heinemann; 2008.

10. Glenner GG, Wong CW. Alzheimer's disease: initial report of the purification and characterization of a novel cerebrovascular amyloid protein. Biochem Biophys Res Commun 1984;120(3):885–90.

11. Maccioni RB, Munoz JP, Barbeito L. The molecular bases of Alzheimer's disease and other neurodegenerative disorders. Arch Med Res 2001;32(5): 367–81.

12. Maccioni RB, Cambiazo V. Role of microtubule-associated proteins in the control of microtubule assembly. Physiol Rev 1995;75(4):835–64.

13. Cruts M, Van Broeckhoven C. Molecular genetics of Alzheimer's disease. Ann Med 1998;30(6):560–5.

14. Kim J, Basak JM, Holtzman DM. The role of apolipoprotein E in Alzheimer's disease. Neuron 2009;63(3):287–303.

15. Raber J, Huang Y, Ashford JW. ApoE genotype accounts for the vast majority of AD risk and AD pathology. Neurobiol Aging 2004;25(5):641–50.

16. Alexopoulos P, Kurz A, Lewczuk P, et al. The sortilin-related receptor SORL1 and the amyloid cascade: a possible explanation for the concurrent elevation of CSF soluble APPalpha and APPbeta in Alzheimer's disease. Int J Geriatr Psychiatry 2010;25(5):542–3.

17. Bettens K, Brouwers N, Engelborghs S, et al. SORL1 is genetically associated with increased risk for late-onset Alzheimer disease in the Belgian population. Hum Mutat 2008;29(5):769–70.

18. Shibata N, Ohnuma T, Baba H, et al. Genetic association between SORL1 polymorphisms and Alzheimer's disease in a Japanese population. Dement Geriatr Cogn Disord 2008;26(2):161–4.

19. Zekanowski C, Styczynska M, Peplonska B, et al. Mutations in presenilin 1, presenilin 2 and amyloid precursor protein genes in patients with early-onset Alzheimer's disease in Poland. Exp Neurol 2003;184(2):991–6.

20. Jun G, Naj AC, Beecham GW, et al. Meta-analysis confirms CR1, CLU, and PICALM as Alzheimer disease risk loci and reveals interactions with APOE genotypes. Arch Neurol 2010;67(12):1473–84.

21. World Population Aging 2007. United Nations, Department of Economic and Social Affairs; 2007. p. 568.

22. Alzheimer's Association. 2010 Alzheimer's disease facts and figures. Alzheimers Dement 2010;6(2):158–94.

23. Prince M, Jackson J, editors. World Alzheimer Report. London (UK): Alzheimer's Disease International; 2009.
24. Kalaria RN, Maestre GE, Arizaga R, et al. Alzheimer's disease and vascular dementia in developing countries: prevalence, management, and risk factors. Lancet Neurol 2008;7(9):812–26.
25. Miech RA, Breitner JC, Zandi PP, et al. Incidence of AD may decline in the early 90s for men, later for women: The Cache County study. Neurology 2002;58(2): 209–18.
26. Plassman BL, Langa KM, Fisher GG, et al. Prevalence of dementia in the United States: the aging, demographics, and memory study. Neuroepidemiology 2007; 29(1–2):125–32.
27. Barnes LL, Wilson RS, Schneider JA, et al. Gender, cognitive decline, and risk of AD in older persons. Neurology 2003;60(11):1777–81.
28. Fitzpatrick AL, Kuller LH, Ives DG, et al. Incidence and prevalence of dementia in the cardiovascular health study. J Am Geriatr Soc 2004;52(2):195–204.
29. Gurland BJ, Wilder DE, Lantigua R, et al. Rates of dementia in three ethnoracial groups. Int J Geriatr Psychiatry 1999;14(6):481–93.
30. Cooper C, Tandy AR, Balamurali TBS, et al. A systematic review and meta-analysis of ethnic differences in use of dementia treatment, care, and research. Am J Geriatr Psychiatry 2010;18(3):193–203.
31. Andersen K, Lolk A, Martinussen T, et al. Very mild to severe dementia and mortality: a 14-year follow-up - The Odense study. Dement Geriatr Cogn Disord 2010;29(1):61–7.
32. Ganguli M, Dodge HH, Shen C, et al. Alzheimer disease and mortality: a 15-year epidemiological study. Arch Neurol 2005;62(5):779–84.
33. Wimo A, Winblad B, Jönsson L. An estimate of the total worldwide societal costs of dementia in 2005. Alzheimers Dement 2007;3(2):81–91 the journal of the Alzheimer's Association.
34. Rabins PV, Lyketsos CG, Steele C. Practical dementia care. 2nd edition. New York: Oxford University Press; 2006. p. xiv, 336.
35. Levy JA, Chelune GJ. Cognitive-behavioral profiles of neurodegenerative dementias: beyond Alzheimer's disease. J Geriatr Psychiatry Neurol 2007;20(4):227–38.
36. Folstein MF, Folstein SE, McHugh PR. "Mini-mental state". A practical method for grading the cognitive state of patients for the clinician. J Psychiatr Res 1975; 12(3):189–98.
37. Teng EL, Chui HC. The modified mini-mental state (3MS) examination. J Clin Psychiatry 1987;48(8):314–8.
38. Manos PJ, Wu R. The ten point clock test: a quick screen and grading method for cognitive impairment in medical and surgical patients. Int J Psychiatry Med 1994;24(3):229–44.
39. Dubois B, Slachevsky A, Litvan I, et al. The FAB: a Frontal Assessment Battery at bedside. Neurology 2000;55(11):1621–6.
40. Salib E, McCarthy J. Mental Alternation Test (MAT): a rapid and valid screening tool for dementia in primary care. Int J Geriatr Psychiatry 2002; 17(12):1157–61.
41. Cullen B, O'Neill B, Evans JJ, et al. A review of screening tests for cognitive impairment. J Neurol Neurosurg Psychiatr 2007;78(8):790–9.
42. Auriacombe S, Lechevallier N, Amieva H, et al. A longitudinal study of quantitative and qualitative features of category verbal fluency in incident Alzheimer's disease subjects: results from the PAQUID study. Dement Geriatr Cogn Disord 2006;21(4):260–6.

43. Baldwin S, Farias ST. Neuropsychological assessment in the diagnosis of Alzheimer's disease. Curr Protoc Neurosci 2009;Chapter 10:Unit10.13.
44. Behl P, Stefurak TL, Black SE. Progress in clinical neurosciences: cognitive markers of progression in Alzheimer's disease. Can J Neurol Sci 2005;32(2): 140–51.
45. Braaten AJ, Parsons TD, Mccue R, et al. Neurocognitive differential diagnosis of dementing diseases: Alzheimer's dementia, vascular dementia, frontotemporal dementia, and major depressive disorder. Int J Neurosci 2006;116(11): 1271–93.
46. Lyketsos CG, Lopez O, Jones B, et al. Prevalence of neuropsychiatric symptoms in dementia and mild cognitive impairment: results from the cardiovascular health study. JAMA 2002;288(12):1475–83.
47. Mayer LS, Bay RC, Politis A, et al. Comparison of three rating scales as outcome measures for treatment trials of depression in Alzheimer disease: findings from DIADS. Int J Geriatr Psychiatry 2006;21(10):930–6.
48. Okura T, Plassman BL, Steffens DC, et al. Prevalence of neuropsychiatric symptoms and their association with functional limitations in older adults in the United States: the aging, demographics, and memory study. J Am Geriatr Soc 2010; 58(2):330–7.
49. Steele C, Rovner B, Chase GA, et al. Psychiatric symptoms and nursing home placement of patients with Alzheimer's disease. Am J Psychiatry 1990;147(8): 1049–51.
50. Stern Y, Tang MX, Albert MS, et al. Predicting time to nursing home care and death in individuals with Alzheimer disease. JAMA 1997;277(10):806–12.
51. Lopez OL, Becker JT, Sweet RA, et al. Psychiatric symptoms vary with the severity of dementia in probable Alzheimer's disease. J Neuropsychiatry Clin Neurosci 2003;15(3):346–53.
52. Cummings JL, Mega M, Gray K, et al. The Neuropsychiatric Inventory: comprehensive assessment of psychopathology in dementia. Neurology 1994;44(12): 2308–14.
53. De Medeiros K, Robert P, Gauthier S, et al. The Neuropsychiatric Inventory-Clinician rating scale (NPI-C): reliability and validity of a revised assessment of neuropsychiatric symptoms in dementia. Int Psychogeriatr 2010;22(6): 1–11.
54. Iverson DJ, Gronseth GS, Reger MA, et al. Practice parameter update: evaluation and management of driving risk in dementia: report of the quality standards subcommittee of the American Academy of Neurology. Neurology 2010;74(16): 1316–24.
55. Dunn LB, Nowrangi MA, Palmer BW, et al. Assessing decisional capacity for clinical research or treatment: a review of instruments. Am J Psychiatry 2006; 163(8):1323–34.
56. Lai JM, Karlawish J. Assessing the capacity to make everyday decisions: a guide for clinicians and an agenda for future research. Am J Geriatr Psychiatry 2007;15(2):101–11.
57. Royall DR, Lauterbach EC, Kaufer D, et al. The cognitive correlates of functional status: a review from the Committee on Research of the American Neuropsychiatric Association. J Neuropsychiatry Clin Neurosci 2007;19(3):249–65.
58. Massoud F. The role of functional assessment as an outcome measure in antidementia treatment. Can J Neurol Sci 2007;34(Suppl 1):S47–51.
59. Pfeffer RI, Kurosaki TT, Harrah CH Jr, et al. Measurement of functional activities in older adults in the community. J Gerontol 1982;37(3):323–9.

60. Fisher A. Assessment of motor and process skills. Development, standardization, and administration manual, vol. 1. 5th edition. Fort Collins (CO): Three Star Press; 2003.

61. Knopman DS, DeKosky ST, Cummings JL, et al. Practice parameter: diagnosis of dementia (an evidence-based review). Report of the Quality Standards Subcommittee of the American Academy of Neurology. Neurology 2001;56(9): 1143–53.

62. Keough J, Huebner RA. Treating dementia: the complementing team approach of occupational therapy and psychology. J Psychol 2000;134(4):375–91.

63. Callahan CM, Boustani MA, Unverzagt FW, et al. Effectiveness of collaborative care for older adults with Alzheimer disease in primary care: a randomized controlled trial. JAMA 2006;295(18):2148–57.

64. Loveman E, Green C, Kirby J, et al. The clinical and cost-effectiveness of donepezil, rivastigmine, galantamine and memantine for Alzheimer's disease. Health Technol Assess 2006;10(1):1–160, iii–iv, ix–xi.

65. Qaseem A, Snow V, Cross JT, et al. Current pharmacologic treatment of dementia: a clinical practice guideline from the American College of physicians and the American academy of family physicians. Ann Intern Med 2008;148(5): 370–8.

66. Birks J, Flicker L. Donepezil for mild cognitive impairment. Cochrane Database Syst Rev 2006;3:CD006104.

67. Birks J, Grimley Evans J, Iakovidou V, et al. Rivastigmine for Alzheimer's disease. Cochrane Database Syst Rev 2009;2:CD001191.

68. McShane R, Areosa Sastre A, Minakaran N. Memantine for dementia. Cochrane Database Syst Rev 2006;2:CD003154.

69. Sano M, Ernesto C, Thomas RG, et al. A controlled trial of selegiline, alpha-tocopherol, or both as treatment for Alzheimer's disease. The Alzheimer's Disease Cooperative Study. N Engl J Med 1997;336(17):1216–22.

70. Suribhatla S, Dennis MS, Potter JF. A study of statin use in the prevention of cognitive impairment of vascular origin in the UK. J Neurol Sci 2005;147–50 229–30.

71. Trompet S, van Vliet P, de Craen AJ, et al. Pravastatin and cognitive function in the elderly. Results of the PROSPER study. J Neurol 2010;257(1):85–90.

72. Mielke MM, Rosenberg PB, Tschanz J, et al. Vascular factors predict rate of progression in Alzheimer disease. Neurology 2007;69(19):1850–8.

73. Cherubini A, Lowenthal DT, Paran E, et al. Hypertension and cognitive function in the elderly. Dis Mon 2010;56(3):106–47.

74. De Vreese LP, Neri M, Fioravanti M, et al. Memory rehabilitation in Alzheimer's disease: a review of progress. Int J Geriatr Psychiatry 2001;16(8):794–809.

75. Woods B, Spector A, Jones C, et al. Reminiscence therapy for dementia. Cochrane Database Syst Rev 2005;2:CD001120.

76. Berg A, Sadowski K, Beyrodt M, et al. Snoezelen, structured reminiscence therapy and 10-minutes activation in long term care residents with dementia (WISDE): study protocol of a cluster randomized controlled trial. BMC Geriatr 2010;10:5.

77. Mittelman MS, Ferris SH, Shulman E, et al. A family intervention to delay nursing home placement of patients with Alzheimer disease. A randomized controlled trial. JAMA 1996;276(21):1725–31.

78. Clare L, Wilson BA, Carter G, et al. Intervening with everyday memory problems in dementia of Alzheimer type: an errorless learning approach. J Clin Exp Neuropsychol 2000;22(1):132–46.

79. Minati L, Edginton T, Grazia Bruzzone M, et al. Reviews: current concepts in Alzheimer's Disease: a multidisciplinary review. Am J Alzheimers Dis Other Demen 2009;24(2):95–121.
80. Spector A, Thorgrimsen L, Woods B, et al. Efficacy of an evidence-based cognitive stimulation therapy programme for people with dementia: randomised controlled trial. Br J Psychiatry 2003;183:248–54.
81. Wilson BA, Evans JJ, Emslie H, et al. Evaluation of NeuroPage: a new memory aid. J Neurol Neurosurg Psychiatry 1997;63(1):113–5.
82. Livingston G, Johnston K, Katona C, et al. Systematic review of psychological approaches to the management of neuropsychiatric symptoms of dementia. Am J Psychiatry 2005;162(11):1996–2021.
83. Moniz-Cook E, Woods RT, Richards K. Functional analysis of challenging behaviour in dementia: the role of superstition. Int J Geriatr Psychiatry 2001;16(1): 45–56.
84. Schneider LS, Tariot PN, Dagerman KS, et al. Effectiveness of atypical antipsychotic drugs in patients with Alzheimer's disease. N Engl J Med 2006;355(15): 1525–38.
85. Rabins PV, Lyketsos CG. Antipsychotic drugs in dementia: what should be made of the risks? JAMA 2005;294(15):1963–5.
86. Sink KM, Holden KF, Yaffe K. Pharmacological treatment of neuropsychiatric symptoms of dementia: a review of the evidence. JAMA 2005;293(5):596–608.
87. Sultzer DL, Davis SM, Tariot PN, et al. Clinical symptom responses to atypical antipsychotic medications in Alzheimer's disease: phase 1 outcomes from the CATIE-AD effectiveness trial. Am J Psychiatry 2008;165(7):844–54.
88. Ballard C, Grace J, McKeith I, et al. Neuroleptic sensitivity in dementia with Lewy bodies and Alzheimer's disease. Lancet 1998;351(9108):1032–3.
89. Lonergan E, Luxenberg J. Valproate preparations for agitation in dementia. Cochrane Database Syst Rev 2009;3:CD003945.
90. Tariot PN, Erb R, Podgorski CA, et al. Efficacy and tolerability of carbamazepine for agitation and aggression in dementia. Am J Psychiatry 1998;155(1):54–61.
91. Starkstein SE, Mizrahi R, Power BD. Depression in Alzheimer's disease: phenomenology, clinical correlates and treatment. Int Rev Psychiatry 2008; 20(4):382–8.
92. Bains J, Birks JS, Dening TR. The efficacy of antidepressants in the treatment of depression in dementia. Cochrane Database Syst Rev 2002;4:CD003944.
93. Drye LT, Martin BK, Frangakis CE, et al. Do treatment effects vary among differing baseline depression criteria in depression in Alzheimer's disease study +/- 2 (DIADS-2)? Int J Geriatr Psychiatry 2010. [Epub ahead of print].
94. Rosenberg PB, Drye LT, Martin BK, et al. Sertraline for the treatment of depression in Alzheimer disease. Am J Geriatr Psychiatry 2010;18(2):136–45.
95. Weintraub D, Rosenberg PB, Drye LT, et al. Sertraline for the treatment of depression in Alzheimer disease: week-24 outcomes. Am J Geriatr Psychiatry 2010;18(4):332–40.
96. Taylor DH Jr, Ezell M, Kuchibhatla M, et al. Identifying trajectories of depressive symptoms for women caring for their husbands with dementia. J Am Geriatr Soc 2008;56(2):322–7.
97. Schulz R, O'Brien AT, Bookwala J, et al. Psychiatric and physical morbidity effects of dementia caregiving: prevalence, correlates, and causes. Gerontologist 1995;35(6):771–91.
98. Luppa M, Luck T, Brahler E, et al. Prediction of institutionalisation in dementia. A systematic review. Dement Geriatr Cogn Disord 2008;26(1):65–78.

99. Gaugler JE, Yu F, Krichbaum K, et al. Predictors of nursing home admission for persons with dementia. Med Care 2009;47(2):191–8.

100. Mittelman MS, Haley WE, Clay OJ, et al. Improving caregiver well-being delays nursing home placement of patients with Alzheimer disease. Neurology 2006; 67(9):1592–9.

101. Norton MC, Piercy KW, Rabins PV, et al. Caregiver-recipient closeness and symptom progression in Alzheimer disease. The Cache County Dementia Progression Study. J Gerontol B Psychol Sci Soc Sci 2009;64(5):560–8.

102. Dubois B, Picard G, Sarazin M. Early detection of Alzheimer's disease: new diagnostic criteria. Dialogues Clin Neurosci 2009;11(2):135–9.

103. Small GW, Kepe V, Ercoli LM, et al. PET of brain amyloid and tau in mild cognitive impairment. N Engl J Med 2006;355(25):2652–63.

104. Rowe CC, Ackerman U, Browne W, et al. Imaging of amyloid beta in Alzheimer's disease with 18F-BAY94-9172, a novel PET tracer: proof of mechanism. Lancet Neurol 2008;7(2):129–35.

105. Wong DF, Rosenberg PB, Zhou Y, et al. In vivo imaging of amyloid deposition in Alzheimer disease using the radioligand 18F-AV-45 (florbetapir [corrected] F 18). J Nucl Med 2010;51(6):913–20.

106. Mielke MM, Kozauer NA, Chan KC, et al. Regionally-specific diffusion tensor imaging in mild cognitive impairment and Alzheimer's disease. Neuroimage 2009;46(1):47–55.

107. Blennow K. Cerebrospinal fluid protein biomarkers for Alzheimer's disease. NeuroRx 2004;1(2):213–25.

108. Marksteiner J, Hinterhuber H, Humpel C. Cerebrospinal fluid biomarkers for diagnosis of Alzheimer's disease: beta-amyloid(1-42), tau, phospho-tau-181 and total protein. Drugs Today (Barc) 2007;43(6):423–31.

109. Landau SM, Harvey D, Madison CM, et al. Comparing predictors of conversion and decline in mild cognitive impairment. Neurology 2010;75(3):230–8.

110. Mangialasche F, Solomon A, Winblad B, et al. Alzheimer's disease: clinical trials and drug development. Lancet Neurol 2010;9(7):702–16.

111. Lilly. Lilly halts development of semagacestat for Alzheimer's disease based on preliminary results of phase III clinical trials. 2010. Available at: http://newsroom.lilly.com/releasedetail.cfm?ReleaseID=499794. Accessed August 27, 2010.

112. McLaurin J, Kierstead ME, Brown ME, et al. Cyclohexanehexol inhibitors of Abeta aggregation prevent and reverse Alzheimer phenotype in a mouse model. Nat Med 2006;12(7):801–8.

113. Pamela G, Martin K, Aleksandra P, et al. Oral amyloid anti-aggregating agent ELND005 is measurable in CSF and brain of healthy adult men. Alzheimers Dement 2009;5(4):P323.

114. Elan. Elan and transition therapeutics announce modifications to ELND005 phase II clinical trials in Alzheimer's disease. Available at: http://newsroom.elan.com/phoenix.zhtml?c=88326&p=irol-pressroomarticle&ID=1365793&highlight. Accessed August 17, 2010.

115. Dodel RC, Du Y, Depboylu C, et al. Intravenous immunoglobulins containing antibodies against beta-amyloid for the treatment of Alzheimer's disease. J Neurol Neurosurg Psychiatry 2004;75(10):1472–4.

116. Pierre NT, Paul A, Jeffrey C, et al. The ADCS valproate neuroprotection trial: primary efficacy and safety results. Alzheimers Dement 2009;5(4):P84–5.

New Wine in Old Bottle: Late-life Psychosis

Alana Iglewicz, MD[a], Thomas W. Meeks, MD[a], Dilip V. Jeste, MD[b],*

KEYWORDS

• Schizophrenia • Psychosis • Late-life • Dementia • Age

Psychosis, most simply defined by the presence of hallucinations and/or delusions, is relatively common in older adults. Multiple etiologies for late-life psychosis exist, as any pathological process affecting the brain can manifest as psychosis. Neuropsychiatric etiologies of psychosis include chronic conditions, such as early-onset schizophrenia, late-onset schizophrenia, delusional disorder, psychosis associated with various dementias, and affective disorders with psychotic features, as well as certain chronic neurological conditions. Additionally, psychosis can be seen in more acute, sometimes reversible conditions, such as delirium, alcohol and/or substance use or withdrawal, and certain neurological diseases. Our review focuses on the nonaffective neuropsychiatric etiologies of late-life psychosis. Within this focus, we distinguish between those conditions that develop in early adulthood and persist into later life versus those with a late-life illness onset.

HISTORY

Much of the research on late-life psychosis, especially that regarding late-life schizophrenia, is predicated on a historical understanding of the longitudinal course of psychosis. Kraepelin is often credited with first conceptualizing and describing schizophrenia as *dementia praecox* in 1896. However, this term was first used by Morel in 1860 to illustrate a case of an adolescent boy with the acute onset of psychotic symptoms and cognitive deterioration.[1,2] The term *dementia praecox* references the course

Financial Disclosure: Dilip V. Jeste: AstraZeneca, Bristol-Myers Squibb, Eli Lilly, and Janssen donate medication to our NIMH-funded research grant, "Metabolic Effects of Newer Antipsychotics in Older Pts."
This work was supported, in part, by the National Institute of Mental Health grant MH080002 and MH01993 and the John A. Hartford Foundation.
[a] Department of Psychiatry, University of California, San Diego, 9500 Gilman Drive, Mail Code 0664, La Jolla, San Diego, CA 92093, USA
[b] Sam and Rose Stein Institute for Research on Aging, University of California, San Diego, 9500 Gilman Drive, # 0664, La Jolla, San Diego, CA 92093, USA
* Corresponding author.
E-mail address: djeste@ucsd.edu

Psychiatr Clin N Am 34 (2011) 295–318
doi:10.1016/j.psc.2011.02.008
0193-953X/11/$ – see front matter © 2011 Elsevier Inc. All rights reserved.

psych.theclinics.com

(progressive) and age of onset (early) of schizophrenia and has laid the foundation for many current conceptualizations and misconceptualizations of late-life psychosis. Jeste and colleagues[3] have summarized this historical background. In contrast to our current conceptualization of dementia, Kraepelin's use of "dementia" suggested a progressive personality deterioration with regard to volition and emotion. Meanwhile, the term "praecox" referenced an age of onset in adolescence or early adulthood.[4] Kraepelin also distinguished between two other phenomenologically distinct groups, which led to his categorical descriptions of *paraphrenia* and *paranoia*. Kraepelin used the term *paraphrenia* to describe patients who had a mostly paranoid presentation and generally a later age of onset.[5] He used the term *paranoia* to depict patients who had chronic, well-organized delusions, but did not manifest perceptual disturbances, personality deterioration, or a formal thought disorder. In many ways, this latter term is similar to the DSM-IV-TR construct of delusional disorder.

More modern concepts of late-life psychosis began to develop with the work of Eugen and Manfred Bleuler. Eugen Bleuler is recognized as being the first scientist to popularize the term *schizophrenia*. In contrast to Kraepelin, he did not believe that the disorder was necessarily characterized by illness course or age of onset.[6] The work of his son, Manfred Bleuler, on late-onset schizophrenia (LOS), demonstrated that the illness could first present later in life.[3,7] A substantial amount of research was completed in the United Kingdom in the mid-20th century on LOS, usually termed *paraphrenia*. Although LOS was initially met with much resistance in the United States, there has been a growing body of literature on LOS in the United States since the late 20th century. The age of onset and the course of the illness have remained centralizing foci of this research.

LATE-LIFE SCHIZOPHRENIA

The term "late-life schizophrenia" refers to schizophrenia in older adults regardless of when their symptoms first manifested. In particular, it is composed of older individuals with schizophrenia who first developed symptoms in early adulthood as well as individuals whose symptoms first emerged in later life.[8] As the aging population rapidly grows, the proportion of older adults with schizophrenia is expected to increase in an unprecedented fashion.[9]

Understanding the epidemiology of late-life schizophrenia is complex, as different nomenclatures, definitions of LOS, diagnostic criteria, and heterogeneity of clinical samples have been applied in the existing literature.[10] The Epidemiologic Catchment Area (ECA) study is most often cited for prevalence rates of late-life schizophrenia. This survey of psychopathology in the general US population reported 1-year schizophrenia prevalence rates of 0.6% among individuals aged 45 to 64 years and 0.2% for individuals aged 65 years and older. The ECA reported a lifetime prevalence of schizophrenia among people aged 45 to 64 of 1.0% and among people aged 65 years and older of 0.3%.[11] Several methodological limitations of this study likely resulted in an underestimation of late-life schizophrenia, including lack of age-appropriate diagnostic interview questions; additionally, there may be a premature death rate among persons with schizophrenia that lowers the prevalence in later life.[8,10,12–14]

The cost of caring for people with late-life schizophrenia is disproportionate to the numbers of individuals with this disorder. The health care costs of late-life schizophrenia are estimated to be at least as much as those among teenagers and young adults with schizophrenia.[8,14] Although the lifetime prevalence of schizophrenia is 1% (vs, for example, 20%–25% in major depression), schizophrenia across all age groups accounts for the greatest proportion of mental health care expenditures.[8,15]

One report comparing the annual health care costs for adults with schizophrenia to adults with dementia, depression, and physical illness found that for individuals older than 65, the annual cost of care for schizophrenia was the most expensive.[16] Nursing home care accounted for the vast majority of such expenditures. Overall, there is an increase in the costs associated with schizophrenia as people age.[17]

The emotional cost of caring for older adults with schizophrenia is also great, especially for spousal caregivers. In a study specifically looking at family caregivers of older adults with psychotic disorders, Patterson and colleagues[18] found that spousal caregivers more frequently provide assistance with instrumental activities of daily living and experience a sense of loss of identity and anticipated lifestyle than do other family member caregivers. Despite the literal and figurative costs of caring for older adults with schizophrenia, there is a relative dearth of research on this important and vulnerable segment of society. Cohen and colleagues[19] found that only 1% of the literature on schizophrenia focuses on late-life schizophrenia.

Early-Onset Schizophrenia in Later Life

Psychiatric symptoms

Historically, people with schizophrenia were thought to have a progressively worsening psychological, functional, and cognitive course as they aged. Much of the literature on community-dwelling individuals with schizophrenia challenges this notion.[1] A pattern of progressive deterioration has been shown in studies examining chronically institutionalized people with schizophrenia.[20,21] However, most individuals with schizophrenia currently do not reside in such institutions and those chronically residing in institutions generally epitomize the most severe manifestations of schizophrenia.[19]

Longitudinal studies examining older adults with early-onset schizophrenia (EOS) living in the community demonstrate a more optimistic prognosis. The Vermont Longitudinal Research Project was a 32-year prospective follow-up study of 118 persons retrospectively diagnosed with schizophrenia. Of the 82 participants who were interviewed 20 to 25 years after the start of the study, 68% no longer experienced signs or symptoms of schizophrenia and 45% no longer experienced any psychiatric symptoms.[22] Harding[23] later summarized 10 longitudinal studies comprising 2429 individuals with schizophrenia followed over an average of 28 years. Forty-six percent to 84% showed significant clinical improvement over time, especially in terms of their positive symptoms, ie, delusions and hallucinations. Similarly, in the World Health Organization (WHO) 15-year and 25-year international prospective study, 48% of the incidence group and 54% of the prevalence group were deemed "globally recovered."[24] In a cross-sectional study comparing a sample of older adults with schizophrenia with a control group of older adults without schizophrenia, Jeste and colleagues[25] found that aging was associated with a decrease in general psychopathology. Aging was not associated with progressive worsening in well-being, psychopathology, or functioning. In contrast to other studies, this study found a relatively stable course for schizophrenia, rather than one hallmarked by striking improvement. Remission rates vary considerably (8%–72%), likely secondary to differing definitions of remission and variations in study populations.[26,27] Overall, the community-based studies summarized previously challenge prior notions that the symptoms of schizophrenia progressively worsen with age.

Cognition

With the exception of chronically institutionalized people with schizophrenia, who are known to have a more deteriorative illness course, the literature supports a remarkably stable pattern of neuropsychological functioning in older individuals with schizophrenia.[17,28–30] For instance, in one study involving 116 community-dwelling individuals with EOS ($\leq$45 years old) versus 122 healthy control participants, no difference in the slope of cognitive decline was seen between the group of individuals with schizophrenia and the healthy controls.[30] In another study comparing dementia screening measures of individuals with EOS, LOS, Alzheimer disease (AD), and healthy controls, a stable cognitive pattern was seen for all groups except for those with AD.[31] Overall, studies involving community-dwelling individuals with schizophrenia support a stable cognitive pattern over time, contrasting with the historical concept of progressive deterioration with *dementia praecox*.

Although the pattern of neuropsychological functioning is stable in later life, the baseline cognition of schizophrenia is generally impaired compared with controls. Schizophrenia is associated with mild to moderate cognitive deficits (approximately 1 standard deviation below the mean of demographically comparable healthy comparison subjects) across a range of cognitive domains.[32] Notably, there is considerable heterogeneity in terms of the level and pattern of cognitive deficits among people with schizophrenia. Thus, there is no specific pattern of cognitive impairment that is either unique to or common among all people with schizophrenia. Nonetheless, deficits are usually found across a range of cognitive abilities, including attention and working memory, learning (but not retention) on measures of episodic memory, executive functions, and psychomotor/processing speed.[32,33] Crystallized verbal knowledge and retention of information once learned tend to be relatively spared. Studies suggest that the memory impairment seen in late-life schizophrenia is the result of poor organization or registration, rather than poor retrieval of information, as is seen in AD.[29,34–36] Elderly people with schizophrenia experience the typical subtle changes in cognitive function that occur with normal aging,[37] but presence of rapid forgetting is atypical and thus warrants further evaluation for possible comorbid factors, such as AD or other cortical dementias.[29]

Function

Likely related to its relatively stable neurocognitive trajectory, the functional course of schizophrenia appears less pessimistic than previously thought. Patterson and colleagues[38] found that the functioning of older adults with schizophrenia was more impaired than that of healthy controls, except with regard to grooming and eating, and that disability was related to greater cognitive impairment, increased extrapyramidal symptoms, and less formal education. In a study comparing middle-aged and older adults with schizophrenia to demographically matched controls, Palmer and colleagues[39] found considerable heterogeneity in the functional status of older adults with schizophrenia. Although the group of people with schizophrenia had a worse functional status than the healthy controls, a substantial number of persons with schizophrenia drove automobiles, lived independently, and had been employed at least half of their adult lives after their schizophrenia was diagnosed. Interestingly, positive symptoms were not correlated with functional status, whereas negative, symptoms (eg, apathy, amotivation) were inversely correlated with functional status. In a qualitative study among 32 adults with chronic schizophrenia aged 50 and older, considerable heterogeneity was found in perceptions of their own functional status, reiterating that statistically significant changes still fail to capture the individual life stories that should always be considered in clinical evaluations.[40]

Life satisfaction and quality of life

Although life satisfaction and quality of life are generally lower among older adults with schizophrenia compared with their peers without schizophrenia, most older adults with schizophrenia report a relatively high level of life satisfaction and deny a worsening in their quality of life associated with aging.[19,41] Life satisfaction is often associated with subjective, rather than objective measures,[41] whereas quality of life has been found to correlate indirectly with positive symptoms.[42] Severity of depressive symptoms, impairment in cognitive functioning, and earlier age of schizophrenia onset influence the mental health quality of life and functioning of older adults with schizophrenia,[43] whereas social functional impairment, psychosocial factors including avoidant coping styles and negative life events, and severity of psychotic symptoms influence the overall health-related quality of life of older adults with schizophrenia.[44] Interestingly, patients with schizophrenia report better subjective well-being than do patients with mood, anxiety, or somatoform disorders,[45] and older individuals with schizophrenia report better mental health quality of life than do younger adults with schizophrenia.[46]

Social connectedness is often related to quality of life. Historically, older adults with schizophrenia were often assumed to be socially isolated. A study comparing middle-aged and older adults with schizophrenia with healthy subjects challenges this belief.[47] Compared with adults without schizophrenia, those with schizophrenia were less likely to be married, have children, and live with others; however, they were still remarkably socially connected—97% had regular contact with family or friends and 62% had been married at some point in their lives. Furthermore, individuals with schizophrenia were similar to those without schizophrenia in terms of presence of a family confidant, frequency of contact with family, extent of interpersonal difficulties, and amount of instrumental support received.

Predictors of outcome

Several factors predict a negative long-term outcome in late-life schizophrenia. These include premorbid deficits in psychosocial and overall function, prominent negative symptoms, and gradual symptom onset.[48] All of the regression models in the WHO 15-year and 25-year international follow-up study indicate that the strongest predictors of long-term outcome in schizophrenia are such measures of the early illness course, with the amount of time experiencing psychotic symptoms in the first 2 years of illness being the strongest predictor of symptoms and disability in later life.[24] In light of the symptomatic improvement seen in many older adults with schizophrenia and the finding that early-onset characteristics best predict long-term outcome, the authors of the WHO international study concluded that the findings "offer robust reasons for therapeutic optimism and point to a critical 'window of opportunity' in the early period of syndromal differentiation."

Late-Onset Schizophrenia and Very-Late-Onset Schizophrenia-Like Psychosis

Background

The nomenclature to describe schizophrenia that first manifests in later life has changed considerably over time. Historically, as previously described, the onset of schizophrenia was thought to be limited to adolescence or early adulthood. Criteria outlined by Feighner and his colleagues[49] in 1972 restricted the diagnosis of schizophrenia to onset before age 40. Similarly, the DSM-III did not allow for the diagnosis if the onset occurred after age 45. Subsequently, the DSM-III-R permitted the diagnosis of schizophrenia late-onset type after age 45, and the DSM-IV contains no diagnostic restrictions for age of onset.[8] An international consensus in 2000 proposed that individuals with onset of schizophrenia after the age of 40 be subdivided into LOS if the symptoms manifested between ages 40 and 60 and very-late-onset schizophrenia-like psychosis (VLOSLP) if the symptoms manifested after age 60.[50] Much of the existing literature does not discern between the latter distinction of LOS and VLOSLP. Rather, onset after age 40 or 45 is often referenced as LOS. As such, this section will summarize what is known about LOS in the broader sense of this definition and will distinguish between LOS and VLOSLP in terms of the international consensus when possible. **Table 1** also summarizes some key differences among various diagnoses of late-life psychosis, with the intent to serve as a quick, somewhat simplified, reference for distinguishing among key clinical differences among these diagnoses based on extant literature.

Epidemiology

The overall epidemiology for late-life schizophrenia (ie, including those with early onsets who have aged) was described previously. Here, we focus on the epidemiology of LOS and VLOSLP. In Manfred Bleuler's study of 459 patients with schizophrenia, 14.8% had onset after age 40.[1,51] Incidence rates for onset after age 44 are 12.6 per 100,000 population per year[50] and incidence rates for VLOSLP increase by 11% every 5 years after age 60.[52] Newer data suggest that the annual incidence for LOS between ages 45 and 64 years in the community is 0.3%.[53]

Clinical features

Several similarities exist between EOS and LOS, including the severity of global psychopathology and positive symptoms, levels of childhood maladjustment, family history of schizophrenia (10%–15% having a first-degree relative with schizophrenia), response to neuroleptics, and chronicity of course.[3,35] Prospective studies indicate that individuals with LOS or EOS have a 2 to 3 times greater mortality rate than various comparison groups, including the general US population aged between 55 and 65 years.[3] Interestingly, individuals with LOS or EOS share an elevated amount of minor physical anomalies compared with healthy subjects, suggesting the possibility of early developmental aberrations.[54] Both groups have higher levels of corrected

Table 1
Comparison of clinical characteristics among various diagnoses of late-life psychosis

	EOS	LOS	VLOSLP	PoD
Schizophrenia family history	↑	↑	Ø	Ø
Dementia-like cognitive decline	Ø	Ø	↑	↑↑
Magnitude of necessary neuroleptic dose	↑↑	↑	↑	↑/Ø
Conclusive/specific brain MRI abnormalities	Ø	Ø	↑	↑/Ø
Female preponderance	Ø	↑	↑↑	Ø
Negative symptoms	↑↑	↑	Ø	Ø
Overall magnitude of cognitive impairment	↑	↑	↑↑	↑↑↑
Presence of minor physical anomalies	↑	↑	Ø	Ø
Preponderance of paranoid subtype	↑	↑↑	↑↑?	N/A
Thought disorder	↑/↑↑	↑	Ø	Ø
Prominence of visual (vs auditory) hallucinations	↑/Ø	↑	↑?	↑↑
Complex (>simple) delusions	↑↑	↑	↑?	↑/Ø

Abbreviations: EOS, early-onset schizophrenia; LOS, late-onset schizophrenia; MRI, magnetic resonance imaging; N/A, not applicable; PoD, psychosis of dementia; VLOSLP, very late-onset schizophrenia-like psychosis; ↑, moderately present; ↑↑, strongly present; Ø, not present; ?, partially supported by the literature.
Data from Palmer BW, McClure F, Jeste DV. Schizophrenia in late-life: findings challenge traditional concepts. Harv Rev Psychiatry 2001;9:51–8.

sensory deficits (eg, wearing eyeglasses and/or hearing aides) compared with controls; however, they have levels of uncorrected sensory impairments similar to age-matched individuals without schizophrenia.[3]

Nonetheless, differences between individuals with EOS and LOS have also been observed in the literature. Phenomenological differences exist between the types of hallucinations and delusions that persons with LOS versus EOS experience. Individuals with LOS more commonly report visual, tactile, and olfactory hallucinations in addition to third-person running commentary and accusatory auditory hallucinations compared with those with EOS.[50,55,56] Individuals with LOS more frequently experience partition (the belief that people, objects, or radiation can pass through what would normally constitute a barrier to such passage), phantom border, and persecutory delusions.[50,57] According to most studies, individuals with LOS less commonly have severe negative symptoms or a formal thought disorder, and thus more commonly present with paranoid-type schizophrenia.[3,35]

However, the most current findings from the research group at the University of California, San Diego (UCSD), synthesizing the data on middle-age and older adults with schizophrenia collected over the past 20 years, challenge some of the accepted similarities and distinctions between individuals with EOS and LOS.[58] Contrasting with previous studies, no statistically significant differences were found between the two groups' severity of negative symptoms or in the proportion of individuals with illness paranoid subtype. More consonant with previous research, the LOS group had less severe positive symptoms and general psychopathology than did the EOS group and were prescribed lower doses of neuroleptics than their EOS peers.[58] Sociodemographic differences were also observed between EOS and LOS patients. LOS patients were more likely to have been married at some point than persons with EOS.[3,58] Women were consistently overrepresented in samples of LOS across multiple studies of LOS. Some investigators hypothesize that this gender difference may reflect psychosocial factors,[50] whereas others theorize that this difference may be hormonally mediated.[1]

Cognition and function

As aforementioned, the Kraepelinian notion of *dementia praecox* fails to capture the stable cognitive trajectory associated with LOS over time.[3,31] In a series of studies completed at UCSD, individuals with LOS were found to be less impaired than were those with EOS in terms of abstraction/flexibility of thinking and semantic memory.[3] Additionally, the newest analyses of the UCSD studies indicated that patients with LOS have better processing speed and verbal memory than do patients with EOS.[58] The San Diego studies also found that individuals with LOS exhibited better premorbid functioning in their adolescent and early adulthood years. Overall, the studies reveal that LOS is certainly not a dementing illness. Nor does EOS appear to be a dementing illness per se in the sense of progressing over time, but it appears possibly to cause more profound baseline cognitive deficits than LOS.

Neuroimaging

Similar to imaging studies in patients with EOS, nonspecific structural abnormalities (eg, higher ventricle-to-brain ratio) and focal structural changes (reductions in the superior temporal gyrus and left temporal lobe) have been seen in imaging studies of patients with LOS.[50,59] Interestingly, larger thalami have been found in imaging studies of patients with LOS compared with patients with EOS, suggesting the theoretical involvement of defective thalamic pruning in the etiology of LOS.[3,60] Although some discrepancies exist in the literature, studies that carefully exclude individuals with organic cerebral illness do not indicate an increase in white matter hyperintensities or tumors in the brains of patients with LOS.[3,61,62]

Very-late-onset schizophrenia-like psychosis

In a prospective study comparing individuals with VLOSLP to a gender-matched sample of individuals with earlier onset schizophrenia, the patients with VLOSLP were distinguished by higher rates of marriage, higher education levels, better responses to treatment with risperidone, and more pronounced cerebellar atrophy.[5,63] A qualitative study examining the subjective experience of individuals with VLOSLP found 4 emerging themes: long-term experience of the self as different, loneliness, solitary coping style, and an attempt to find meaning in the manifestation of the psychosis.[40] Overall, VLOSLP may be a neurodegenerative process in contrast to LOS that develops before age 60, which is theorized to be a neurodevelopmental process.[1,50] However, more research is needed to substantiate these theories. In a case report, Cervantes and colleagues[64] propose that a 100-year-old woman meets the criteria for LOS, challenging our reluctance to diagnose schizophrenia when the symptoms emerge after age 60. Much research remains to be conducted to better characterize this syndrome currently labeled as VLOSLP.

DELUSIONAL DISORDER

A dearth of literature exists about delusional disorder in older adults. Studies often do not distinguish between delusions in general, which can be present in a multitude of disorders, and delusional disorder more specifically. Further complicating the picture, the nosology of delusional disorder has shifted over time. Historically, delusional disorder has been referenced as paranoia, paranoid reaction, paraphrenia, paranoid psychosis, paranoid condition, paranoid state, and paranoid disorder.[65]

According to DSM-IV-TR, delusional disorder generally manifests in middle to late adulthood, with women presenting later than men. The prevalence is 0.03% and is somewhat higher in women.[66] De Portugal and colleagues[67] found a female-to-male ratio of 1.6:1.0, with men experiencing more severe symptoms and worse functional outcomes. Meanwhile, the incidence of delusional disorder is 15.6 per 100,000.[68]

Delusional disorder accounts for 1% to 4% of inpatient psychiatric hospital admissions and is seen more frequently in lower socioeconomic status and immigrant populations.[65] In a study comparing patients with late-onset psychosis with somatic delusions to both controls and late-onset psychotic patients without somatic delusions, most participants with somatic delusions met criteria for delusional disorder.[69] Additionally, those with somatic delusions were more commonly female, had been sick longer, had lower IQs, were often immigrants or first generation, poorly complied with psychotropic treatment, sought repeated medical evaluations, and presented with varied somatic delusions. Although admitted to hospitals less frequently, people with delusional disorder often have more severe psychopathology than individuals with schizophrenia.[70] Risk factors for delusional disorder for the general adult population include a family history of schizoid, avoidant, or paranoid personality disorder or schizophrenia.[71] Considering the symptomatic severity associated with delusional disorder, the related cost from extensive use of medical services, the decrease in patient quality of life, and the limited extant data on delusional disorder, there is an unambiguous need for increased research into the optimal identification of and treatment for older adults with delusional disorder. These efforts may entail training and interventions in primary care and other nonpsychiatric settings.

PSYCHOSIS OF ALZHEIMER DISEASE
Epidemiology

In their extensive review of 55 studies on the psychosis of Alzheimer disease (AD), Ropacki and Jeste[72] found the median prevalence of psychotic symptoms was 41.1%, the median prevalence of delusions was 36.0%, and the median prevalence of hallucinations was 18.0%. Prevalence was affected by setting, with higher rates of psychosis in inpatient settings than in outpatient settings. Prevalence rates of psychotic symptoms in 85-year-old individuals with AD have recently been found to be 36%.[73] One-year incidence rates for the development of psychosis in patients with AD range from 20.0% to 25.0%, whereas 2-year incidence rates range from 32.5% to 36.1%.[74–76] Incidence seemingly levels off after 3 years.[72]

Clinical Features

Several differences distinguish the psychosis seen in AD from that in late-life schizophrenia. Visual hallucinations are more common than are auditory hallucinations in AD, contrasting the pattern seen in schizophrenia.[72] Schneiderian first-rank symptoms (eg, auditory hallucinations commenting on actions, thought insertion, thought withdrawal) are exceedingly rare in AD.[77]

The delusions seen in AD often have distinguishing characteristics from those in schizophrenia. The delusions are typically simple, nonbizarre, and paranoid.[77] They often relate to memory deficits, as exemplified by delusions of theft occurring after individuals with AD misplace items. Misidentification delusions, the false belief that close loved ones are not who they say they are, are frequent in the psychosis seen in AD. In fact, a recent study examining late-onset AD found that misidentification delusions were the most common psychotic symptom reported (23.4% had misidentification delusions, 21.1% had paranoid delusions, 3.1% had imposter delusions).[78]

Also in contrast to the pattern with schizophrenia, a past history of psychosis is rare for patients with AD with psychotic symptoms.[79] Hallucinations and delusions often appear to remit in the later stages of AD, but it is unclear if this pattern reflects an artifact secondary to patients being unable to communicate their psychotic symptoms in the later stages of their illness or a natural resolution of the symptoms; nonetheless, the psychosis of AD does appear to have a more fluctuant course with remissions and recurrences than that seen in late-life schizophrenia.[77]

Risk Factors and Associations

The association between psychosis in AD and several demographic variables is equivocal. In their review of the literature, Ropacki and Jeste[72] noted that 5 of 7 studies examining the relationship between psychosis with AD and ethnicity found an association with being African American. Meanwhile, family history of dementia, older age, and female gender are weakly associated with an increased risk for psychosis of AD.[72,80] Psychosis of AD inconsistently relates to older age, duration of AD, and later age of onset of AD.[72,74]

Bassiony and colleagues[81] determined different associations and risk markers for the delusions and hallucinations of AD. Delusions and combined delusions and hallucinations in individuals with AD were associated with older age, increased depression, more aggression, and worse general health. In contrast, hallucinations in individuals with AD were associated with having more severe dementia, being African American, having less formal education, and having gait impairment. Antihypertensive use was associated with delusions, whereas anxiolytic use was associated with hallucinations.

However, these data are limited, as they were not analyzed with multiple regression analysis.

Newer data indicate that psychosis in AD may have genetic determinants. Psychosis with AD is thought to represent a distinct phenotype.[82] Sweet and colleagues[78] found that psychosis aggregates with late-onset AD families, suggesting a possible genetic basis. Apolipoprotein E4 (APO E4) genotype, dopamine and serotonin receptor gene polymorphisms, serotonin and dopamine transporter gene polymorphisms, as well as nicotinic acetylcholine receptor, interleukin-1β gene promoter, catecholamine-O-methyl-transferase (COMT), and neuregulin-1 (NRG1) genetic polymorphisms are being analyzed as possible correlates with psychosis of AD.[73,83] The extant literature on APO E4 genotype and psychosis of AD is remarkably equivocal,[73,83] and data on other genes are quite premature, making it difficult to discern any clear genetic determinants of psychosis in AD at this time.

In summarizing the neuropathological, neurochemical, and neuroimaging correlates of psychosis in AD, Jeste and Finkel[77] reported that researchers have found an association between delusions in dementia and frontotemporal cortex dysfunction in addition to an association between psychosis in dementia and increased subcortical norepinephrine levels, greater cortical neurodegenerative changes, and decreased cortical and subcortical serotonin/5-HIAA levels. Lee and colleagues[84] describe a correlation between psychotic symptoms in AD and white matter changes in the frontal, left basal ganglia, and parieto-occipital brain regions. More specifically, the white matter changes are associated with delusional misidentification, but not hallucinations or paranoid delusions.

Clinical Sequelae

The clinical and psychosocial consequences of psychosis in AD and other dementias are profound. In distinction from AD without psychotic symptoms, psychosis with AD is associated with greater cognitive impairment and more rapid cognitive decline.[74,79,85,86] Psychosis in dementia is linked to greater caregiver distress,[87,88] poorer quality of life,[89] greater prevalence of extrapyramidal signs,[90] decreased physical health,[81] and increased mortality (specifically associated with hallucinations as opposed to delusions).[91,92] Psychosis of dementia has also been linked with other neuropsychiatric disturbances, such as anxiety, agitation, and aggression.[72,93–96] For example, 85% of patients with dementia who were selected to participate in a study based on their problematic behaviors had psychotic symptoms. Behavioral disturbances and agitation are often inciting factors for institutionalization in general. It is thus not surprising that psychosis of AD is a significant predictor of functional decline and institutionalization.[89,91,97]

Psychosis Associated with Other Dementias

Psychosis frequently complicates various other non-AD dementias. Three common disorders in that category are vascular dementia (VaD), Parkinson disease dementia (PDD), and Lewy body dementia (LBD). In their population-based study of 85-year-old individuals with dementia, Ostling and colleagues[73] found that a higher percentage of people with VaD had psychotic symptoms than did people with AD (54% vs 36% respectively). They also observed that delusions were nearly twice as common in VaD than in AD. No association was found between degree of dementia severity and presence of psychotic symptoms in VaD, contrasting the pattern found in AD wherein the probability of psychosis increases with worsening severity of AD up to a certain stage of illness. The manifestation of psychosis in VaD likely depends on the brain region(s) affected by the vascular insult(s), eg, well-formed visual hallucinations in an occipital lobe infarct.

Psychosis commonly occurs in both PDD and LBD. The clinical characteristics of PDD and LBD are similar, but the timing of dementia onset relative to the onset of parkinsonism symptoms helps differentiate PDD from LBD. PDD is diagnosed when the dementia onset is 1 year or more after the onset of parkinsonism. In contrast, LBD is diagnosed when the dementia onset occurs within 1 year after the onset of motor symptoms of parkinsonism.[98] Patients with parkinsonism and psychosis (both LBD and PDD) can be categorized as experiencing "benign hallucinosis" or complex psychotic symptoms. "Benign hallucinosis," which often occurs in PD without dementia, implies nontroubling mild visual perceptual disturbances for which patients usually maintain insight and often do not warrant treatment.[99] In contrast, people with PDD and LBD more often experience frightening complex psychotic symptoms for which they lack insight, are associated with behavioral changes, and often warrant treatment.[99]

In a prospective study of 239 community-based patients with PD followed over 12 years,[100] 60% had psychotic symptoms and the incidence rate of psychosis was 79.7 per 1000 person-years. Psychosis in PD is associated with increased odds of dementia, increased disability, older age at onset of PD, presence of REM sleep behavior disorder, and higher doses of dopaminergic treatment, suggesting that psychosis of PD indicates a more malignant course of the illness.[100]

Proposed diagnostic criteria for psychosis in PD include having at least illusions, hallucinations, delusions, or a false sense of presence on a recurrent or continuous basis for 1 month with possible associated features of insight, dementia, and treatment for PD.[101] Visual hallucinations are the most frequent psychotic symptom present in PDD,[102] occurring in nearly half of patients.[103] Delusions are usually in the presence of comorbid hallucinations in PDD and are seen in up to 10% of patients.[104,105] Similar to AD, persistence of psychosis in PD and PDD is associated with caregiver distress, institutionalization, and functional impairment.[99,106]

Psychotic symptoms in LBD can be classified as hallucinations, delusions, or misidentifications.[107] As with PDD, visual hallucinations are the most frequent psychotic symptom in LBD and serve as one of the core diagnostic features.[97] Systematized delusions and hallucinations in other modalities occur less frequently than do visual hallucinations, but are not uncommon, and are thus supportive diagnostic features. Misidentifications in LBD range from simple misidentifications of people to "delusional misidentification syndromes," such as Capgras syndrome and the "phantom boarder" delusion.[108,109] A recent study found that 78% of patients with LBD had hallucinations, 56% had misidentifications, and 25% had delusions.[107] Individuals with LBD have higher rates of hallucinations and delusions than do individuals with either PDD or PD without dementia.[103] Because the psychotic symptoms with LBD occur earlier in the course of the disease and are more frequent than in AD, they tend to cause more caregiver distress at the early stages of illness.[110] Interestingly, neural correlates to the psychotic symptoms in LBD have been discovered recently.[111] Visual hallucinations, delusions, and misidentifications respectively relate to dysfunction in the cortical occipital and parietal association areas, frontal cortex, and limbic-paralimbic areas.

Treatment

Schizophrenia
Pharmacotherapy Most of the studies of pharmacotherapy treatments for late-life schizophrenia focus on individuals with EOS, rather than LOS or VLOSLP. Although

certain discrepancies exist, these studies overall support the efficacy of various atypical antipsychotics, including clozapine, risperidone, olanzapine, and aripiprazole, in the treatment of older adults with schizophrenia.[112–114] Use of low-dose risperidone has relatively more positive data in controlled trials.[115,116] Similar rates of efficacy for the treatment of older persons with chronic schizophrenia were found between risperidone (average dose 2 mg) and olanzapine (average dose 10 mg) in a randomized controlled trial (RCT), but olanzapine was associated with greater metabolic side effects.[117] Jeste and colleagues[114] recommend that when used, risperidone should be started at 0.25 to 0.50 mg/day and increased no more than 0.50 mg/day to a maximum dosage of 3.00 mg/day or less. Risperidone 1.25 to 3.50 mg/day was the first-line recommendation according to expert consensus for the treatment of late-life schizophrenia, followed closely by quetiapine 100 to 300 mg/day, olanzapine 7.5 to 15.0 mg/day, and aripiprazole 15 to 30 mg/day in a survey completed by 48 American experts in geriatric medicine and geriatric psychiatry.[118] A recent Cochrane review[119] concluded that there is no current evidence base specifically for antipsychotic drug treatment for older people with LOS or VLOSLP. Open studies of typical antipsychotics used for the treatment of LOS and VLOSLP indicated that 48% to 61% of patients demonstrated full remission of psychotic symptoms.[50]

When treating older adults with antipsychotic medications, it is imperative to consider various side effects. These include cardiovascular, sedative, anticholinergic, and metabolic effects, in addition to extrapyramidal symptoms (EPS), tardive dyskinesia (TD), hyperprolactinemia, agranulocytosis, and neuroleptic malignant syndrome (NMS).[112] Orthostatic hypotension commonly occurs in older adults treated with medications that block α-1 adrenoreceptors (eg, conventional low-potency antipsychotics, risperidone, quetiapine, and clozapine)[112] and is associated with falls and hip fractures.[120] Meanwhile, the use of typical antipsychotics is limited by the dramatically increased risk of TD in older adults treated with typical antipsychotics. Jeste[121] determined that the cumulative annual incidence of TD in older adults treated with low-dose typical antipsychotics was 26.1%, which is 5 to 6 times the rate of that observed in younger adults. Atypical antipsychotics are associated with significantly lower rates of TD in older adults than are typical antipsychotics, as demonstrated by a prospective study comparing risperidone to haloperidol.[122] However, adverse metabolic effects associated with atypical antipsychotics, including weight gain, dyslipidemia, and glucose intolerance/diabetes mellitus, are concerning. In an analysis of 45 cases of new-onset diabetes and diabetic ketoacidosis associated with atypical antipsychotic use, Jin and colleagues[123] reported that 44% were related to clozapine, whereas 42% were related to olanzapine. In light of their potential adverse metabolic consequences, close monitoring in older adults prescribed atypical antipsychotics remains important. Jin and colleagues[124] determined that the triglyceride–high-density lipoprotein ratio, waist circumference, and body mass index were each independent risk markers for metabolic syndrome in antipsychotic-treated adults aged 40 and older. The underlying mechanisms of metabolic syndrome associated with atypical antipsychotic use are unknown, but hypothetically may involve alterations in ghrelin and adiponectin levels.[125] In summary, antipsychotics are useful in controlling the symptoms of late-life schizophrenia, but their use can be problematic in older adults because of their proclivity to cause side effects. As such, one should heed caution when using these medications in this population.

Psychosocial interventions Growing evidence supports the adjunctive use of psychosocial interventions to treat late-life schizophrenia. Pharmacologic treatments aim to reduce symptom burden. However, a reduction in psychotic symptoms does not necessarily translate into improved functioning.[126] In the arena of functional improvement, psychosocial interventions, used in conjunction with pharmacotherapy, show promise as an adjunctive treatment modality in older adults with schizophrenia. For example, Functional Adaptation Skills Training (FAST), a group-format manualized therapy that targets everyday life skills, improves the functional adaptation of older adults with schizophrenia[126,127] and decreases their short-term use of emergency medical services.[128] Meanwhile, a pilot study of Programa de Entrenamiento para el Desarrollo de Aptitudes para Latinos (PEDAL [A Training Program to Develop Skills for Latinos]),[129] a culturally modified version of FAST for older Latinos with chronic psychosis, indicates that PEDAL helps improve the everyday living skills of older Latino patients with chronic psychotic disorders up to 6 to 12 months.

Cognitive-behavioral therapy (CBT) and social skills training (SST) are evidence-based adjunctive therapies to psychopharmacologic treatment in younger adults with schizophrenia.[130] RCTs of the combination of CBT and SST, called cognitive behavioral social skills training (CBSST), for adults with late-life schizophrenia indicated that CBBST led to better skills acquisition and self-reported functioning than did participation in standard care,[131] with benefits persisting at 1-year follow-up.[132] Participants' neuropsychological test results did not mediate the improvement in functioning observed with CBSST.[133] A decrease in personal sense of hopelessness may explain the efficacy of CBSST in older adults with schizophrenia, suggesting that hopelessness might be a promising target in CBT for late-life schizophrenia.[134]

Cognitive training (CT), also referenced as cognitive remediation, aims to improve the neuropsychological functioning of individuals with schizophrenia. Reviews of the literature on CT conclude that this treatment modality helps improve the everyday functioning, symptoms, and cognitive performance of adults with schizophrenia, especially when combined with pharmacologic and psychosocial interventions.[135,136] Additionally, employment can add meaning and quality to life and many middle-aged and older adults with schizophrenia, often to many people's surprise, desire to work or volunteer. Research shows that supported employment, based on the principle of "place then train" is more successful than is conventional work rehabilitation, based on the principle of "train then place."[137] Supported employment is effective at helping middle-aged and older people with schizophrenia obtain competitive employment with respective improvement in their quality of life.[138] Overall, numerous evidence-based psychosocial interventions help improve the quality of life and functional status of older adults with schizophrenia when used in conjunction with pharmacotherapy.

Treating the psychosis of AD

Pharmacotherapy interventions Much of the evidence-based research on the treatment of psychosis in dementia focuses on pharmacotherapy, despite a general consensus that trials of psychosocial interventions are preferred before initiating medications because of the general lack of favorable risk-benefit profiles for pharmacotherapy in psychosis of dementia.[139] As older adults are more susceptible to extrapyramidal side effects and tardive dyskinesia caused by typical antipsychotics,[121] atypical antipsychotics have become widely used in the treatment of psychosis with AD over the past decade; yet, the evidence to support their use is mixed.[140] The Clinical Antipsychotic Trials of Intervention Effectiveness for Alzheimer Disease (CATIE-AD) is the largest nonindustry-sponsored study of the use of atypical antipsychotics to treat psychosis and/or agitation/aggression in individuals with dementia[140] and its primary outcome measure was one of effectiveness (vs efficacy)—time to medication discontinuation for any reason. The authors of CATIE-AD[141] found no significant difference between placebo, risperidone, quetiapine, and olanzapine for all-cause discontinuation rate, but found that fewer people taking risperidone and olanzapine discontinued because of lack of efficacy. However, several studies more clearly support the efficacy of low-dose risperidone (1 mg–2 mg) and olanzapine (5 mg–10 mg) in treating AD with psychosis.[93,142–144] It is difficult to generalize the findings from these studies, as most were conducted in nursing homes, many contained patients with forms of dementia other than AD, and most were not designed explicitly to examine psychotic symptoms.[145] Not all studies have found risperidone and olanzapine to be efficacious in this population. For example, Deberdt and colleagues[146] found no difference in efficacy among placebo, olanzapine, and risperidone, but did find that risperidone was associated with increased frequency of elevated prolactin levels (78% compared with 16.7% for olanzapine and 5% for placebo) and that olanzapine was associated with increased frequency of weight gain. Meanwhile, a review of the literature on aripiprazole for psychosis of AD indicates that only 1 of 3 existing RCTs found that aripiprazole was significantly more efficacious for addressing psychosis of AD than placebo.[113] Similarly, the data on cholinesterase inhibitors for the treatment of psychosis of AD are mixed, and even less sound in their clinical trial design.[72] The efficacy of atypical antipsychotics may be no different from that of typical antipsychotics, as evidenced by similar effect sizes (about 18%) found in meta-analyses of atypical and typical antipsychotics.[147,148] In the survey previously described, the experts' first-line recommendation for the treatment of agitated dementia with delusions was risperidone 0.5 to 2.0 mg/day followed by olanzapine 5.0 to 7.5 mg/day and quetiapine 50 to 150 mg/day.[118]

In addition to their mixed efficacy, use of atypical antipsychotics is complicated by their side-effect profile and respective black-box warnings issued by the Food and Drug Administration (FDA). The FDA first issued a warning about atypical antipsychotics in 2003 entitled "Cerebrovascular Adverse Events, Including Stroke, in Elderly Patients with Dementia." An avalanche of similar warnings for various atypical antipsychotics including olanzapine and aripiprazole ensued, followed by warnings for an increased risk of mortality in patients receiving atypical antipsychotics. A meta-analysis of the data[147] indicated that the overall rates of cerebrovascular events (CVAEs) in patients treated with atypical antipsychotics was 1.9% versus 0.9% in placebo-treated individuals, with a respective odds ratio of 2.1. Meanwhile, another meta-analysis[149] determined that the risk of mortality in patients receiving atypical antipsychotics was 3.5% compared with 2.3% in the placebo group, yielding an odds ratio of 1.5. Limitations in the data used to formulate the black-box warnings abound. The studies were designed to determine efficacy, not CVAEs or mortality; the category of CVAEs was not operationally defined; substantial information regarding the specifics of the deaths was not available; and no clear differences between the risks of atypical and typical antipsychotics have been discerned.[140] Yet, the known side effects, including metabolic symptoms, are alarming. In lieu of these adverse events and the lack of solid evidence-based research regarding the treatment of psychosis in AD, Meeks and Jeste[150] conclude "When treatment becomes necessary, atypical antipsychotics are one of several off-label treatment options but, if chosen, should be used judiciously in the context of shared-decision making, close monitoring, and minimization of dose/treatment duration." When antipsychotics are used, the treatment should be individualized. Low doses should be used over short periods of time with the eventual goal of discontinuation when possible.

Treatment considerations for the psychosis of PDD and LBD Special pharmacologic treatment decisions need to be considered with the psychosis of PDD and LBD. Worsening parkinsonism with the use of antipsychotics merits careful attention, especially because sensitivity to antipsychotic medications is one of the suggestive diagnostic features of LBD[98] and dopaminergic blockade can worsen parkinsonian symptoms in both conditions. For the psychosis of PDD, RCTs indicate that low-dose clozapine (25 to 150 mg) is efficacious without worsening parkinsonism symptoms, although clozapine is challenging to use in older adults because of its risk for agranulocytosis (necessitating frequent laboratory draws) and its potent anticholinergic properties.[102,151,152] Quetiapine is anecdotally the first-line treatment for psychosis in PD, but interestingly, RCTs comparing it to placebo do not strongly support its efficacy.[153,154] Quetiapine was found to be just as effective as clozapine in one study[155] and its use has been supported by open-label trials.[99] Although not commonly considered for treating the psychosis associated with PD, small doses of risperidone (0.25 to 1.25 mg per day) have been shown to improve hallucinations without worsening parkinsonism in a limited number of patients.[156] In a meta-analysis of studies on the treatment of psychosis in PD,[157] only clozapine was clearly recommended as an evidence-based treatment. Nevertheless, clozapine is often not chosen first clinically because of the possibility for serious adverse events and the required close monitoring. Some evidence suggests that cholinesterase inhibitors may have antipsychotic properties in PD.[99]

For the psychosis of LBD, cholinesterase inhibitors are the recommended first-line treatment considering their possible cognitive symptom benefit and relative lack of toxicity compared with antipsychotic medications.[99] In addition to worsening parkinsonism, neuroleptic use in patients with LBD has been associated with life-threatening adverse events in approximately half of exposed individuals.[158] In a very recent RCT of citalopram and risperidone for the treatment of neuropsychiatric symptoms in LBD, both citalopram and risperidone were poorly tolerated and lacked clear efficacy.[159] As with PDD, when antipsychotics are used in LBD, quetiapine is often a first-line therapy, despite the overwhelming lack of supportive empirical evidence.

Psychosocial interventions In light of the black-box warnings and the conflicting efficacy data on the use of antipsychotics to address psychosis of dementia, psychosocial interventions are of particular interest. Yet, there is a clear dearth of literature guiding clinicians on the systematic use of psychosocial interventions.[160,161] Ayalon and colleagues[162] organized nonpharmacologic interventions for dementia into 3 categories, which each assume a different etiology for the presenting neuropsychiatric symptoms. These include learning and behavioral (eg, a patient's screaming behaviors become reinforced as they attract desired attention), unmet needs (eg, repetitive vocalizations serve as auditory stimulation), and environmental vulnerability and reduced stress-threshold (eg, too much noise results in agitation).

In their systematic review of the evidence-based literature on nonpharmacologic interventions, Ayalon and colleagues[162] found only 3 RCTs meeting the strict inclusion criteria outlined by the American Psychological Association, all of which examined caregiving interventions. The results of these studies were inconclusive. Livingston and colleagues[160] also reviewed nonpharmacologic treatments for the neuropsychiatric symptoms of dementia and similarly found a paucity of high-quality studies. Of the 162 reviewed studies, they found that behavioral management and caregiver psycho-education techniques were efficacious over several months, whereas music therapy and sensory stimulation were useful only during the session, but lacked enduring efficacy. In contrast, repetitive exercise, reality orientation therapy, Montessori activities, and validation therapy did not improve the neuropsychiatric symptoms of dementia, at least based on the criteria used in the studies. Of course, as wisely quoted, absence of evidence is not evidence of absence [of efficacy].[140,160]

Despite the dearth of evidence-based research into psychosocial interventions for dementia, lessons gleaned from clinical experience and the extant clinical research suggest clinicians first identify and address the potential underlying triggers for the psychosis and/or problematic behaviors. Physical symptoms (eg, pain, urinary infections, or constipation), environmental triggers, and understimulation or overstimulation can all serve as inciting factors.[139,162] Underlying medical etiology and delirium always need to be considered when evaluating psychosis in people with dementia.[161] Cohen-Mansfield[161] cautions clinicians against assuming that individuals with dementia are experiencing psychosis when their behavior may actually be reflecting misinterpretations of reality based on memory deficits, sensory impairments, inappropriate sensory stimulation, or underlying medical causes. Overall, the approach should be individualized and patient-centered.

FUTURE RESEARCH DIRECTIONS

With the exponential aging of the population, the numbers of older individuals experiencing psychosis will likewise expand. As outlined in this article, late-life psychosis is associated with decreased quality of life, caregiver distress, institutionalization, and increased health care costs. Existing pharmacotherapy for late-life psychosis is far from ideal in light of its risky side-effect profile, especially for the psychosis of dementia. Existing psychosocial therapies for psychosis of dementia are promising, but more evidence-based data on these therapies are needed to merit widespread implementation. There is thus a call for research into novel safe, well-tolerated, and efficacious pharmacotherapies for psychosis in late life. There is also a call for research into psychosocial interventions, especially for dementias, because the high-quality empirical evidence base is notably sparse. Recent research challenges the Kraepelinian notion of *dementia praecox* and should help dispel some of the stigma associated with the long-term prognosis of schizophrenia. Efforts to educate the public and health care providers to dispel myths about aging with schizophrenia would be worthwhile causes. Similarly, intergenerational dialogues between younger individuals with new-onset schizophrenia and older individuals who have aged with schizophrenia in the community may be fruitful. A prophylactic model is also warranted. The consistent finding that the best predictor of the long-term consequences of schizophrenia is the severity of symptoms in the first 2 years of illness should inspire continued research into early interventions for schizophrenia. Finally, clinicians who are providing pharmacotherapy to older adults with schizophrenia need better education about existing adjunctive evidence-based psychosocial interventions and how to integrate and implement these treatments. By building on the existing and future research, and ensuring we provide individualized, patient-centered care grounded in common sense principles, we can optimize the care of older adults with psychosis.

REFERENCES

1. Palmer BW, McClure F, Jeste DV. Schizophrenia in late-life: findings challenge traditional concepts. Harv Rev Psychiatry 2001;9:51–8.
2. Wender PH. Dementia praecox: the development of the concept. Am J Psychiatry 1963;119:1143–51.
3. Jeste DV, Symonds LL, Harris MJ, et al. Non-dementia non-praecox dementia praecox? Late-onset schizophrenia. Am J Geriatr Psychiatry 1997;5:302–17.
4. Kraepelin E. Dementia praecox and paraphrenia [Translated in 1919 from the eighth German edition of the 'Text-book of Psychiatry,' vol. iii, part ii, section on Endogenous Dementias published in 1913]. Huntington (NY): Krieger; 1971.

5. Seeman M, Jeste DV. Historical perspective. In: Hassett A, Ames D, Chiu E, editors. Psychosis in the elderly. New York: Taylor & Francis Group; 2005. p. 1–9.
6. Bleuler E. Dementia praecox or the group of schizophrenias [Zinkin J, Trans]. New York: International Universities Press; 1950.
7. Bleuler M. Late schizophrenic clinical pictures. Fortschr Neurol Psychiatr 1943; 15:259–90.
8. Palmer BW, Heaton SC, Jeste DV. Older patients with schizophrenia: challenges in the coming decades. Psychiatr Serv 1999;50:1178–83.
9. Jeste DV, Alexopoulos GS, Bartels SJ, et al. Consensus statement on the upcoming crisis in geriatric mental health: research agenda for the next two decades. Arch Gen Psychiatry 1999;56:848–53.
10. Castle DJ. Epidemiology of late onset schizophrenia. In: Howard R, Rabins PV, Castle DJ, editors. Late onset schizophrenia. Philadelphia: Wrightson Biomedical Publishing Ltd; 1999. p. 139–46.
11. Robins LN, Regier DA. Psychiatric disorders in America: the epidemiologic catchment area study. New York: The Free Press; 1991.
12. Regier DA, Kaelber CT, Rae DS, et al. Limitations of diagnostic criteria and assessment instruments for mental disorders. Implications for research and policy. Arch Gen Psychiatry 1998;55:109–15.
13. Auquier P, Lançon C, Rouillon F, et al. Mortality in schizophrenia. Pharmacoepidemiol Drug Saf 2007;16:1308–12.
14. Cuffel BJ, Jeste DV, Halpain M, et al. Treatment costs and use of community mental health services for schizophrenia by age cohorts. Am J Psychiatry 1996;153:870–6.
15. Wasylenki DA. The cost of schizophrenia. Can J Psychiatry 1994;39:65–9.
16. Bartels SJ, Clark RE, Peacock WJ, et al. Medicare and Medicaid costs for schizophrenia patients by age cohort compared with costs for depression, dementia, and medically ill patients. Am J Geriatr Psychiatry 2003;11:648–57.
17. Folsom DP, Lebowitz BD, Lindamer LA, et al. Schizophrenia in late life: emerging issues. Dialogues Clin Neurosci 2006;8:45–52.
18. Patterson TL, Semple SJ, Shaw WS, et al. Researching the caregiver: family members who care for older psychotic patients. Psychiatr Ann 1996;26:772–84.
19. Cohen CI, Cohen GD, Blank K, et al. Schizophrenia and older adults: an overview: directions for research and policy. Am J Geriatr Psychiatry 2000;8:19–28.
20. Davidson M, Harvey PD, Powchik P, et al. Severity of symptoms in chronically institutionalized geriatric schizophrenic patients. Am J Psychiatry 1995;152: 197–207.
21. Harvey PD, Silverman JM, Mohs RC, et al. Cognitive decline in late-life schizophrenia: a longitudinal study of geriatric chronically hospitalized patients. Biol Psychiatry 1999;45:32–40.
22. Harding C, Brooks G, Ashikaga T, et al. The Vermont longitudinal study of persons with severe mental illness II: long-term outcome of subjects who retrospectively met DSM-III criteria for schizophrenia. Am J Psychiatry 1987;144: 727–35.
23. Harding CM. Changes in schizophrenia across time: paradoxes, patterns and predictors. In: Cohen CI, editor. Schizophrenia into later life. Washington, DC: American Psychiatric Publishing Inc; 2003. p. 19–42.
24. Harrison G, Hopper K, Craig T, et al. Recovery from psychotic illness: a 15- and 25-year international follow-up study. Br J Psychiatry 2001;178:506–17.
25. Jeste DV, Twamley EW, Eyler Zorrilla LT, et al. Aging and outcome in schizophrenia. Acta Psychiatr Scand 2003;107:336–43.

26. Cohen CI, Vahia I, Reyes P, et al. Focus on geriatric psychiatry: schizophrenia in later life: clinical symptoms and social well-being. Psychiatr Serv 2008;59: 232–4.

27. Auslander LA, Jeste DV. Sustained remission of schizophrenia among community-dwelling older outpatients. Am J Psychiatry 2004;161:1490–3.

28. Heaton RK, Gladsjo JA, Palmer BW, et al. Stability and course of neuropsychological deficits in schizophrenia. Arch Gen Psychiatry 2001;58:24–32.

29. Heaton R, Paulsen J, McAdams LA, et al. Neuropsychological deficits in schizophrenia: relationship to age, chronicity and dementia. Arch Gen Psychiatry 1994;51:469–76.

30. Eyler-Zorrilla LT, Heaton RK, McAdams LA, et al. Cross-sectional study of older outpatients with schizophrenia and healthy comparison subjects: no difference in age-related cognitive decline. Am J Psychiatry 2000;157:1324–6.

31. Palmer BW, Bondi MW, Twamley EW, et al. Are late-onset schizophrenia-spectrum disorders a neurodegenerative condition? Annual rates of change on two dementia measures. J Neuropsychiatry Clin Neurosci 2003;15:45–52.

32. Palmer BW, Dawes SE, Heaton RK. What do we know about neuropsychological aspects of schizophrenia? Neuropsychol Rev 2009;19:365–84.

33. Heinrichs RW, Zakzanis KK. Neurocognitive deficit in schizophrenia: a quantitative review of the evidence. Neuropsychology 1998;12:426–45.

34. Ting C, Rajji TK, Ismail Z, et al. Differentiating the cognitive profile of schizophrenia from that of Alzheimer disease and depression in late life. PLos One 2010;5:e10151.

35. Jeste DV, Harris MJ, Krull A, et al. Clinical and neuropsychological characteristics of patients with late-onset schizophrenia. Am J Psychiatry 1995;152:722–30.

36. Paulsen JS, Heaton RK, Sadek JR, et al. The nature of learning and memory impairments in schizophrenia. J Int Neuropsychol Soc 1995;1:88–99.

37. Palmer BW, Dawes SE. Cognitive aging: from basic skills to scripts and schemata. In: Jeste DV, Depp CD, editors. Handbook of successful cognitive and emotional aging. Arlington (VA): American Psychiatric Publishing, Inc; 2010. p. 37–54.

38. Patterson TL, Klapow JC, Eastham J, et al. Correlates of functional status in older patients with schizophrenia. Psychiatry Res 1998;80:41–52.

39. Palmer BW, Heaton RK, Gladsjo JA, et al. Heterogeneity in functional status among older outpatients with schizophrenia: employment history, living situation, and driving. Schizophr Res 2002;55:205–15.

40. Shepherd S, Depp CA, Harris G, et al. Perspectives on schizophrenia over the lifespan: a qualitative study. Schizophr Bull 2010 Jul 5. [Epub ahead of print].

41. Cohen CI, Talavera N, Hartung R. Predictors of subjective well-being among older, community-dwelling persons with schizophrenia. Am J Geriatr Psychiatry 1997;5:145–55.

42. Patterson TL, Kaplan RM, Grant I, et al. Quality of well-being in late life psychosis. Psychiatry Res 1996;63:169–81.

43. Sciolla A, Patterson TL, Wetherell J, et al. Functioning and well-being of middle-aged and older patients with schizophrenia; measurement with the 36-item short-form (SF-36) health survey. Am J Geriatr Psychiatry 2003;11:629–37.

44. Patterson TL, Shaw W, Semple SJ, et al. Health-related quality of life in older patients with schizophrenia and other psychoses: relationships among psychosocial and psychiatric factors. Int J Geriatr Psychiatry 1997;12:452–61.

45. Priebe S, Reininghaus U, McCabe R, et al. Factors influencing subjective quality of life in patients with schizophrenia and other mental disorders: a pooled analysis. Schizophr Res 2010;121:251–8.

46. Folsom DP, Depp C, Palmer BW, et al. Physical and mental health-related quality of life among older people with schizophrenia. Schizophr Res 2009; 108:207–13.
47. Semple SJ, Patterson TL, Shaw WS, et al. The social networks of older schizophrenia patients. Int Psychogeriatr 1997;9:84–94.
48. Ram R, Bromet EJ, Eaton WW, et al. The natural course of schizophrenia: a review of first-admission studies. Schizophr Bull 1992;18:185–207.
49. Feighner JP, Robins E, Guze SB, et al. Diagnostic criteria for use in psychiatric research. Arch Gen Psychiatry 1972;26:57–63.
50. Howard R, Rabins PV, Seeman MV, et al. Late-onset schizophrenia and very-late-onset schizophrenia-like psychosis: an international consensus. Am J Psychiatry 2000;157:172–8.
51. Bleuler M. The schizophrenic disorders: long-term patient and family studies [Translated by S.M. Clemens]. New Haven (CT); London: Yale University Press; 1978.
52. van Os J, Howard R, Takei N, et al. Increasing age is a risk factor for psychosis in the elderly. Soc Psychiatry Psychiatr Epidemiol 1995;30:161–4.
53. Köhler S, van Os J, de Graaf R, et al. Psychosis risk as a function of age at onset: a comparison between early- and late-onset psychosis in a general population sample. Soc Psychiatry Psychiatr Epidemiol 2007;42:288–94.
54. Lohr JB, Alder M, Flynn K, et al. Minor physical anomalies in older patients with late-onset schizophrenia, early-onset schizophrenia, depression, and Alzheimer's disease. Am J Geriatr Psychiatry 1997;5:318–23.
55. Pearlson GD, Kreger L, Rabins RV, et al. A chart review study of late-onset and early-onset schizophrenia. Am J Psychiatry 1989;146:1568–74.
56. Howard R, Castle D, Wessely S, et al. A comparative study of 470 cases of early and late-onset schizophrenia. Br J Psychiatry 1993;163:352–7.
57. Hassett A. Defining psychotic disorders in an aging population. In: Hassett A, Ames D, Chiu E, editors. Psychosis in the elderly. Oxford (UK): Taylor and Francis; 2005. p. 11–24.
58. Vahia IV, Palmer BW, Depp C, et al. Late-onset schizophrenia: a subtype of schizophrenia? Acta Psychiatr Scand 2010;122(5):414–26.
59. Howard R, Mellers J, Petty R, et al. Magnetic resonance imaging volumetric measurements of the superior temporal gyrus, hippocampus, parahippocampal gyrus, frontal and temporal lobes in late paraphrenia. Psychol Med 1995;25: 495–503.
60. Corey-Bloom J, Jernigan T, Archibald S, et al. Quantitative magnetic resonance imaging of the brain in late-life schizophrenia. Am J Psychiatry 1995;152:447–9.
61. Symonds LL, Olichney JM, Jernigan TL, et al. Lack of clinically significant structural abnormalities in MRIs of older patients with schizophrenia and related psychoses. J Neuropsychiatry Clin Neurosci 1997;9:251–8.
62. Howard R, Cox T, Almeida O, et al. White matter signal hyperintensities in the brains of patients with late paraphrenia and the normal community-living elderly. Biol Psychiatry 1995;38:86–91.
63. Barak Y, Aizenberg D, Mirecki I, et al. Very late-onset schizophrenia-like psychosis: clinical and imaging characteristics in comparison with elderly patients with schizophrenia. J Nerv Ment Dis 2002;190:733–6.
64. Cervantes AN, Rabins PV, Slavney PR. Onset of schizophrenia at age 100. Psychosomatics 2006;47:356–9.
65. Kendler KS. Demography of paranoid psychosis (delusional disorder): a review and comparison with schizophrenia and affective illness. Arch Gen Psychiatry 1982;39:890–902.

66. American Psychiatric Association. Diagnostic and statistical manual of mental disorders [text revision]. 4th edition. Washington, DC: American Psychiatric Association; 2000.

67. de Portugal E, González N, Miriam V, et al. Gender differences in delusional disorder: evidence from an outpatient sample. Psychiatry Res 2010;177:235–9.

68. Copeland JR, Dewey ME, Scott A, et al. Schizophrenia and delusional disorder in older age: community prevalence, incidence, comorbidity and outcome. Schizophr Bull 1998;19:153–61.

69. Rockwell E, Krull AJ, Dimsdale J, et al. Late-onset psychosis with somatic delusions. Psychosomatics 1994;35:66–72.

70. Evans JD, Paulsen JS, Harris MJ, et al. A clinical and neuropsychological comparison of delusional disorder and schizophrenia. J Neuropsychiatry Clin Neurosci 1996;8:281–6.

71. Kendler S, Davis KL. The genetics and biochemistry of paranoid schizophrenia and other paranoid psychoses. Schizophr Bull 1981;7:689–709.

72. Ropacki SA, Jeste DV. Epidemiology of and risk factors for psychosis of Alzheimer's disease: a review of 55 studies published from 1990 to 2003. Am J Psychiatry 2005;162:2022–30.

73. Ostling S, Gustafson D, Blennow K, et al. Psychotic symptoms in a population-based sample of 85-year-old individuals with dementia. J Geriatr Psychiatry Neurol 2011;24(1):3–8.

74. Levy ML, Cummings JL, Fairbanks LA, et al. Longitudinal assessment of symptoms of depression, agitation, and psychosis in 181 patients with Alzheimer's disease. Am J Psychiatry 1996;153:1438–43.

75. Paulsen JS, Salmon DP, Thal LJ, et al. Incidence of and risk factors for hallucinations and delusions in patients with probable AD. Neurology 2000;54:1965–71.

76. Caligiuri MP, Peavy G, Salmon DP, et al. Neuromotor abnormalities and risk for psychosis in Alzheimer's disease. Neurology 2003;61:954–8.

77. Jeste DV, Finkel SI. Psychosis of Alzheimer's disease and related dementias: diagnostic criteria for a distinct syndrome. Am J Geriatr Psychiatry 2000;8:29–34.

78. Sweet RA, Bennett DA, Graff-Radford NR, et al. Assessment and familial aggregation of psychosis in Alzheimer's disease from the National Institute on Aging Late Onset Alzheimer's Disease Family Study. Brain 2010;133:1155–62.

79. Jeste DV, Wragg RE, Salmon DP, et al. Cognitive deficits of patients with Alzheimer's disease with and without delusions. Am J Psychiatry 1992;149:184–9.

80. Schneider LS, Dagerman KS. Psychosis of Alzheimer's disease: clinical characteristics and history. J Psychiatr Res 2004;38:105–11.

81. Bassiony MM, Steinberg MS, Warren A, et al. Delusions and hallucinations in Alzheimer's disease: prevalence and clinical correlates. Int J Geriatr Psychiatry 2000;15:99–107.

82. Sweet RA, Nimgaonkar VL, Devlin B, et al. Psychotic symptoms in Alzheimer disease: evidence for a distinct phenotype. Mol Psychiatry 2003;8:383–92.

83. DeMichele-Sweet MA, Sweet RA. Genetics of psychosis in Alzheimer's disease: a review. J Alzheimers Dis 2010;19:761–80.

84. Lee DY, Choo IH, Kim KW, et al. White matter changes associated with psychotic symptoms in Alzheimer's disease patients. J Neuropsychiatry Clin Neurosci 2006;18:191–8.

85. Wilkosz PA, Miyahara S, Lopez OL, et al. Prediction of psychosis onset in Alzheimer disease: the role of cognitive impairment, depressive symptoms, and further evidence for psychosis subtypes. Am J Geriatr Psychiatry 2006;14:352–60.

86. Weamer EA, Emanuel JE, Varon D, et al. The relationship of excess cognitive impairment in MCI and early Alzheimer's disease to the subsequent emergence of psychosis. Int Psychogeriatr 2009;21:78–85.

87. Kaufer DI, Cummings JL, Christine D, et al. Assessing the impact of neuropsychiatric symptoms in Alzheimer's disease: the neuropsychiatry inventory caregiver distress scale. J Am Geriatr Soc 1998;46:210–5.

88. Matsumoto N, Ikeda M, Fukuhara R, et al. Caregiver burden associated with behavioral and psychological symptoms of dementia in elderly people in the local community. Dement Geriatr Cogn Disord 2007;23:219–24.

89. Cummings JL, Diaz C, Levy ML, et al. Neuropsychiatric syndromes in neurodegenerative diseases: frequency and significance. Semin Clin Neuropsychiatry 1996;1:241–7.

90. Stern Y, Albert M, Brandt J, et al. Utility of extrapyramidal signs and psychosis as predictors of cognitive and functional decline, nursing home admission, and death in Alzheimer's disease: prospective analyses from the predictors study. Neurology 1994;44:2300–7.

91. Magni E, Binetti G, Bianchetti A, et al. Risk of mortality and institutionalization in demented patients with delusions. J Geriatr Psychiatry Neurol 1996;9:123–6.

92. Wilson RS, Krueger KR, Kamenetsky JM, et al. Hallucinations and mortality in Alzheimer disease. Am J Geriatr Psychiatry 2005;13:984–90.

93. Schneider LS, Katz IR, Park S, et al. Psychosis of Alzheimer disease: validity of the construct and response to risperidone. Am J Geriatr Psychiatry 2003;11:414–25.

94. Kotrla KJ, Chacko RC, Harper RG, et al. Clinical variables associated with psychosis in Alzheimer's disease. Am J Psychiatry 1995;152:1377–9.

95. Gilley DW, Whalen ME, Wilson RS, et al. Hallucinations and associated factors in Alzheimer's disease. J Neuropsychiatry Clin Neurosci 1991;3:371–6.

96. Gilley DW, Wilson RS, Beckett LA, et al. Psychotic symptoms and physically aggressive behavior in Alzheimer's disease. J Am Geriatr Soc 1997;45:1074–9.

97. Rabins PV, Mace NL, Lucas MJ. The impact of dementia on the family. JAMA 1982;248:333–5.

98. McKeith IG, Dickson DW, Lowe J, et al. Consortium on DLB. Diagnosis and management of dementia with Lewy bodies: third report of the DLB Consortium. Neurology 2005;65:1863–72.

99. Weintraub D, Hurtig HI. Presentation and management of psychosis in Parkinson's disease and dementia with Lewy bodies. Am J Psychiatry 2007;164:1491–8.

100. Forsaa EB, Larsen JP, Wentzel-Larsen T, et al. A 12-year population-based study of psychosis in Parkinson disease. Arch Neurol 2010;67:996–1001.

101. Ravina B, Marder K, Fernandez HH, et al. Diagnostic criteria for psychosis in Parkinson's disease: report of an NINDS, NIMH work group. Mov Disord 2007;22:1061–8.

102. Marti MJ, Tolosa E, de la Cerda A. Dementia in Parkinson's disease. J Neurol 2007;254:41–8.

103. Aarsland D, Ballard C, Larsen JP, et al. A comparative study of psychiatric symptoms in dementia with Lewy bodies and Parkinson's disease with and without dementia. Int J Geriatr Psychiatry 2001;16:528–36.

104. Aarsland D, Larsen JP, Cummins JL, et al. Prevalence and clinical correlates of psychotic symptoms in Parkinson disease: a community-based study. Arch Neurol 1999;56:595–601.

105. Marsh L, Williams JR, Rocco M, et al. Psychiatric comorbidities in patients with Parkinson disease and psychosis. Neurology 2004;63:293–300.

106. Aarsland D, Larsen JP, Tandberg E, et al. Predictors of nursing home placement in Parkinson's disease: a population-based, prospective study. J Am Geriatr Soc 2000;48:938–42.

107. Nagahama Y, Okina T, Suzuki N, et al. Classification of psychotic symptoms in dementia with Lewy bodies. Am J Geriatr Psychiatry 2007;15:961–7.

108. Ballard C, Holmes C, McKeith IG, et al. Psychiatric morbidity in dementia with Lewy bodies: a prospective clinical and neuropathological comparative study with Alzheimer's disease. Am J Psychiatry 1999;156:1039–45.

109. Hirono N, Cummings JL. Neuropsychiatric aspects of dementia with Lewy bodies. Curr Psychiatry Rep 1999;1:85–92.

110. Ricci M, Guidoni SV, Sepe-Monti M, et al. Clinical findings, functional abilities and caregiver distress in the early stage of dementia with Lewy bodies (DLB) and Alzheimer's disease (AD). Arch Gerontol Geriatr 2009;49:e101–4.

111. Nagahama Y, Okina T, Suzuki N, et al. Neural correlates of psychotic symptoms in dementia with Lewy bodies. Brain 2010;133:557–67.

112. Sable JA, Jeste DV. Antipsychotic treatment for late-life schizophrenia. Curr Psychiatry Rep 2002;4:299–306.

113. Kohen I, Lester PE, Lam S. Antipsychotic treatments for the elderly: efficacy and safety of aripiprazole. Neuropsychiatr Dis Treat 2010;24:47–58.

114. Jeste DV, Eastham JH, Lacro JP, et al. Management of late-life psychosis. J Clin Psychiatry 1996;57:39–45.

115. Madhusoodanan S, Brecher M, Brenner R, et al. Risperidone in the treatment of elderly patients with psychotic disorders. Am J Geriatr Psychiatry 1999;7:132–8.

116. Davidson M, Harvey PD, Vervarcke J, et al. A long-term, multicenter, open-label study of risperidone in elderly patients with psychosis. On behalf of the Risperidone Working Group. Int J Geriatr Psychiatry 2000;15:506–14.

117. Jeste DV, Barak Y, Madhusoodanan S, et al. International multisite double-blind trial of the atypical antipsychotics risperidone and olanzapine in 175 elderly patients with chronic schizophrenia. Am J Geriatr Psychiatry 2003;11:638–47.

118. Alexopoulos GS, Streim JE, Carpenter D. Expert consensus guidelines for using antipsychotic agents in older patients. J Clin Psychiatry 2004;65:5–99.

119. Arunpongpaisal S, Ahmed I, Aqeel N, et al. Antipsychotic drug treatment for elderly people with late-onset schizophrenia. Cochrane Database Syst Rev 2009;2:CD004162.

120. Campbell AJ. Drug treatment as a cause of falls in old age: a review of the offending agents. Drugs Aging 1991;1:289–302.

121. Jeste DV. Tardive dyskinesia in older patients. J Clin Psychiatry 2000;61:27–32.

122. Jeste DV, Lacro JP, Bailey A, et al. Lower incidence of tardive dyskinesia with risperidone compared with haloperidol in older patients. J Am Geriatr Soc 1999;47:716–9.

123. Jin H, Meyer JM, Jeste DV. Phenomenology of and risk factors for new-onset diabetes mellitus and diabetic ketoacidosis associated with atypical antipsychotics: an analysis of 45 published cases. Ann Clin Psychiatry 2002;14:59–64.

124. Jin H, Meyer J, Mudaliar S, et al. Use of clinical markers to identify metabolic syndrome in antipsychotic-treated patients. J Clin Psychiatry 2010;71(10):1273–8.

125. Jin H, Meyer JM, Mudaliar S, et al. Impact of atypical antipsychotic therapy on leptin, ghrelin, and adiponectin. Schizophr Res 2008;100:70–85.

126. Patterson TL, McKibbin CL, Taylor MJ, et al. Functional Adaptation Skills Training (FAST): a pilot psychosocial intervention study in middle-aged and

older patients with chronic psychotic disorders. Am J Geriatr Psychiatry 2003; 11:17–23.

127. Patterson TL, McKibbin C, Mausbach BT, et al. Functional Adaptation Skills Training (FAST): a randomized trial of a psychosocial intervention for middle-aged and older patients with chronic psychotic disorders. Schizophr Res 2006;86:291–9.

128. Mausbach BT, Cardenas V, McKibbin CL, et al. Reducing emergency medical service use in patients with chronic psychotic disorders: results from the FAST intervention study. Behav Res Ther 2008;46:145–53.

129. Patterson TL, Bucardo J, McKibbin CL, et al. Development and pilot testing of a new psychosocial intervention for older Latinos with chronic psychosis. Schizophr Bull 2005;31:922–30.

130. McQuaid JR, Granholm E, McClure FS, et al. Development of an integrated cognitive-behavioral, social skills training intervention for older patients with schizophrenia. J Psychother Pract Res 2000;9:1–8.

131. Granholm E, McQuaid JR, McClure FS, et al. A randomized, controlled trial of cognitive behavioral social skills training for middle-aged and older outpatients with chronic schizophrenia. Am J Psychiatry 2005;162:520–9.

132. Granholm E, McQuaid JR, McClure FS, et al. Randomized controlled trial of cognitive behavioral social skills training for older people with schizophrenia: 12-month follow-up. J Clin Psychiatry 2007;68:730–7.

133. Granholm E, McQuaid JR, Link PC, et al. Neuropsychological predictors of functional outcome in Cognitive Behavioral Social Skills Training for older people with schizophrenia. Schizophr Res 2008;100:133–43.

134. Emmerson LC, Granholm E, Link PC, et al. Insight and treatment outcome with cognitive-behavioral social skills training for older people with schizophrenia. J Rehabil Res Dev 2009;46:1053–8.

135. Twamley EW, Jeste DV, Bellack AS. A review of cognitive training in schizophrenia. Schizophr Bull 2003;29:359–82.

136. McGurk SR, Twamley EW, Sitzer DI, et al. A meta-analysis of cognitive remediation in schizophrenia. Am J Psychiatry 2007;164:1791–802.

137. Twamley EW, Padin DS, Bayne KS, et al. Work rehabilitation for middle-aged and older people with schizophrenia: a comparison of three approaches. J Nerv Ment Dis 2005;193:596–601.

138. Twamley EW, Narvaez JM, Becker DR, et al. Supported employment for middle-aged and older people with schizophrenia. Am J Psychiatr Rehabil 2008;11:76–89.

139. Salzman C, Jeste DV, Meyer RE, et al. Elderly patients with dementia-related symptoms of severe agitation and aggression: consensus statement on treatment options, clinical trials methodology, and policy. J Clin Psychiatry 2008;69:889–98.

140. Jeste DV, Blazer D, Casey DE, et al. ACNP white paper: update on the use of antipsychotic drugs in elderly persons with dementia. Neuropsychopharmacology 2008;33:957–70.

141. Schneider LS, Ismail MS, Dagerman K, et al. Clinical antipsychotic trials of intervention effectiveness (CATIE): Alzheimer's disease trial. Schizophr Bull 2003;29:57–72.

142. Katz IR, Jeste DV, Mintzer JE, et al. Comparison of risperidone and placebo for psychosis and behavioral disturbances associated with dementia: a randomized, double-blind trial. J Clin Psychiatry 1999;60:107–15.

143. DeDeyn PP, Rabheru K, Rasmussen A, et al. A randomized trial of risperidone, placebo, and haloperidol for behavioral symptoms of dementia. Neurology 1999;53:946–55.

144. Street JS, Clark WS, Gannon KS, et al. Olanzapine treatment of psychotic and behavioral symptoms in patients with Alzheimer disease in nursing care facilities: a double-blind randomized, placebo-controlled trial. The HGEU Study Group. Arch Gen Psychiatry 2000;57:968–76.

145. Hoeh N, Gyulai L, Weintraub D, et al. Pharmacologic management of psychosis in the elderly: a critical review. J Geriatr Psychiatry Neurol 2003;16:213–8.

146. Deberdt WG, Dysken MW, Rappaport SA, et al. Comparison of olanzapine and risperidone in the treatment of psychosis and associated behavioral disturbances in patients with dementia. Am J Geriatr Psychiatry 2005;13:722–30.

147. Schneider LS, Dagerman K, Insel PS. Efficacy and adverse effects of atypical antipsychotics for dementia: meta-analysis of randomized, placebo-controlled trials. Am J Geriatr Psychiatry 2006;14:191–210.

148. Schneider LS, Pollock VE, Lyness SA. A meta-analysis of controlled trials of neuroleptic treatment in dementia. J Am Geriatr Soc 1990;38:553–63.

149. Schneider LS, Dagerman KS, Insel P. Risk of death with atypical antipsychotic drug treatment for dementia: meta-analysis of randomized placebo-controlled trials. JAMA 2005;294:1934–43.

150. Meeks TW, Jeste DV. Beyond the black box: what is the role for antipsychotics in dementia? Curr Psychiatr 2008;7:50–65.

151. The French Clozapine Parkinson Study Group. Clozapine in drug-induced psychosis in Parkinson's disease. Lancet 1999;353:2041–2.

152. Parkinson Study Group. Low-dose clozapine for the treatment of drug-induced psychosis in Parkinson's disease. N Engl J Med 1999;340:757–63.

153. Rabey JM, Prokhorov T, Miniovitz A, et al. Effect of quetiapine in psychotic Parkinson's disease patients: a double-blind labeled study of 3 months' duration. Mov Disord 2007;22:313–8.

154. Ondo WG, Tintner R, Voung KD, et al. Double-blind, placebo-controlled, unforced titration parallel trial of quetiapine for dopaminergic-induced hallucinations in Parkinson's disease. Mov Disord 2005;20:958–63.

155. Morgante L, Epifanio A, Spina E, et al. Quetiapine and clozapine in parkinsonian patients with dopaminergic psychosis. Clin Neuropharmacol 2004;27:153–6.

156. Meco G, Alessandria A, Bonifati V, et al. Risperidone for hallucinations in levodopa-treated Parkinson's disease patients. Lancet 1994;343:1370–1.

157. Frieling H, Hillemacher T, Ziegenbein M, et al. Treating dopamimetic psychosis in Parkinson's disease: structured review and meta-analysis. Eur Neuropsychopharmacol 2007;17:165–71.

158. McKeith I, Fairbaim A, Perry R, et al. Neuroleptic sensitivity in patients with senile dementia of Lewy body type. BMJ 1992;305:673–8.

159. Culo S, Mulsant BH, Rosen J, et al. Treating neuropsychiatric symptoms in dementia with Lewy bodies: a randomized controlled-trial. Alzheimer Dis Assoc Disord 2010 Jul 9. [Epub ahead of print].

160. Livingston G, Johnston K, Katona C, et al. Systematic review of psychological approaches to the management of neuropsychiatric symptoms of dementia. Am J Psychiatry 2005;162:1996–2021.

161. Cohen-Mansfield J. Nonpharmacologic interventions for psychotic symptoms in dementia. J Geriatr Psychiatry Neurol 2003;16:219–24.

162. Ayalon L, Gum AM, Feliciano L, et al. Effectiveness of nonpharmacological interventions for the management of neuropsychiatric symptoms in patients with dementia: a systematic review. Arch Intern Med 2006;166:2182–8.

Geriatric Bipolar Disorder

Martha Sajatovic, MD[a,b,*], Peijun Chen, MD, PhD, MPH[c]

KEYWORDS
- Bipolar disorder • Geriatric • Elderly • Diagnosis • Treatment
- Mania • Depression

Whereas older adults comprised nearly one-third of the sample reported in the first article by Cade[1] on the use of lithium for treatment of mania, subsequent decades saw very few publications on late-life bipolar disorder. Fortunately, and in concert with global demographic trends, there has been recent growth in the awareness of and research on late-life bipolar disorder.[2] Bipolar disorder in geriatric patients includes illness of new-onset (late-onset bipolar disorder), as well as bipolar disorder which first manifested in earlier life and which has persisted. This article focuses on the epidemiology, phenomenology, assessment, diagnosis, and treatment of geriatric bipolar disorder. It provides suggestions for future directions in research on late-life bipolarity.

EPIDEMIOLOGY

Reports on the prevalence of geriatric bipolar disorder varies across studies, likely attributable to the complexity and heterogeneity of bipolar illness; issues related to case identification, case classification, and variability in settings; and study methodologies. The Epidemiologic Catchment Area (ECA) Survey (1988) reported a 12-month prevalence rate of 0.1% of bipolar disorder among those aged 65 years or older

Dr Chen has nothing to disclose.

Dr Sajatovic has received research grants from GlaxoSmithKline and AstraZeneca and is a consultant to Cognition Group, United BioSource Corporation (UBC), ePharma Solutions, and Medco. Dr Sajatovic receives royalties from Springer Press, Johns Hopkins University Press, Oxford Press, and Lexi-Comp. Dr Sajatovic has also received research grants from Pfizer and from Merck.

[a] Department of Psychiatry, Case Western Reserve University School of Medicine, 11100 Euclid Avenue, Cleveland, OH 44106, USA

[b] Neurological Outcomes Center, Neurological Institute, University Hospitals of Cleveland, Case Western Reserve University School of Medicine, 11100 Euclid Avenue, Cleveland, OH 44106, USA

[c] Geriatric Psychiatry, Department of Psychiatry, Louis Stokes Cleveland VA Medical Center, Case Western Reserve University School of Medicine, 10000 Brecksville Road, Brecksville, OH 44141, USA

* Corresponding author. Department of Psychiatry, Case Western Reserve University School of Medicine 11100 Euclid Avenue, Cleveland, OH 44106.
E-mail address: Martha.sajatovic@uhhospitals.org

Psychiatr Clin N Am 34 (2011) 319–333
doi:10.1016/j.psc.2011.02.007
0193-953X/11/$ – see front matter © 2011 Elsevier Inc. All rights reserved.

according to the *Diagnostic and Statistical Manual of Mental Disorders* (DSM) Third Edition (III) criteria.[3] For individuals aged 65 years and greater, Unutzer and colleagues[4] reported a prevalence rate of 0.25%, whereas Hirschfeld and colleagues[5] reported a prevalence rate of 0.5%. The highest lifetime prevalence rate (1%) was reported by Kessler and colleagues[6] in the US National Comorbidity Survey Replication (NCS-R) among those aged 60 years or older according to the DSM Fourth Edition (IV) criteria. It thus seems that geriatric bipolar disorder is relatively rare in the community, with a point prevalence rate in the order of 0.1% to 0.5% and an estimated lifetime prevalence rate in the order of 0.5% to 1%.

In contrast to relative rarity in the community, data from clinical settings suggest that geriatric bipolar disorder is relatively common. Yassa and colleagues[7] found a relatively high treated prevalence ranging from 4% to 8% in geriatric psychiatry inpatient units. A North American report noted that 17% of elders presenting to psychiatric emergency rooms have bipolar disorder.[8]

The growing absolute numbers and proportion of older adults in the population may be swelling the number of elders seeking care for bipolar disorder. This group of elders would be expected to include some individuals seeking care for the first time. An Australian study revealed an increase in the number of individuals older than 65 years with bipolar disorder from 2% in 1980 to 10% in 1998.[9] A report from Finland suggested that 20% of first admissions with the diagnosis of bipolar disorder occur after the age of 60 years.[10] The limited data on age of onset among older adults with bipolar disorder suggest that most patients manifest their first episode of depression or mania as young adults[6,8,9,11] and only a relatively small fraction of older adults have illness with onset in later life.[12]

Case classification of geriatric bipolar disorder can be extremely challenging. The presence of comorbid medical and neurologic conditions in geriatric patients may potentially result in true bipolar disorder cases being classified in the category of bipolar disorder not otherwise specified (NOS) (DSM-IV, 296.80) or mood disorder due to general medical condition (DSM-IV, 293.83) if general medical conditions or substance use as contributing factors cannot be entirely ruled out. Further, the historical category of secondary mania implies that central nervous system (CNS) injury is responsible for the syndrome.[13] The neurologic literature uses the term disinhibition syndrome to describe a presentation identical to what is considered mania in the psychiatric literature. These inconsistencies create uncertainty regarding the true incidence and prevalence of the geriatric bipolar disorder. It also raises the question of whether bipolar disorders in late-life are qualitatively different than those in younger adults.

Age of onset of the index episode of bipolar disorder is an important variable in estimating the incidence of disease (ie, new occurrence of bipolar disorder) and may help to distinguish subtypes of bipolar disorder.[14] There is growing consensus for a cutoff age of 50 years as a distinguishing feature of early- versus late-onset bipolar disorder. In a retrospective study of 20 patients aged 65 years or older who were admitted to a university hospital because of mania, Benedetti and colleagues[15] found the mean age of onset at 49 years. Moorhead and Young[16] used a UK psychiatric case registry to retrospectively evaluate the age of onset in patients with bipolar I disorder and found that those subjects without a family history tended to have a later age of onset, with a modal age of onset at 49 years.[16]

However, even in those patients with mania or bipolar disorder with evidence of comorbid neurologic lesions, familial vulnerability remains a contributory factor in geriatric bipolar disorder patients, and studies show that even in the neurologic subgroup of older bipolar disorder patients, the prevalence of a positive family history in first-degree relatives remains quite high.[17-19]

Retrospective studies of geriatric bipolar disorder found that about half of all patients experience depression as their first mood episode.[17,18,20,21] After the first episode of depression, many patients tend to experience a very long latency (mean of 15 years) before their first manic episode became evident.[18,22]

Determinants of expression of geriatric bipolar disorder seem multifactorial and may include genetics, medical comorbidity, neurologic injury, lifestyle, and stress. Genetic vulnerability is suggested in studies of subgroups with high familial prevalence of mood disorder (50%–80%) among first-degree relatives.[18,23] Cerebrovascular disease and other neurologic conditions may also contribute to bipolar disorder vulnerability, especially when brain lesions compromise the integrity of limbic, striatal, and prefrontal cortical neuronal circuits in the elderly.[18,24–27] Psychosocial factors including negative life events, such as early loss and trauma in childhood, and adolescence may increase bipolar disorder vulnerability later in life.[28]

It is unclear whether the rate of functional recovery among individuals with bipolar disorder varies with age. In a longitudinal study of 219 patients with bipolar I disorder over a period of up to 25 years, Solomon and colleagues[29] reported that the probability of recovery was significantly decreased for subjects with cycling episodes, mood episodes with severe onset, and greater cumulative morbidity. Depp and colleagues[30] noted that psychotic depressive symptoms as well as cognitive impairment in elderly adults with bipolar disorder contributed to the finding of a lower health-related quality of life and functioning. In 33 older adults with bipolar disorder aged 50 years or older (mean, 69.7; SD, 7.9), Gildengers and colleagues[31] reported that older adults with bipolar disorder had more cognitive dysfunction and more rapid cognitive decline than expected given their age and education, which may lead to decreased independence and increased reliance on family and community supports. In contrast to the apparent cognitive and functional decline seen with aging for patients with bipolar disorder, the risk of completed suicide in bipolar disorder is highest among patients younger than 35 years, suggesting that older patients with early onset of bipolar disorder have a decreased rate of suicide.[32] Presumably, older adults included in bipolar disorder studies represent a survivor cohort.[11]

Elderly bipolar disorder individuals are disproportionately affected by medical burden, particularly cardiovascular disease, diabetes, hypertension, hyperlipidemia, and obesity.[33,34] Medical comorbidity is associated with a more disabling course of bipolar illness,[35] and there is an association between the cumulative number of illnesses and the estimated relative risk of suicide.[36] Gildengers and colleagues[37] compared medical burden in 54 bipolar disorder elders and 108 elders with major depression matched on age, sex, race, and lifetime duration of mood disorder and found that whereas overall medical burden was comparable in the 2 groups, individuals with bipolar disorder had a higher body mass index, defined as the weight in kilograms divided by the height in meters squared, and a greater burden from endocrine/metabolic and cardiovascular diseases.

Gildengers and colleagues[38] found that approximately half of older adults with bipolar disorder scored at least 1 SD below the mean of the comparison subjects on the Mini-Mental State Examination and the Mattis Dementia Rating Scale. Bipolar disorder might increase the risk of late-life dementia.[39] Kessing and colleagues[40] studied patients discharged from a first-ever psychiatric hospitalization with a diagnosis of bipolar disorder or mania and found that this cohort had an increased risk of a dementia diagnosis on subsequent hospital readmission compared with patients with medical conditions and with the general population.[41]

Several possible abnormalities flowing from neuronal dysfunction may be responsible for both the deteriorating course of illness in patients with bipolar disorder as well as the tremendous medical comorbidity seen in bipolar disorder populations.[42] These abnormalities include dysregulation of hypothalamic-pituitary-adrenal axis, glutamate toxicity, abnormalities in calcium signaling, and glial cell pathology. Berk[43] has described a neuroprogression model of bipolarity in which biochemical mechanisms include inflammatory cytokines, neurotrophins, and oxidative stress. Whereas some individuals with bipolar disorder go on to develop substantial and clinically significant cognitive impairment later in life, others do not,[31] and it is not clear if this is because of the differences in underlying bipolar disorder pathophysiology, medical comorbidity, or unrelated factors.

In contrast to comorbid medical and neurologic abnormalities, psychiatric comorbidity may be somewhat lower for geriatric patients with bipolar disorder than for younger populations. Using the Veterans Affairs National Database, Sajatovic and Kales[44] identified psychiatric comorbidity in 4668 geriatric patients with bipolar disorder and found that the prevalence of substance abuse was 8.9% and that of anxiety disorders was 15.2%, including 5.4% cases of posttraumatic stress disorder and dementia in 741 (4.5%) cases. Using data on geriatric bipolar disorder from the National Epidemiology Survey on Alcohol Related Conditions (NESARC), Goldstein and colleagues[45] reported lifetime and 12-month prevalence of alcohol use disorder (38.1% and 38.1%, respectively), dysthymia (15.5% and 7.1%, respectively), generalized anxiety disorder (20.5% and 9.5%, respectively), and panic disorder (19.0% and 11.9%, respectively).

Older adults with bipolar disorder tend to have substantial use of both hospital and ambulatory care services. Sajatovic and colleagues[46] found that older patients with bipolar disorder had a similar frequency of hospitalization as older patients with schizophrenia. Bartels and colleagues[47] found that elderly patients with bipolar disorder used almost 4 times the total amount of mental health services and were 4 times more likely to have had a psychiatric hospitalization over the previous 6 months compared with elderly patients with unipolar disorder.

PHENOMENOLOGY, ASSESSMENT, AND DIAGNOSIS

In general, patients with bipolar disorder may manifest with variable clinical presentations, including bipolar I mania, bipolar I hypomania, bipolar I depression, bipolar mixed states, bipolar II hypomania, bipolar II depression, bipolar cyclothymia, bipolar NOS, and mood disorder due to a general medical condition. Misdiagnosis of bipolar disorder has been reported as one of major factors that may delay treatment and functional recovery.[5,48]

The phenomenology of geriatric bipolar disorder has not been well studied, and diagnosis based on clinical presentation is difficult because of comorbid medical disorders. Kessing[49] reported that compared with a young cohort aged 50 years or less (n = 867), those aged 50 years or more (n = 852), presented more often with severe depressive episodes and psychotic symptoms (32.0% vs 17.0%), as well as hypomania (16.4% vs 12.7%), or manic episode without psychosis (37.5% vs 28.7%). In contrast, other studies report no differences in symptomsbetween patients older than 60 years and those younger than 40 years.[50]

Oostervink and colleagues[51] compared elderly patients aged 60 years or more (n = 475, including 141 subjects with an age of onset of 50 years or more) with patients younger than 50 years (n = 2286) and found that in the year before enrolment, elderly patients, especially those with an early onset, more frequently reported a rapid cycling course of illness and fewer suicide attempts. At baseline, elderly patients were on more psychotropic medications and demonstrated less severe manic and psychiatric symptoms but had no difference in depressive symptoms.[51]

An assessment of older adults presenting with symptoms of mania, depression, or mixed states requires a thorough examination and differential diagnostic evaluation, including identifying any potentially treatable medical conditions that may contribute to the manic/depressive symptoms, and establishing a baseline from which to monitor treatment response and adverse effects. Assessment should include family history and careful characterization of prior mood episodes. A complete physical and neurologic examination should be conducted. Laboratory workup should include a comprehensive metabolic panel, complete blood cell count, thyroid function, toxicology screen, and more specialized assessments as may be indicated by the history, physical, or neurologic examination. Neuroimaging to rule out acute CNS pathology should be complemented by specialized studies (ie, electroencephalogram, lumbar puncture) as indicated. A significant overlap in symptom presentation between mania and delirium in the geriatric patient requires close observation over time to identify symptoms such as fluctuating level of consciousness and sudden change in orientation, memory, and language, all of which are more characteristic of delirium than mania. Agitation or disinhibition of dementia must also be considered as part of the differential diagnosis. New-onset mania in an older individual may be directly related to a medical or neurologic disorder as well as medications such as corticosteroids and dopamine-related drugs (secondary mania).

TREATMENT

Given the complex nature of geriatric bipolar disorder, comorbidity, and behavioral disturbances, inpatient intervention may be required for stabilization, safety, and medical and psychiatric diagnostic workup. Other options include intensive outpatient treatment, care in a day hospital, and enhanced outpatient follow-up. As in mixed-age bipolar disorder patients, treatments may differ depending on illness polarity, symptom severity, and phase (acute vs stabilization vs maintenance treatment).

Drug Treatment of Acute Mania

An open-label trial involving 31 patients aged 60 years or older with bipolar disorder illustrated the feasibility of treating older adults with bipolar disorder with lithium or valproate under protocolized conditions.[52] A National Institute of Mental Health, multisite randomized controlled trial (RCT) of lithium versus valproate for short-term treatment of bipolar mania/hypomania in adults aged 60 years and older (GERI-BD) with a targeted total of 258 subjects is currently being conducted in the United States and is anticipated to more clearly identify tolerability and efficacy of lithium versus valproate in the treatment of acute mania, hypomania, or mixed episode in geriatric bipolar I disorder patients.[53]

Lithium may be less prescribed in the elderly because of concerns regarding tolerability and multiple medical comorbidities.[54] However, lithium may be the preferred choice for older adults with classic mania and minimal neurologic impairment.[55] Lithium may have additional benefit for reducing suicide risk[56] and may reduce the risk of dementia or Alzheimer disease.[57] It has been suggested that geriatric bipolar disorder patients may respond to lower lithium levels compared with younger adults.[58] In the elderly, side effects of lithium include cognitive impairment, ataxia or gait abnormalities, tremor, urinary frequency or renal deterioration, hypothyroidism, weight gain, rash or cutaneous abnormalities, worsening of arthritis, and peripheral edema.[55] Older adults are more prone to acute lithium toxicity because of reduced renal clearance, vulnerability to medical comorbidity (especially cardiovascular abnormalities), and drug-drug interactions with angiotensin-converting enzyme inhibitors, calcium antagonists, thiazide and loop diuretics, and nonsteroidal antiinflammatory drugs.[59]

Valproate has been suggested to be effective in geriatric bipolar disorder.[55,60] Valproate may also be associated with more risk in the elderly than in mixed-age patients. The free serum valproate level should be checked, in addition to total levels in geriatric patients, especially in patients being coadministered aspirin, warfarin, digitoxin, and phenytoin, wherein protein displacement can occur. Pancreatitis and fatal hepatotoxicity are rare side effects associated with valproate, but these seem to be lessened with age.[61] Valproate may occasionally cause encephalopathy, especially in patients with urea cycle disorder.[62]

Carbamazepine has been used as an off-label alternative to lithium for decades. Its extended-release form received US Food and Drug Administration (FDA) approval in 2004 for the treatment of bipolar disorder. Carbamazepine may offer some advantage in patients with atypical bipolar disorder or secondary mania.[63,64] However, there are no controlled clinical trials of carbamazepine specifically in geriatric bipolar disorder. In geriatric patients, carbamazepine titration should be slow, given reduced drug metabolic rates[65] and clearance.[66]

All the second-generation antipsychotics except for clozapine are FDA approved for acute bipolar mania. Data on use of antipsychotic compounds in geriatric bipolar disorder populations are limited. In a secondary data analysis of 94 patients aged 50 years or older, patients treated with olanzapine demonstrated an improvement in manic symptoms when compared with patients treated with divalproex.[67] Risperidone was effective in elderly bipolar disorder patients in case series reports,[68,69] and clozapine has demonstrated some benefit in treating elderly bipolar disorder patients.[24] Quetiapine (QTP) is a potentially useful treatment option among older adults with bipolar I mania, compared with younger adults, as suggested by a recent posthoc analysis of 2 QTP monotherapy clinical trials comparing those aged 55 years or greater (n = 59) with younger adults (n = 344).[70] This study demonstrated that both older and younger patients treated with QTP had significant improvement from baseline on Young Mania Rating Scale (YMRS) scores compared with placebo-treated patients. QTP-treated older patients (n = 28; mean age, 62.9 years; range, 55–79 years) demonstrated a sustained reduction in the YMRS score compared with placebo-treated patients (n = 31; mean age, 61.3 years; range, 55–72 years) that was apparent by day 4 of treatment.

Side effects of particular concern with antipsychotic treatment in the elderly include weight gain, metabolic abnormalities, sedation, extrapyramidal symptoms, fall risk, and neuroleptic malignant syndrome. Reflecting their increased use in clinical settings, antipsychotics have become the most costly class of drug for Medicaid programs, exceeding the runner-up (antidepressants) by a wide margin.[71] A 2009 report noted that 65% of bipolar disorder elders in nursing homes receive antipsychotics.[72] A particular concern in geriatric patients is the potentially increased mortality associated with antipsychotic medications. The FDA has placed a black box warning on all atypical and typical agents warning of the significant increased risk of death in elderly patients with dementia.[73] Although the atypical antipsychotic drugs are an extremely useful and important part of treatment in younger patients with bipolar disorder, and are considered the first-line treatment,[74] their role in treatment for elders with bipolar disorder needs further study.[75]

Drug Treatment of Bipolar Depression

Lithium, the anticonvulsant lamotrigine, and selected atypical antipsychotics, including QTP and olanzapine/fluoxetine combination, have demonstrated efficacy in the treatment of bipolar depression in mixed-age bipolar disorder populations.[76–78] Sajatovic and colleagues[79] have recently conducted a multisite, 12-week, open-label trial of add-on lamotrigine in 57 elderly adults with bipolar I and II depressions. Lamotrigine was added on to current maintenance mood-stabilizing medication, initiated at 25 mg/d, and titrated to a target dose of 200 mg/d. Primary study outcome was change from baseline on the Montgomery-Åsberg Depression Rating Scale (MADRS). Secondary outcomes included depressive symptoms as evaluated with the Hamilton Depression Rating Scale (HAMD), manic symptoms as evaluated with the YMRS, global psychopathology as evaluated with the Clinical Global Impression (CGI), and the general health status as evaluated with the World Health Organization Disability Assessment Schedule II (WHODAS). Side effects were documented using the Udvalg for Kliniske Undersøgelser (UKU) Side Effect Rating Scale, and medical illness burden with the Cumulative Illness Rating Scale for Geriatrics (CIRS-G). All subjects met depressive symptom severity criteria of 18 or more on the Hamilton Depression Rating Scale (HAMD-24). The mean age of the sample was 66.5 years and the range was 60 to 90 years; bipolar I disorder accounted for 77.2% of subjects. The mean CIRS-G score was 9.4 (SD ± 4.7), which is consistent with other reports of geriatric bipolar disorder samples. The mean lamotrigine dose was 150.9 mg/d, range 25 to 200 mg/d. The mean (SD, range) primary outcome measure (MADRS) decreased significantly from 25.3 (8.3, 9–48) at baseline to 9.8 (8.3, 0–38) at end point ($t = 12.1$, $df = 53$, $P<.01$).Similarly, the mean (SD, range) HAMD-24 decreased significantly from 27.1 (6.7, 18–49) to 11.9 (9.8, 0–46), ($t = 13.2$, $df = 53$, $P<.01$). For the 54 patients for whom the final MADRS scores were available, 35 (64.8%) met depression response criteria, whereas 31 (57.4%) met remission criteria. There was significant improvement in the overall CGI ($t = 10.09$, $df = 52$, $P<.01$). Functional status, as measured by subscales of the WHODAS II, was significantly improved in most domains including self-care ($t = 2.93$, $df = 46$, $P<.01$), life activities ($t = 2.94$, $df = 46$, $P<.01$), ability to understand and communicate ($t = 4.08$, $df = 46$, $P<.01$), participation in society ($t = 6.03$, $df = 46$, $P<.01$), and getting along with people ($t = 3.89$, $df = 46$, $P<.01$). There were 19 of 57 (33.3%) individuals who dropped out of the study prematurely, with 6 of them dropping out because of adverse events (4 cases of rash, 1 case of hyponatremia, and 1 case of manic switch). The 2 cases of rash were possibly drug-related and resolved with study drug discontinuation. Physical parameters showed no significant change in the group means from baseline.

A recent meta-analysis of placebo-controlled trials in bipolar depression suggested that QTP and olanzapine are effective and rapidly acting as both adjunct therapies and monotherapies in bipolar depression.[80] However, the risk of metabolic effects is particularly high with olanzapine, and may be worse in elderly populations because of their already increased propensity for weight gain, metabolic syndrome, and diabetes. Correll and colleagues[81] reported that among patients treated with atypical antipsychotics, older age is significantly associated with metabolic syndrome and that patients with metabolic syndrome have a doubled 10-year coronary heart disease risk.

QTP may be an effective treatment of older adult bipolar depression.[82] A posthoc analysis combined results from two 8-week, double-blind, randomized, placebo-controlled studies of QTP in fixed doses (300 or 600 mg/d) in bipolar depression. The primary outcome was change from baseline on the MADRS. Samples included 72 older adults aged 55 to 65 years (mean ± SD, 58.4 ± 2.6 years; n = 23 on QTP, 300 mg/d; n = 23 on QTP, 600 mg/d; and n = 26 on placebo) and 906 younger adults aged 18 to 55 years (mean 35.7 ± 9.9 years; n = 304, 298, and 304 on QTP, 300 mg/d, QTP, 600 mg/d, and placebo, respectively). Illness baseline characteristics were broadly similar between older and younger adults. In older adults, the MADRS score decreased (mean ± SE) to 13.4 ± 2.4 with QTP, 300 mg/d; to 14.2 ± 2.5 with QTP, 600 mg/d; and to 8.0 ± 2.3 with placebo. Although the original study was not powered to detect differences in younger versus older adults, mean treatment group differences with the placebo were similar in magnitude in older and younger adults. Median times to first response in older adults were 16 days for QTP, 300 mg/d; 17 days for QTP, 600 mg/d; and 16 days for placebo (observed cases, intention-to-treat population, based on change from baseline in total MADRS), whereas respective times in younger adults were 15, 15, and 22 days. For both age groups, discontinuation rates were similar between QTP, 300 mg/d, and placebo groups and elevated in individuals who received QTP, 600 mg/d. Study discontinuation rates were similar between age groups at 29.2% for QTP, 300 mg/d; 48.1% for QTP, 600 mg/d; and 29.6% for placebo in older adults, compared with 37.1%, 45.8%, and 38.1%, respectively, in younger adults. The most common reasons for discontinuation were adverse events in groups treated with QTP (most frequently sedation, somnolence, and dizziness) and lack of efficacy in groups treated with placebo, with no age-related differences.

The role of antidepressant drugs as part of the bipolar treatment is controversial. However, the overall risk may be relatively low in geriatric bipolar disorder patients. Schaffer and colleagues[83] conducted population-based retrospective cohort design study that used the administrative databases for all individuals aged 66 years and older in a Canadian health care network. Bipolar disorder patients who received a prescription for an antidepressant medication (n = 1072) were compared with a control group (n = 3000) of randomly selected subjects from the eligible bipolar disorder population who did not receive a prescription for an antidepressant medication during the same surveillance period. During a total of 5135 person-years of follow-up, antidepressant use among elderly bipolar disorder patients was associated with decreased rates of hospitalization for manic/mixed episodes. Aizenberg and colleagues[84] reported on a retrospective case-controlled evaluation over a 10-year period evaluating suicide attempts among elderly bipolar disorder patients in relation to exposure to psychotropic medications. Although the sample size was relatively small (16 patients with attempted suicide), the investigators noted that elderly bipolar disorder patients who received treatment with mood stabilizers and antidepressants seemed to be at a reduced risk for suicide.

Maintenance Drug Treatment of Bipolar Disorder

Data from the NIHM-funded Systematic Treatment Enhancement Program for Bipolar Disorder (STEP-BD) study on prescription patterns and recovery status,[85] in younger subjects (n = 3364) aged 20 to 59 years and older subjects (n = 246) aged 60 years and older, showed that 78.5% of older patients versus 66.8% of younger patients achieved a recovered status. Those who achieved a recovered status took an average of 2.05 medications, with no difference between the age groups. The older group had 29.5% of patients on lithium versus 37.8% of younger patients. Lithium dosing was lower among individuals aged 50 years and older, but 42.1% of recovered bipolar disorder elders achieved recovery with lithium alone compared with only 21.3% of the younger group.

Lamotrigine received FDA approval for the maintenance treatment of bipolar disorder in 2003 based on data from mixed-age bipolar disorder patient populations.[86,87] A secondary analysis of 86 bipolar disorder adults aged 55 years and older suggested that overall, lamotrigine was more effective in delaying bipolar depressive relapse and lithium was more effective in delaying mania.[88] In a recent retrospective analysis of older adults with unipolar depression and bipolar disorder, which compared each patient to his or her own clinical course before and after lithium treatment, the probability of relapse and recurrence, suicidal behavior, and severity of mood disturbance was significantly decreased by lithium maintenance.[89]

Olanzapine, aripiprazole, QTP, and ziprasidone as well as risperidone long-acting injection have received FDA approval for the maintenance treatment of bipolar disorder in general adult bipolar disorder patients. However, their efficacy and tolerability have not been established in older adults.

A large randomized open-label study compared lithium and valproate monotherapies and combination treatment (The BALANCE trial) in bipolar maintenance in mixed-age patients (no upper age restriction, n = 330).[90] Combination treatment or lithium monotherapy seemed superior to treatment with valproate alone in prevention of relapse over a 2-year study period.[90] Although older and younger subgroups did not seem to differ with respect to treatment response to monotherapy versus combination therapy, the numbers of older adults were relatively small.

Electroconvulsive Therapy

Electroconvulsive therapy (ECT) remains a safe and often effective treatment of acute mania and severe depression with 80% response rate in the general population.[91,92] ECT demonstrated efficacy and safety in the treatment of 211 older adults with depression,[93] although the antimanic efficacy of ECT has not been studied in geriatric patients. ECT is often considered when patients require rapid and definitive clinical response, such as bipolar disorder patients at immediate suicidal or homicidal risk; in catatonic, psychotic or agitated states; or in medically compromised states. However, the possible long-term cognitive effects of ECT remain unclear.

Psychosocial Interventions

Psychosocial intervention is an essential part of the treatment of patients with bipolar disorder in addition to biological interventions. This may be especially true for older adults with complex biopsychosocial stress. Psychosocial interventions could play an important role in improving short-term outcome including symptom and stress reduction, as well as long-term outcomes including adherence enhancement, relapse prevention, functional recovery, and reduction of medical comorbidity. Common intervention models include cognitive-behavioral therapy (CBT), interpersonal social rhythm therapy (IPSRT), family-focused therapy (FFT), psychoeducation model, and an integrated care model.[94,95] In a 1-year randomized trial from the systematic treatment enhancement program comparing the effectiveness of CBT, FTT, IPSRT, and collaborative care (control intervention consisting of 3 sessions) as adjuncts to medications (n = 293, mean age = 40.1 years, SD = 11.8, range 17–65 years), Miklowitz and colleagues[96] found that patients receiving intensive psychotherapy (CBT, FTT, or IPSRT) had significantly higher year-end recovery rates than patients receiving collaborative care (64.4% vs 51.5%, respectively), and that patients in the FFT group had the best outcome, followed by those in the IPSRT and CBT (76.9%, 64.5%, and 60.0%, respectively) groups, even though no statistically significant difference was observed among the 3 intensive psychotherapies.

Psychosocial interventions focusing on medication adherence and ways of reducing relapse have shown promising benefits though implementing these approaches in real-world settings, and in older adults, need further study.[97,98] A small pilot study of a medication adherence skills training for bipolar disorder (MAST-BD) for older adults with bipolar disorder (n = 21, mean age = 60 years, SD = 6), demonstrated that the MAST-BD intervention was feasible, acceptable to patients, and associated with improvement mean in medication adherence, medication management ability, depressive symptoms, and selected indices of health-related quality of life.[99]

Kilbourne and colleagues[33] demonstrated that a bipolar disorder medical care model (BCM) when compared with usual care, may improve physical and mental health–related quality of life over a 6-month period. These investigators also demonstrated in a subsequent study that BCM is a feasible model for older medically ill patients with bipolar disorder.[100]

AREAS FOR FUTURE STUDY

Given that the elderly are the fastest growing segment of the United States population, that the number of bipolar disorder elders are increasing, and that bipolar disorder elders are disproportionately affected by illness complexity and comorbidity,[9,53] a better understanding of phenomenology, pathophysiology, and treatment of late-life bipolar disorder is of substantial public health importance. Areas that deserve particular focus and study include medical comorbidity and the relationship between shared or overlapping contributors and specific treatment approaches that may differ from recommendations in current bipolar disorder treatment guidelines. Geriatric patients with bipolar disorder are typically excluded from RCTs. However, simply extrapolating findings from young adult bipolar disorder populations as a standard on which to base clinical care may lead to incorrect assumptions regarding treatment needs and treatment response. Prospective studies focused specifically on geriatric bipolar disorder patients are urgently needed. Finally, an integrated neuroscience approach that includes and evaluates multiple relevant clinical and neurobiological domains such as clinical subtypes, cognitive status, neuroimaging, and genetics may help to predict individual treatment response.[101–105]

REFERENCES

1. Cade JF. Lithium salts in the treatment of psychotic excitement. Med J Aust 1949;2(10):349–52.
2. Gyulai L, Young RC. New research perspectives in the treatment of bipolar disorder in older adults. Bipolar Disord 2008;10(6):659–61.
3. Weissman MM, Leaf PJ, Tischler GL, et al. Affective disorders in five United States communities. Psychol Med 1988;18(1):141–53.
4. Unutzer J, Simon G, Pabiniak C, et al. The treated prevalence of bipolar disorder in a large staff-model HMO. Psychiatr Serv 1998;49(8):1072–8.
5. Hirschfeld RM, Calabrese JR, Weissman MM, et al. Screening for bipolar disorder in the community. J Clin Psychiatry 2003;64(1):53–9.
6. Kessler RC, Berglund P, Demler O, et al. Lifetime prevalence and age-of-onset distributions of DSM-IV disorders in the National Comorbidity Survey Replication. Arch Gen Psychiatry 2005;62(6):593–602.
7. Yassa R, Nair V, Nastase C, et al. Prevalence of bipolar disorder in a psychogeriatric population. J Affect Disord 1988;14(3):197–201.
8. Depp CA, Lindamer LA, Folsom DP, et al. Differences in clinical features and mental health service use in bipolar disorder across the lifespan. Am J Geriatr Psychiatry 2005;13(4):290–8.
9. Almeida OP, Fenner S. Bipolar disorder: similarities and differences between patients with illness onset before and after 65 years of age. Int Psychogeriatr 2002;14(3):311–22.
10. Rasanen P, Tiihonen J, Hakko H. The incidence and onset-age of hospitalized bipolar affective disorder in Finland. J Affect Disord 1998;48(1):63–8.

11. Depp CA, Jeste DV. Bipolar disorder in older adults: a critical review. Bipolar Disord 2004;6(5):343–67.
12. Sajatovic M, Blow FC, Ignacio RV, et al. New-onset bipolar disorder in later life. Am J Geriatr Psychiatry 2005;13(4):282–9.
13. Krauthammer C, Klerman GL. Secondary mania: manic syndromes associated with antecedent physical illness or drugs. Arch Gen Psychiatry 1978;35(11): 1333–9.
14. Leboyer M, Henry C, Paillere-Martinot ML, et al. Age at onset in bipolar affective disorders: a review. Bipolar Disord 2005;7(2):111–8.
15. Benedetti A, Scarpellini P, Casamassima F, et al. Bipolar disorder in late life: clinical characteristics in a sample of older adults admitted for manic episode. Clin Pract Epidemiol Ment Health 2008;4:22.
16. Moorhead SR, Young AH. Evidence for a late onset bipolar-I disorder sub-group from 50 years. J Affect Disord 2003;73(3):271–7.
17. Snowdon J. A retrospective case-note study of bipolar disorder in old age. Br J Psychiatry 1991;158:485–90.
18. Shulman KI, Tohen M, Satlin A, et al. Mania compared with unipolar depression in old age. Am J Psychiatry 1992;149(3):341–5.
19. Tohen M, Shulman KI, Satlin A. First-episode mania in late life. Am J Psychiatry 1994;151(1):130–2.
20. Stone K. Mania in the elderly. Br J Psychiatry 1989;155:220–4.
21. Broadhead J, Jacoby R. Mania in old age: a first prospective study. Int J Geriatr Psychiatry 1990;5(4):215–22.
22. Shulman K, Post F. Bipolar affective disorder in old age. Br J Psychiatry 1980; 136:26–32.
23. Hays JC, Krishnan KR, George LK, et al. Age of first onset of bipolar disorder: demographic, family history, and psychosocial correlates. Depress Anxiety 1998;7(2):76–82.
24. Shulman RW, Singh A, Shulman KI. Treatment of elderly institutionalized bipolar patients with clozapine. Psychopharmacol Bull 1997;33(1):113–8.
25. Pearlson GD. Structural and functional brain changes in bipolar disorder: a selective review. Schizophr Res 1999;39(2):133–40 [discussion: 162].
26. Zald DH, Kim SW. Anatomy and function of the orbital frontal cortex, I: anatomy, neurocircuitry; and obsessive-compulsive disorder. J Neuropsychiatry Clin Neurosci 1996;8(2):125–38.
27. Starkstein SE, Robinson RG. Mechanism of disinhibition after brain lesions. J Nerv Ment Dis 1997;185(2):108–14.
28. Beyer JL, Kuchibhatla M, Cassidy F, et al. Stressful life events in older bipolar patients. Int J Geriatr Psychiatry 2008;23(12):1271–5.
29. Solomon DA, Leon AC, Coryell WH, et al. Longitudinal course of bipolar I disorder: duration of mood episodes. Arch Gen Psychiatry 2010;67(4):339–47.
30. Depp CA, Davis CE, Mittal D, et al. Health-related quality of life and functioning of middle-aged and elderly adults with bipolar disorder. J Clin Psychiatry 2006; 67(2):215–21.
31. Gildengers AG, Mulsant BH, Begley A, et al. The longitudinal course of cognition in older adults with bipolar disorder. Bipolar Disord 2009;11(7):744–52.
32. Tsai SY, Kuo CJ, Chen CC, et al. Risk factors for completed suicide in bipolar disorder. J Clin Psychiatry 2002;63(6):469–76.
33. Kilbourne AM, Post EP, Nossek A, et al. Improving medical and psychiatric outcomes among individuals with bipolar disorder: a randomized controlled trial. Psychiatr Serv 2008;59(7):760–8.

34. McIntyre RS, Konarski JZ, Soczynska JK, et al. Medical comorbidity in bipolar disorder: implications for functional outcomes and health service utilization. Psychiatr Serv 2006;57(8):1140–4.

35. Brown SL. Variations in utilization and cost of inpatient psychiatric services among adults in Maryland. Psychiatr Serv 2001;52(6):841–3.

36. Juurlink DN, Herrmann N, Szalai JP, et al. Medical illness and the risk of suicide in the elderly. Arch Intern Med 2004;164(11):1179–84.

37. Gildengers AG, Whyte EM, Drayer RA, et al. Medical burden in late-life bipolar and major depressive disorders. Am J Geriatr Psychiatry 2008;16(3):194–200.

38. Gildengers AG, Butters MA, Seligman K, et al. Cognitive functioning in late-life bipolar disorder. Am J Psychiatry 2004;161(4):736–8.

39. Kessing LV, Andersen PK. Does the risk of developing dementia increase with the number of episodes in patients with depressive disorder and in patients with bipolar disorder? J Neurol Neurosurg Psychiatry 2004;75(12):1662–6.

40. Kessing LV, Olsen EW, Mortensen PB, et al. Dementia in affective disorder: a case-register study. Acta Psychiatr Scand 1999;100(3):176–85.

41. Kessing LV, Nilsson FM. Increased risk of developing dementia in patients with major affective disorders compared to patients with other medical illnesses. J Affect Disord 2003;73(3):261–9.

42. Schloesser RJ, Huang J, Klein PS, et al. Cellular plasticity cascades in the pathophysiology and treatment of bipolar disorder. Neuropsychopharmacology 2008;33(1):110–33.

43. Berk M. Neuroprogression: pathways to progressive brain changes in bipolar disorder. Int J Neuropsychopharmacol 2009;12(4):441–5.

44. Sajatovic M, Kales HC. Diagnosis and management of bipolar disorder with comorbid anxiety in the elderly. J Clin Psychiatry 2006;67(Suppl 1):21–7.

45. Goldstein BI, Herrmann N, Shulman KI. Comorbidity in bipolar disorder among the elderly: results from an epidemiological community sample. Am J Psychiatry 2006;163(2):319–21.

46. Sajatovic M, Popli A, Semple W. Ten-year use of hospital-based services by geriatric veterans with schizophrenia and bipolar disorder. Psychiatr Serv 1996;47(9):961–5.

47. Bartels SJ, Forester B, Miles KM, et al. Mental health service use by elderly patients with bipolar disorder and unipolar major depression. Am J Geriatr Psychiatry 2000;8(2):160–6.

48. Wang PS, Schneeweiss S, Avorn J, et al. Risk of death in elderly users of conventional vs. atypical antipsychotic medications. N Engl J Med 2005; 353(22):2335–41.

49. Kessing LV. Diagnostic subtypes of bipolar disorder in older versus younger adults. Bipolar Disord 2006;8(1):56–64.

50. Van Gerpen MW, Johnson JE, Winstead DK. Mania in the geriatric patient population: a review of the literature. Am J Geriatr Psychiatry 1999;7(3):188–202.

51. Oostervink F, Boomsma MM, Nolen WA, et al. Bipolar disorder in the elderly; different effects of age and of age of onset. J Affect Disord 2009;116(3): 176–83.

52. Gildengers AG, Mulsant BH, Begley AE, et al. A pilot study of standardized treatment in geriatric bipolar disorder. Am J Geriatr Psychiatry 2005;13(4): 319–23.

53. Young RC, Schulberg HC, Gildengers AG, et al. Conceptual and methodological issues in designing a randomized, controlled treatment trial for geriatric bipolar disorder: GERI-BD. Bipolar Disord 2010;12(1):56–67.

54. Shulman KI, Rochon P, Sykora K, et al. Changing prescription patterns for lithium and valproic acid in old age: shifting practice without evidence. BMJ 2003;326(7396):960–1.
55. Sajatovic M. Treatment of bipolar disorder in older adults. Int J Geriatr Psychiatry 2002;17(9):865–73.
56. Kessing LV, Sondergard L, Kvist K, et al. Suicide risk in patients treated with lithium. Arch Gen Psychiatry 2005;62(8):860–6.
57. Kessing LV, Sondergard L, Forman JL, et al. Lithium treatment and risk of dementia. Arch Gen Psychiatry 2008;65(11):1331–5.
58. Schaffer CB, Garvey MJ. Use of lithium in acutely manic elderly patients. Clin Gerontol 1984;3:58–60.
59. Eastham JH, Jeste DV, Young RC. Assessment and treatment of bipolar disorder in the elderly. Drugs Aging 1998;12(3):205–24.
60. Chen ST, Altshuler LL, Melnyk KA, et al. Efficacy of lithium vs. valproate in the treatment of mania in the elderly: a retrospective study. J Clin Psychiatry 1999;60(3):181–6.
61. Bowden CL, Lawson DM, Cunningham M. The role of divalproex in the treatment of bipolar disorder. Psychiatr Ann 2002;32(12):742–50.
62. Abbott Laboratories. Depakote tablet [product information]. Divalproex sodium delayed-release tablets. Abbott Park (IL): Abbott; 2001.
63. Greil W, Kleindienst N, Erazo N, et al. Differential response to lithium and carbamazepine in the prophylaxis of bipolar disorder. J Clin Psychopharmacol 1998; 18(6):455–60.
64. Evans DL, Byerly MJ, Greer RA. Secondary mania: diagnosis and treatment. J Clin Psychiatry 1995;56(Suppl 3):31–7.
65. Cates M, Powers R. Concomitant rash and blood dyscrasias in geriatric psychiatry patients treated with carbamazepine. Ann Pharmacother 1998;32(9):884–7.
66. Battino D, Croci D, Rossini A, et al. Serum carbamazepine concentrations in elderly patients: a case-matched pharmacokinetic evaluation based on therapeutic drug monitoring data. Epilepsia 2003;44(7):923–9.
67. Bayer JL, Siegal A, Kennedy JS. Olanzapine, divalproex and placebo treatment, non-head to head comparisons of older adults acute mania. 10th Congress of the International Psychogeriatric Association. Nice (France), September 9–14, 2001.
68. Madhusoodanan S, Brenner R, Araujo L, et al. Efficacy of risperidone treatment for psychoses associated with schizophrenia, schizoaffective disorder, bipolar disorder, or senile dementia in 11 geriatric patients: a case series. J Clin Psychiatry 1995;56(11):514–8.
69. Madhusoodanan S, Suresh P, Brenner R, et al. Experience with the atypical antipsychotics–risperidone and olanzapine in the elderly. Ann Clin Psychiatry 1999; 11(3):113–8.
70. Sajatovic M, Calabrese JR, Mullen J. Quetiapine for the treatment of bipolar mania in older adults. Bipolar Disord 2008;10(6):662–71.
71. Centers for Medicare and Medicaid Services, Chartbook: Medicaid Pharmaceutical Benefit Use and Reimbursement in 2003. Available at: http://www.cms.hhs. gov/MedicaidDataSourcesGenInfo/downloads/Pharmacy_RX_Chartbook_2003. pdf. Accessed August 1, 2009.
72. Crystal S, Olfson M, Huang C, et al. Broadened use of atypical antipsychotics: safety, effectiveness, and policy challenges. Health Aff (Millwood) 2009;28(5): w770–81.
73. Center for Drug Evaluation and Research. Deaths with antipsychotics in elderly patients with behavioral disturbances [FDA public health advisory]. Rockville

(MD): US Food and Drug Administration; 2005. Available at: www.fda.gov/cder/drug/advisory/antipsychotics.htm. Accessed February 16, 2011.

74. American Psychiatric Association. Practice guideline for the treatment of patients with bipolar disorder [revision]. Am J Psychiatry 2002;159(4 Suppl):1–50.

75. Aziz R, Lorberg B, Tampi RR. Treatments for late-life bipolar disorder. Am J Geriatr Pharmacother 2006;4(4):347–64.

76. International Consensus Group on the evidence-based pharmacologic treatment of bipolar I and II depression. J Clin Psychiatry 2008;69(10):1632–46.

77. Fountoulakis KN, Vieta E. Treatment of bipolar disorder: a systematic review of available data and clinical perspectives. Int J Neuropsychopharmacol 2008; 11(7):999–1029.

78. Kennedy GJ. Bipolar disorder in late life: depression. Prim Psychiatr 2008;15: 30–4.

79. Sajatovic M, Gildengers A, Al Jurdi R, et al. Multi-site, open-label, prospective trial of lamotrigine for geriatric bipolar depression. Hollywood (FL): American College of Neuropsychopharmacology (ACNP); 2009.

80. Cruz N, Sanchez-Moreno J, Torres F, et al. Efficacy of modern antipsychotics in placebo-controlled trials in bipolar depression: a meta-analysis. Int J Neuropsychopharmacol 2010;13(1):5–14.

81. Correll CU, Frederickson AM, Kane JM, et al. Metabolic syndrome and the risk of coronary heart disease in 367 patients treated with second-generation antipsychotic drugs. J Clin Psychiatry 2006;67(4):575–83.

82. Sajatovic M. Quetiapine for the treatment of depressive episodes in adults aged 55 to 65 years with bipolar disorder. New Orleans (LA): American Association of Geriatric Psychiatry (AAGP); 2007.

83. Schaffer A, Mamdani M, Levitt A, et al. Effect of antidepressant use on admissions to hospital among elderly bipolar patients. Int J Geriatr Psychiatry 2006; 21(3):275–80.

84. Aizenberg D, Olmer A, Barak Y. Suicide attempts amongst elderly bipolar patients. J Affect Disord 2006;91(1):91–4.

85. Al Jurdi RK, Marangell LB, Petersen NJ, et al. Prescription patterns of psychotropic medications in elderly compared with younger participants who achieved a "recovered" status in the systematic treatment enhancement program for bipolar disorder. Am J Geriatr Psychiatry 2008;16(11):922–33.

86. Calabrese JR, Bowden CL, Sachs G, et al. A placebo-controlled 18-month trial of lamotrigine and lithium maintenance treatment in recently depressed patients with bipolar I disorder. J Clin Psychiatry 2003;64(9):1013–24.

87. Bowden CL, Calabrese JR, Sachs G, et al. A placebo-controlled 18-month trial of lamotrigine and lithium maintenance treatment in recently manic or hypomanic patients with bipolar I disorder. Arch Gen Psychiatry 2003;60(4): 392–400.

88. Sajatovic M, Gyulai L, Calabrese JR, et al. Maintenance treatment outcomes in older patients with bipolar I disorder. Am J Geriatr Psychiatry 2005;13(4): 305–11.

89. Lepkifker E, Iancu I, Horesh N, et al. Lithium therapy for unipolar and bipolar depression among the middle-aged and older adult patient subpopulation. Depress Anxiety 2007;24(8):571–6.

90. BALANCE investigators and collaborators, Geddes JR, Goodwin GM, et al. Lithium plus valproate combination therapy versus monotherapy for relapse prevention in bipolar I disorder (BALANCE): a randomised open-label trial. Lancet 2010;375(9712):385–95.

91. American Psychiatric Association. The practice of ECT: recommendations for treatment, training and privileging. Washington, DC: American Psychiatric Press; 2001.

92. Mukherjee S, Sackeim HA, Schnur DB. Electroconvulsive therapy of acute manic episodes: a review of 50 years' experience. Am J Psychiatry 1994; 151(2):169–76.

93. van der Wurff FB, Stek ML, Hoogendijk WJ, et al. The efficacy and safety of ECT in depressed older adults: a literature review. Int J Geriatr Psychiatry 2003; 18(10):894–904.

94. Castle DJ, Berk L, Lauder S, et al. Psychosocial interventions for bipolar disorder. Acta Neuropsychiatr 2009;21:275–84.

95. Miklowitz DJ, Otto MW. Psychosocial interventions for bipolar disorder: a review of literature and introduction of the systematic treatment enhancement program. Psychopharmacol Bull 2008;40(4):116–31.

96. Miklowitz DJ, Otto MW, Frank E, et al. Psychosocial treatments for bipolar depression: a 1-year randomized trial from the Systematic Treatment Enhancement Program. Arch Gen Psychiatry 2007;64(4):419–26.

97. Sajatovic M, Chen P, Dines P, et al. Psychoeducational approaches to medication adherence in patients with bipolar disorder. Dis Manag Health Outcome 2007;15(3):181–92.

98. Bauer MS, Biswas K, Kilbourne AM. Enhancing multiyear guideline concordance for bipolar disorder through collaborative care. Am J Psychiatry 2009; 166(11):1244–50.

99. Depp CA, Lebowitz BD, Patterson TL, et al. Medication adherence skills training for middle-aged and elderly adults with bipolar disorder: development and pilot study. Bipolar Disord 2007;9:636–45.

100. Kilbourne AM, Post EP, Nossek A, et al. Service delivery in older patients with bipolar disorder: a review and development of a medical care model. Bipolar Disord 2008;10(6):672–83.

101. Gordon E. Integrating genomics and neuromarkers for the era of brain-related personalized medicine. Personalized Medicine 2007;4(2):201–15.

102. Gordon E, Barnett KJ, Cooper NJ, et al. An "integrative neuroscience" platform: application to profiles of negativity and positivity bias. J Integr Neurosci 2008; 7(3):345–66.

103. Mulert C, Juckel G, Augustin H, et al. Comparison between the analysis of the loudness dependency of the auditory N1/P2 component with LORETA and dipole source analysis in the prediction of treatment response to the selective serotonin reuptake inhibitor citalopram in major depression. Clin Neurophysiol 2002;113(10):1566–72.

104. Simons AD, Gordon JS, Monroe SM, et al. Toward an integration of psychologic, social, and biologic factors in depression: effects on outcome and course of cognitive therapy. J Consult Clin Psychol 1995;63(3):369–77.

105. Kemp AH, Gordon E, Rush AJ, et al. Improving the prediction of treatment response in depression: integration of clinical, cognitive, psychophysiological, neuroimaging, and genetic measures. CNS Spectr 2008;13(12):1066–86.

Late-life Depression: Evidence-based Treatment and Promising New Directions for Research and Clinical Practice

Carmen Andreescu, MD[a], Charles F. Reynolds III, MD[b],*

KEYWORDS

- Late-life depression • Treatment algorithms
- Novel treatment modalities

OVERVIEW

Depression results in more years lived with disability than any other disease, and ranks fourth in terms of disability-adjusted life years.[1–3] Projections are that, by 2020, depression will be second only to heart disease in its contribution to the global burden of disease (measured by disability-adjusted life years).[4] As the population ages, successive cohorts of older adults will experience depressive disorders.[4] Late-life depression (LLD) carries additional risk for suicide, medical comorbidity, disability, and family caregiving burden.[5–7] Although treatment is effective in reducing symptoms, it is less successful in achieving and maintaining remission and in averting years

Supported in part by P30 MH71944, K23 MH 086686, R01 MH 083660, the John A. Hartford Foundation Center of Excellence in Geriatric Psychiatry, and the UPMC Endowment in Geriatric Psychiatry.
Financial disclosure: Carmen Andreescu has no conflict of interest to report. Charles F. Reynolds III has received pharmaceutical supplies for his NIH-sponsored research from GlaxoSmithKline, Pfizer Inc, Eli Lilly and Co, Bristol Meyers Squibb, Wyeth Pharmaceuticals, and Forest Pharmaceuticals.
[a] Department of Psychiatry, Western Psychiatric Institute and Clinic, University of Pittsburgh, 3811 O'Hara Street, 247 Sterling Plaza, Pittsburgh, PA 15213, USA
[b] Department of Psychiatry, Western Psychiatric Institute and Clinic, University of Pittsburgh, 3811 O'Hara Street, 758 Bellefield Towers, Pittsburgh, PA 15213, USA
* Corresponding author.
E-mail address: reynoldscf@upmc.edu

Psychiatr Clin N Am 34 (2011) 335–355
doi:10.1016/j.psc.2011.02.005
0193-953X/11/$ – see front matter © 2011 Elsevier Inc. All rights reserved.

lived with disability. Although response and remission rates to pharmacotherapy and electroconvulsive therapy (ECT) are comparable with those in midlife depression, relapse rates are higher,[8] underscoring the challenge not only to achieve but also to maintain wellness.

This article reviews the evidence base for LLD treatment options and provides a more in-depth analysis of treatment options for difficult-to-treat LLD variants (eg, psychotic depression, vascular depression). Treatment algorithms are also reviewed based on predictors of response and novel treatment options that represent promising leads.

Standard Treatment

Pharmacotherapy

Approximately two-thirds of patients presenting with severe forms of depression respond to antidepressant treatment. However, older, frail people are particularly vulnerable to antidepressant side effects, especially cardiovascular and anticholinergic side effects, and this can compromise compliance and effectiveness of treatment.[9]

Acute Treatment

A recent meta-analysis of acute pharmacological trials revealed a paucity of placebo-controlled trials in older depressed populations.[10] Using a 50% reduction in the Hamilton Rating Scale for Depression (HRSD) as the primary outcome measure, the meta-analysis reported an overall number needed to treat (NNT) of 8 (95% confidence interval [CI] 5,11) when all antidepressant classes were collapsed together.[10] The analysis of each class was similar: for tricyclic antidepressants (TCAs) the NNT was 5 (95% CI 3,9) and for selective serotonin reuptake inhibitors (SSRIs) the NNT was 8 (95% CI 5,11). Because the confidence intervals between TCAs and SSRIs overlap substantially, these data do not support that one drug class is more effective than another.[10] A limitation of the studies examined in this meta-analysis is that they were efficacy trials, excluding subjects with comorbid psychiatric illnesses, medical comorbidity and poor treatment response history, thus limiting generalizability.[10] Moreover, the largest trials conducted so far showed a large placebo response rate and a significant number of subjects who do not respond or who have residual depressive symptoms.[10]

In a large (N = 728) trial, Nelson and colleagues[11] used the HRSD to determine the symptoms that showed the greatest improvement during treatment: depressed mood (effect size [ES] 0.93), decreased interest and activity (ES 0.86), psychic anxiety (ES 0.65), guilt (ES 0.63), suicidal ideation/behavior (ES 0.6). Consequently, the investigators compared the results with those obtained using 5 other scales (Montgomery Asberg Depression Rating Scale, the Keller Brief Depression Rating Scale, Yale Depression Inventory, Quick Inventory of Depressive Symptoms, Inventory of Depressive Symptoms) and reported that there is considerable agreement among the scales with regard to symptoms sensitive to change during treatment of LLD.[11]

LLD is also more varied in its clinical presentations than its midlife equivalent. Thus, instruments currently used to define depression might not capture the entire spectrum or phenotype of depressive disorders in the elderly. Moreover, instruments such as HRSD or Montgomery Asberg Depression Rating Scale are difficult to use on a regular base in the real-life environment of the currently overcrowded outpatient clinics. Self-report measures, such as PHQ9, provide a more practical, easy-to-use tool for measure-based care, and fit in well with the strategies of depression care management.[10]

An effectiveness trial of older depressed outpatients reported a post hoc analysis for participants treated with citalopram in the Sequenced Treatment Alternatives to Relieve Depression (STAR*D) analyzing the correlation between age of onset of the first MD episode and clinical outcome.[12] Remission rates (defined by a 16-item Quick Inventory of Depressive Symptomatology-Self-rated) were not statistically different between earlier onset (age of onset <55 years; 30.8%) and late onset (31.9%).[12]

A 2006 Cochrane Review on the use of antidepressants in the elderly examined the efficacy of antidepressant classes, compared the withdrawal rates associated with each class, and described the side effect profile of antidepressants for treating depression in patients age 55 years and older.[9] The review did not find any differences in efficacy between classes of antidepressants, although it reported that TCAs are associated with a higher withdrawal rate because of side effect experiences (**Table 1**).[9] The small number of studies restricted the validity of subgroup analysis on different populations (outpatient/inpatients/community volunteers/nursing home residents).[9] Because few trials used standardized instruments to report side effects, the Cochrane Review used an analysis of withdrawal rates and described the ratios of the number of side effects experienced by patients treated with each antidepressant class. Thus, TSA recipients experienced more gastrointestinal side effects (4.6 side effects experienced by 10 TCA recipients compared with 2.9/10 SSRI recipients) and more neuropsychiatric side effects (4.1 side effects experienced by 10 TCA recipients compared with 2.3/10 SSRI recipients). However, nausea and vomiting were experienced by a greater percentage of SSRI recipients.[9] A STAR*D report on melancholiform depression in midlife reported that the presence of melancholic features was associated with significantly reduced remission rates to SSRI (8.4% compared with 24.1% in nonmelancholiform depression).[13]

Overall, these studies underscore the similar incomplete response to antidepressant treatment across the life cycle and highlight the challenge to develop novel, more efficacious treatment strategies, especially for patients who do not respond fully to first-line treatments. The goal of acute, or short-term, treatment is full remission of symptoms. The goal of longer-term treatment is prevention of recurrence. Getting well is important but not enough . It is staying well that counts.

Table 1
Comparing antidepressants for acute treatment of LLD: duration of treatment

Antidepressant Classes Compared	Primary Outcome Efficacy (Change in HDRS)		Secondary Outcome (Withdrawal Rates)	
	No. of Trials	RR	No. of Trials	Withdrawal Rates
	16		26	
TCAs vs SSRIs	9 trials	No difference (RR 1.07, CI 0.94–1.22)	14	SSRI<TCAs (RR 1.36, CI 1.09–1.70)
TCAs vs MAOIs	2 studies	RR 1.16, CI 0.74–1.83	3	ND (RR 0.91, CI 0.64–1.29)
TCAs vs atypicals[a]	4 trials	RR 0.84, CI 0.51–1.38	8	ND (RR 0.96, CI 0.75–1.24)
SSRIs vs MAOIs	1 trial	RR 0.81, CI 0.55–1.20	1	ND (RRs not given)
MAOIs vs atypical	No trial		No trial	
SSRIs vs atypicals	No trial		No trial	

Abbreviations: CI, confidence interval; RR, risk ratio; HDRS, Hamilton Depression Rating Scale; MAOI, monoamine oxidase inhibitors.
[a] Atypical antidepressants: tianeptine, mirtazepine, reboxetine, buspirone, milnaciprin, bupropion.
Data from Mottram P, Wilson K, Strobl J. Antidepressants for depressed elderly. Cochrane Database Syst Rev 2006;1:CD003491.

Maintenance Treatment

There is limited consensus about the length of long-term maintenance pharmaco-therapy after a first episode of depression, most experts recommending 6 to 12 months of pharmacotherapy after a first episode of depression in old age.[14] Recurrence rates in LLD range from 50% to 90% in a period of 2 to 3 years.[15] Thus, the goal of the treatment is not only acute recovery but also prevention of recurrence.[16] There are few controlled studies on the efficacy of maintenance antidepressant medication. Maintenance nortriptyline (plasma steady-state level 80–120 ng/mL), monthly interpersonal therapy (IPT), and the combination of the 2 were superior to placebo in preventing recurrence for 3 years among patients with LLD with a history of multiple episodes.[17] Citalopram (dose 20–40 mg/d)[18] but not sertraline (50–100 mg/d)[19] have differed from placebo in 2 randomized trials following subjects for 48 and 100 weeks respectively. The most recent study to date to test the efficacy of an SSRI in maintenance treatment of LLD tested the efficacy of 2-year maintenance treatment with paroxetine and monthly interpersonal therapy.[16] Major depression recurred in 35% of the patients receiving paroxetine and psychotherapy, 37% of those receiving paroxetine and clinical management sessions (30-minute visits with no specific therapy, questions about symptoms and possible side effects), 68% of those receiving placebo and psychotherapy, and 58% of those receiving placebo and clinical management sessions.[16] The relative risk of recurrence among patients receiving placebo was 2.4 times that among those receiving paroxetine (dose 10–40 mg/d).[16] Moreover, patients treated with paroxetine for 2 years were less likely to have recurrent depression, whereas maintenance psychotherapy did not prevent recurrences.[16] Patients in their first lifetime episodes also benefited from maintenance treatment of 2 years, thus not supporting the conventional wisdom and practice of limiting continuation treatment to 6 to 12 months following remission from acute treatment.[16]

Another important and clinically relevant aspect of maintenance treatments is that the NNT is around 4, in contrast with an NNT of 7 to 8 in acute treatment. In comparison, 4 large trials of statins found that the number of patients needed to be treated with statins for 5 years to prevent another myocardial infarction was 21,[16] indicating a larger clinical effect size for maintenance antidepressant pharmacotherapy.

Psychotherapy

Given the propensity to multiple side effects noticed in the elderly, psychotherapy may represent a safer alternative. Most guidelines advocate the additional benefit of supporting antidepressant medication with psychosocial interventions.[6,17,20] An expert-consensus guideline from 2001 considered cognitive behavioral therapy (CBT), problem-solving therapy (PST), IPT, and supportive therapy as first-line psychosocial interventions, whereas psychodynamic therapy received a more controversial rating (26% of the experts rated this as first line and 36% as third line).[14] Overall, the expert consensus recommended psychotherapy as an adjunctive treatment to medication, except for mild depression or dysthymia, for which psychotherapy alone was considered an alternate initial treatment strategy.[14] The more commonly prescribed psychotherapies are developed from cognitive therapy, which focuses on dysfunctional beliefs; they include CBT, PST, and behavioral activation. Numerous descriptive studies have examined the technical issues in adapting these therapies to aging populations: emphasizing behavioral techniques, repeating information, a slower pace, and using different sensory modalities.[21] Thus, given the executive dysfunctions described in LLD,[22] several experts advocated for the use of PST[23,24] that uses behavioral activation and explicitly trains patients to select and solve daily problems as a way of increasing self-efficacy and overcoming the feelings of helplessness at the core of depression.

However, there is little evidence based on randomized controlled trials that specifically examines the efficacy of various types of psychotherapy in older people.

A Cochrane Review from 2007 identified 9 trials of CBT and psychodynamic therapy, 7 of these providing comparison data between CBT and controls.[20] CBT was more effective than waiting list controls, whereas there was no difference in treatment effect between CBT and psychodynamic therapy. However, the superiority CBT to waiting list was maintained only when assessed via the HRSD; it disappeared when using the Geriatric Depression Scale (GDS).[20] All the trials analyzed had small sample sizes, the inclusion criteria allowed for both major depression and dysthymia, included both clinical populations as well as community volunteers,[25] with duration varying from 4 to 24 weeks.[20] The investigators concluded that, although CBT-derived therapies seem to be superior to waiting list control, the small size of the meta-analysis, the high dropout rates, and the heterogeneity of the study populations and the interventions limited the ability to generalize these findings to clinical populations.[20]

One more recent randomized, controlled trial reported that in 4 months, CBT was more effective than treatment as usual or talking control (supportive therapy) for late-life depressed subjects (total N = 204).[26] Another randomized, controlled trial showed that, in a period of 12 weeks, PST was superior to supportive therapy in older adults with major depression and executive dysfunction.[27] Integrating the results of 89 controlled studies of LLD acute treatment, a recent meta-analysis[28] reported that both pharmacotherapy and psychotherapy render comparable, moderate-to-large effect sizes (Cohen d 0.62–0.69 for pharmacotherapy studies and 0.83–1.09 for psychotherapy studies).

ECT

Older depressed patients are often frailer and particularly prone to the side effects of antidepressants. ECT has been established as particularly effective in LLD.[29] Although it is still controversial, ECT seems to be a safe treatment even in elderly with comorbid cardiovascular illness, dementia, or Parkinson disease.[30]

From the various randomized controlled trials of ECT for elderly people (>60 years old), only 4 trials were eligible for inclusion in the Cochrane meta-analysis, 1 comparing the efficacy of real ECT versus simulated ECT, 2 comparing the efficacy of unilateral versus bilateral ECT, and the other comparing the efficacy of weekly ECT with three times weekly ECT. However, the various methodological problems did not allow the investigators to perform a quantitative comparative analysis of these studies.[31] The investigators concluded that neither the efficacy of unilateral compared with bilateral ECT, nor of the 3-week ECT compared with weekly ECT, has been convincingly proved.[31] Moreover, studies that establish the long-term effects of ECT or those comparing the safety and efficacy of ECT with antidepressants in subpopulations such as elderly depressed with dementia or vascular disease are still needed.[31]

Post-ECT maintenance treatment with pharmacotherapy are discussed later.

Difficult-to-treat LLD

In general, the pharmacological treatment of LLD is only partially successful, with about 50% of patients improving with antidepressant monotherapy to the point of full response or remission. Many factors predict a difficult-to-treat depression, including clinical profile (comorbid anxiety, psychotic symptoms, poor sleep, low self-esteem), high medical burden, coexisting cognitive impairment.[32] Partial response poses the risk of chronic relapsing depression, nonadherence to other treatments for coexisting medical disorders, family caregiver burden, and suicide.

Treatment-resistant Depression

Treatment-resistant depression reportedly affects up to one-third of older depressed patients.[33] Before labeling an episode of depression as treatment resistant, it is important to ensure that the diagnosis is correct and that the patient has received an adequate dose of treatment, for an appropriate length of time, to assess the presence of comorbid physical and psychiatric conditions.[34] Pharmacological options of treatment-resistant depression can be grouped in 2 categories: switching or combining. In the first case, treatment is switched within or between classes of antidepressants and thus avoids polypharmacy and potential increased side effects and medication costs.[35] Combination strategies have the advantage of building on achieved improvements and are recommended when partial response has already been obtained. The most frequently used augmenting agents are lithium, atypical antipsychotics, and thyroid hormones. A sequential treatment protocol compared augmentation with lithium, switching to monoamine oxidase inhibitors (MAOI) or to ECT in elderly with partial acute response to either venlafaxine or nortriptyline.[36] Augmentation with lithium was the best treatment option in this group for both efficacy and tolerability.[36] So far, the combination of antidepressants and atypical antipsychotics (aripiprazole and olanzapine) are the only approved augmenting agents for treatment-resistant depression. A recent pilot study in older adults using aripiprazole augmentation reported that 50% of the 24 incomplete responders to prior sequential treatment with SSRI and serotonin-norepinephrine reuptake inhibitor pharmacotherapy remitted in 12 weeks with the addition of aripiprazole (mean daily dose 10 mg) and remission was sustained during 6 months of continuation treatment.[37]

Several experimental, less well studied alternatives use central nervous system stimulants such as methylphenidate, modafinil, ω-3 fatty acids, lamotrigine, topiramate, herbal supplements, or β-blockers.[38–40]

Although there is no equivalent in the elderly of the STAR*D trial in midlife adults, Dew and colleagues[41] reported a cumulative response rate of more than 80% to successive augmentation strategies, a rate similar to that reported in the STAR*D trials.

Therefore, if patients stay the course in depression care management with evidence-based pharmacotherapy, most eventually reach full response or remission. Eliciting treatment adherence is an important part of depression care management and usually involves working with family care givers in building a therapeutic alliance.[42]

Anxious Depression

Comorbid anxiety is common in late-life depression, having a prevalence of up to 65% in clinical samples.[43,44] Several studies reported that greater severity of anxiety is associated with increased risk of withdrawal from treatment, decreased response to acute antidepressant treatment, and a longer time to both response and remission.[45] In a controlled, randomized trial, we reported that high pretreatment levels of anxiety symptoms increased not only the risk of nonresponse in acute treatment but also the risk of recurrence of depression in the first 2 years after response to antidepressant treatment.[45] Also, persistent severe symptoms of anxiety after 6 weeks of treatment were associated with longer time and lower rates of remission of LLD.[46] Among anxiety symptoms, worry more than panic predicted longer time to response and earlier recurrence in subjects with LLD treated with paroxetine (**Fig. 1**).[47]

Psychotic Depression

High rates of major depressive disorder (MDD) with psychotic features (as high as 45%) have been reported in elderly inpatients with depression.[48,49] Psychotic

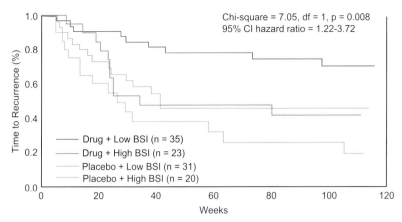

Fig. 1. Comorbid anxiety symptoms and time to recurrence of late-life depression. (*From* Andreescu C, Lenze EJ, Dew MA, et al. Effect of comorbid anxiety on treatment response and relapse risk in late-life depression: controlled study. Br J Psychiatry 2007;190:347; with permission.)

depression is associated with poorer short-term outcome, longer time to recovery, greater disability, and greater mortality than MDD without psychosis.[50] There have been only 2 randomized controlled pharmacotherapy trials of psychotic depression in older people. The first examined the efficacy of an antidepressant alone (nortriptyline, target plasma level 100 ng/mL) versus a combination of antidepressant and antipsychotic (notriptyline plus placebo/perphenazine, mean does 18.9 mg/d).[51] The categorical response was mediocre with both the antidepressant alone and with the combination (44% and 50% respectively), the investigators hypothesizing that the low response rate might have been caused by the heterogeneity of pathogenesis of psychotic depression in older patients, some of whom might have had incipient dementia.[51] The higher frailty of older patients often leads to the use of ECT early in the course of the treatment.[52] The second controlled trial examined for 12 weeks the efficacy of olanzapine (dose 5–20 mg/d) plus placebo or a combination of olanzapine and sertraline (50–150 mg/d) in patients with psychotic depression, and reported the results in the subgroup (more than 60 years old).[53] The combination of olanzapine plus sertraline was associated with a greater remission rate than olanzapine monotherapy (41.9% vs 23.9%, $\chi^2 = 9.53$, $P = .02$).[53]

Although practice guidelines recommend the use of an antidepressant and an antipsychotic for the treatment of psychotic depression, an analysis regarding the use of pharmacotherapy in psychotic depression revealed that, with usual care, only 5% of subjects received an adequate dose of an antidepressant and a high dose of an antipsychotic.[54] The intensity of pharmacotherapy in the combination trials was significantly associated only with the duration of current depressive episode. Most subjects (84%) received no antipsychotic or, at best, subtherapeutic doses of antipsychotics, and only about half of them (48%) received therapeutic doses of antidepressants.[54] The high proportions of patients who did not receive antipsychotics or received low doses of antipsychotics may be to the result of a lack of recognition of psychotic features.[54]

ECT has been reported to show a response rate of 87% in a mixed sample of psychotic and nonpsychotic depressed subjects[55] but there is a rapid increase in depressive symptoms after ECT.[55] However, pharmacotherapy may be more practical in community settings. Post-ECT maintenance treatment seems to be more effective when Li is combined with an antidepressant than when the antidepressant (nortriptyline) is used alone (39% relapse rate for the combination versus 60% relapse rate for antidepressant monotherapy).[55]

Vascular Depression

The vascular depression hypothesis was formulated in 1997 and postulates that cerebrovascular disease can predispose, precipitate, or perpetuate a depressive syndrome in older adults.[55] Depressed older adults with subcortical ischemic lesions often have a distinct clinical presentation with motor retardation, apathy, disability, increased risk of dementia, and a low familial load of depression.[55] Most,[56–58] but not all,[59] studies documented poorer response to antidepressants for patients with depression and subcortical vascular lesions. SSRIs have so far been of limited efficacy in depressed patients with subcortical vascular lesions. Some experts recommended the use of dopamine-acting agents (especially in depressed subjects with frontostriatal impairment) or psychotropics with cathecholaminergic activity that might promote recovery following ischemic events.[60] Two studies examined the advantages of using adjuvant calcium channel blockers, concluding that the augmentation of fluoxetine treatment with nimodipine leads to better treatment results and lower rates of recurrence at 8 months.[61,62]

Depression in the Context of Cognitive Impairment

Cognitive impairment in LLD is a core feature of the illness, contributing to disability and impaired quality of life. In a recent randomized controlled trial, the investigators tested the efficacy of added donepezil to antidepressant treatment in improving cognitive performance and reducing recurrences of depression in 2 years of maintenance treatment.[63] The overall response rate to open escitalopram (followed by duloxetine and duloxetine plus aripiprazole as needed) was about 65%. During double-blind, placebo-controlled maintenance treatment for 2 years (with adjunctive donepezil or placebo), patients randomly assigned to donepezil had small improvement in cognitive function but substantially greater rates of recurrent major depressive episodes, compared with placebo. In the subgroup of patients with mild cognitive impairment (MCI) at the start of maintenance treatment (n = 57), 3 of 30 patients on donepezil (10%) converted to dementia within 2 years, versus 9 of 27 (33%) on placebo (Fisher exact P = .05). The investigators concluded that augmentation of maintenance pharmacotherapy with cholinesterase inhibitors in older adults with depression depends on a careful weighing of benefits and risks, especially in those with MCI. There seems to be no benefit in patients without MCI.[63]

Major depression affects about 25% of patients with Alzheimer disease (AD) and it is a major cause of disability, being associated with increased impairment in the quality of life and activities in daily life (ADLs), greater caregiver burden, increased physical aggression, and increased risk of suicide.[64] Various studies have investigated the treatment response in depression comorbid with cognitive impairment but most included subjects with major depression but also with depressive symptoms, or subjects with various grades of cognitive impairment. Few studies focused on patients with MDD and AD. Moclobemid, citalopram, and clomipramine were found to be superior to placebo in the short-term treatment of depression in AD.[65–67] A 12-week randomized controlled trial showed that sertraline (mean dose 95 mg/d) was superior to placebo (effect size 0.85) in treating MDD in patients with AD.[64] Sertraline-treated patients also had a trend toward less ADL decline, although there was no benefit to cognition as assessed by the Mini Mental State Examination at 12 weeks.[64] However, a follow-up report examining the week 24 outcome of patients who participated in the trial found no between-groups differences in depression response or remission rates or secondary outcomes (such as ADL decline), concluding that sertraline may not be beneficial for long-term treatment of depression in AD.[68] The association between damage to the locus coeruleus and depression in AD suggests a better efficacy of noradrenergic than serotoninergic antidepressants. We only found 1 study comparing the efficacy of citalopram and mianserin in elderly depressed subjects with dementia.[69] On balance, the evidence supporting the efficacy of antidepressant pharmacotherapy for depression in AD is mixed and inconclusive.

Bipolar Depression

Manic and bipolar depressed patients represent 5% to 15% of patients presenting for acute treatment at geriatric psychiatry services.[70] There are no systematic studies of the treatment of bipolar depression in the elderly,[70] and clinicians usually rely on data from mixed-age studies, case reports, or uncontrolled trials.[71] Various strategies have been proposed, including combinations of paroxetine and lithium[72] and the preferred use of SSRIs and bupropion rather than tricyclics.[70] Optimal mood-stabilizer dosing for lithium in bipolar elderly patients has not been assessed, and its tolerability in the elderly is a particular concern (increased cognitive impairment, neurological side effects, delirium, sick sinus syndrome, hypothyroidism, polyuria, edema).[73] Experts recommend lower doses than for mixed-age patients (0.5–0.8 mEq/L), but lithium toxicity has been reported in the elderly even at moderate concentrations (0.5–0.8 mEq/L).[70] Other recommendations include combination of lithium and an SSRI, the use of lamotrigine or other anticonvulsants, or the addition of an atypical antipsychotic.[70] ECT should also be considered in patients with bipolar depression or rapid cycling symptoms refractory to pharmacotherapy, in suicidal patients, or those with inadequate food and fluid intake.[70]

A retrospective analysis of the efficacy of lithium (mean dose 750 mg/d) and lamotrigine (mean dose 240 mg/d) in the maintenance treatment geriatric bipolar disorder reported that lamotrigine but not lithium maintenance therapy significantly delayed time to intervention for a depressive episode.[71]

At this time there are no studies exploring the impact of cognitive impairment or of comorbid medical conditions on acute/long-term treatment of bipolar depression in the elderly.

Predictors of Treatment Response: Use of Treatment Decision-making Trees

Successful antidepressant treatment is one of the most effective ways to reduce disability, prevent morbidity, and improve quality of life in older depressed patients. However, LLD is often resistant to treatment and may exhibit a slower resolution of symptoms than midlife depression.[74] The identification of predictors of treatment response would allow the clinicians to modify treatment options earlier in the course of the treatment.

Several studies explored the biological, clinical, and psychosocial predictors of treatment response in LLD (**Table 2**).

However, it may be difficult for clinicians to integrate the various predictors reported in the literature into a practical treatment strategy. In an analysis that pooled data from the acute treatment phase of 3 National Institute of Mental Health–funded treatment studies, we attempted to integrate and develop a hierarchy of clinical predictors of treatment response.[75] Using signal detection theory,[76] we built 2 different models

Table 2
Predictors of treatment response in LLD

Predictors of Treatment Response		Role	Study
Biologic predictors	Serotonin transporter	S allele increases treatment resistance	Lotrich et al,[110] 2008
	REM sleep latency	Decreased REM sleep latency correlates with poor response	Reynolds et al,[102] 1991
	Glucose cerebral metabolism	Reduced glucose metabolism in ACC and mPFC correlated with better response	Smith et al,[103] 1999
	Increased metabolism in ACC	Predicts response to rTMS in vascular depression	Narushima et al,[81] 2010
Clinical predictors	Medical burden	Greater medical burden predicted slower recovery	Dew et al,[41] 2007
	Early symptom improvement	Predicted faster response	Mulsant et al,[104] 2006
	Age of onset of first episode	Younger age at onset predicted poorer response	Dew et al,[78] 1997
	Sleep disturbances	Baseline sleep disturbance predicted poorer response	Reynolds et al,[102] 1991 Dew et al,[78] 1997
	Baseline HDRS scores	Higher score correlated with slower response	Gildengers et al,[105] 2005
	Baseline anxiety	Increased baseline anxiety correlated with slower response	Andreescu et al,[45] 2007
	Suicidal ideation	Baseline suicidal ideation correlated with longer time to response	Szanto et al,[106] 2003
	Response to previous antidepressant treatment	Poor previous antidepressant response correlated with decrease rate of response	Tew et al,[107] 2006
Psychosocial predictors	Social support	Poor social support and poor family support correlated with poor response	Dew et al,[78,108] 1997 Martire et al,[108] 2007
	Social inequalities	Low income correlated with poorer response	Cohen et al,[109] 2006
	Self-esteem	Higher self-esteem correlated with faster response	Gildengers et al,[105] 2005

Abbreviations: ACC, anterior cingulate cortex; HDRS, Hamilton Depression Rating Scale; mPFC, medial prefrontal cortex; REM, rapid eye movement.

by modulating the sensitivity threshold for each predictor of treatment response to obtain hierarchies of risk correlates with different patients' characteristics.

Thus, for patients requiring an aggressive treatment approach (eg, patients with a high risk of suicide or severely disabled by their symptoms), the most significant predictor of treatment response was early symptom improvement (40% drop in

Hamilton scores by 4 weeks), followed by lower levels of baseline anxiety and later age of onset of first episode of depression.[75] No other clinical predictors, including adequacy of previous treatment (as measured by the antidepressant treatment history form [ATHF] score),[77] race, recurrence, or baseline sleep disturbance reached significance levels (**Fig. 2**).

For patients requiring a more conservative treatment approach (eg, patients with a history of multiple, unsuccessful, underdosed trials), the most significant predictor of treatment response was again early symptom improvement, followed by baseline anxiety and adequacy of previous antidepressant trials (**Fig. 3**).

These reports confirmed earlier work on the trajectory of acute response that emphasized that early symptom resolution predicts more stable long-term treatment response.[78,79] Higher levels of acute or chronic stressors, poorer social support, younger age at onset, melancholiform features, older current age, and higher current anxiety also predicted a poorer response profile.[78] The importance of early symptom resolution was further emphasized by the 2006 Maintenance Treatment Trial[16] that noted that patients who needed adjunctive medication in acute treatment to get well also had a more brittle long-term response.

CHALLENGES AND FUTURE DIRECTIONS
Novel Treatment Options

Advances in LLD treatment include novel treatments, personalized treatment (according to depression type, individual characteristics), and strategies to improve access to and delivery of care.[2]

- Novel treatments include transcranial magnetic stimulation (TMS), deep brain stimulation, vagus nerve stimulation (VNS), and magnetic seizure therapy.

TMS has been approved since 2008 as treatment of depression resistant to pharmacotherapy. High-frequency pulse (>1 Hz) repetitive TMS (rTMS) is usually applied to the left dorsolateral prefrontal cortex.[80] A recent randomized, placebo-controlled trial indicated that rTMS may be beneficial for vascular depression (response 39%, remission 27% vs sham 7% and 4% respectively). Subgenual cingulate θ activity predicts treatment response in rTMS in vascular depression.[81]

Deep brain stimulation delivers a continuous train of repetitive, brief small voltage pulses mainly to the subgenual anterior cingulate cortex (ACC), an area that has been associated with treatment-resistant depression.[82] More recent case reports delivered the voltage pulses to either deep brain structures such as nucleus accumbens and ventral striatum.[83]

VNS was approved for treatment-resistant depression in 2005. The procedure stimulates the left cervical vagus nerve through low-frequency, chronic, intermittent-pulsed electric signals, stimulates areas involved in mood regulation (locus coeruleus, nucleus raphe magnus), and seems to modulate hippocampal neurogenesis.[84] To our knowledge, there are no trials of VNS in LLD.

Several small trials examined the safety and efficacy of magnetic seizure therapy in depression. Its antidepressant effect seems to be less robust than that of ECT.[2]

- Informed/personalized treatment uses neuroimaging techniques such as blood oxygenation level–dependent (BOLD) functional magnetic resonance imaging (fMRI) or diffusion tensor imaging (DTI).

In the last decade, there has been a rapid increase in the availability of magnetic resonance imaging (MRI), and it is likely that, in the near future, MRI accessibility

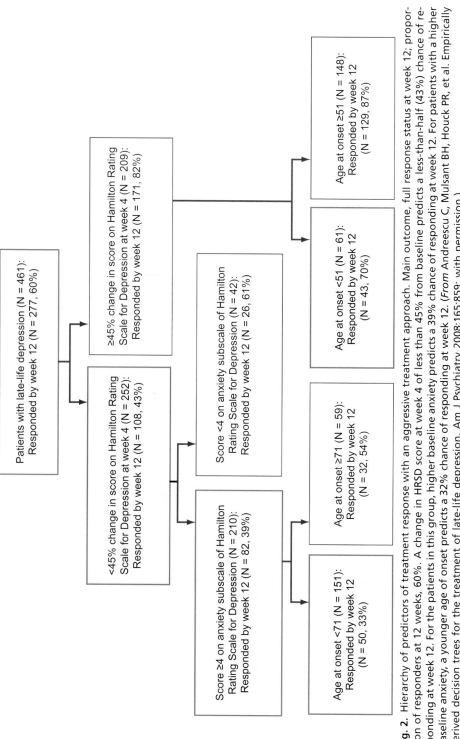

Fig. 2. Hierarchy of predictors of treatment response with an aggressive treatment approach. Main outcome, full response status at week 12; proportion of responders at 12 weeks, 60%. A change in HRSD score at week 4 of less than 45% from baseline predicts a less-than-half (43%) chance of responding at week 12. For the patients in this group, higher baseline anxiety predicts a 39% chance of responding at week 12. For patients with a higher baseline anxiety, a younger age of onset predicts a 32% chance of responding at week 12. (*From* Andreescu C, Mulsant BH, Houck PR, et al. Empirically derived decision trees for the treatment of late-life depression. Am J Psychiatry 2008;165:859; with permission.)

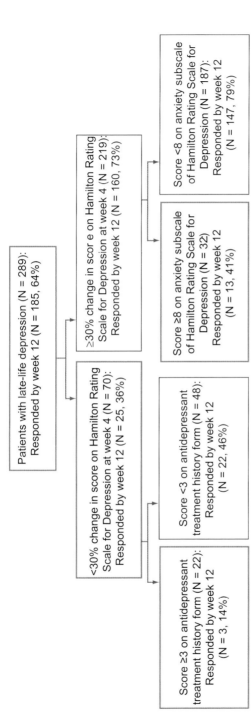

Fig. 3. Hierarchy of predictors of treatment response with a conservative treatment approach. Main outcome, full response status at week 12; proportion of responders at 12 weeks, 64%. For the ATHF, a score greater than or equal to 3 indicates probably adequate antidepressant treatment history (trial of more than 4 weeks of an antidepressant at an adequate dose); ATHF les than 3 indicates inadequate antidepressant treatment history (trial of less than 4 weeks, or of more than 4 weeks but with an inadequate dose). High anxiety, at least moderate anxiety symptoms; low anxiety, mild or no anxiety symptoms. Change in HRSD at week 4 of less than 30% from baseline predicts a 35% chance of responding at week 12. For those subjects with a change in HRSD at week 4 of less than 30%, a history of at least 1 adequate antidepressant trial predicts a 13% chance of responding at week 12. For those subjects with a change in HRSD at week 4 higher than 30%, the next predictor is baseline anxiety. A higher baseline anxiety score predicts a lower chance of responding at 12 weeks (40%), whereas a lower baseline anxiety score predicts a 79% chance of responding at week 12. (*From* Andreescu C, Mulsant BH, Houck PR, et al. Empirically derived decision trees for the treatment of late-life depression. Am J Psychiatry 2008;165:860; with permission.)

will continue to increase, along with a decrease in scanning costs. If this trend continues, then using MRI to optimize the choice of medications for an individual with depression is possible. The identification of magnetic resonance (MR) markers of treatment response would allow for faster and more efficient trial rather than waiting 3 to 6 weeks to determine whether a new intervention is effective. Several MR markers of treatment response have been identified: lower activation of the rostral ACC at baseline, increased burden of white matter hyperintensities in the frontal regions, and lower fractional anisotropy in frontolimbic areas were associated with poor treatment response in either midlife[85,86] or late-life studies of depression.[87,88]

Pharmacogenetics involves the use of molecular genetic information to assist in the prediction of drug efficacy and drug-induced adverse events. In a heterogeneous disorder such as LLD, pharmacogenetic data could be paramount for the development of individualized treatment approaches.[89] Although the neuroimaging prediction of antidepressant response is not yet refined/cheap enough for clinical applications, genotyping assays are easy to do and their costs have rapidly decreased. Various candidate genes in the serotoninergic system (most notably the serotonin transporter polymorphism) have been associated with treatment response.[90] The serotonin transporter gene (SLC6A4) also influences treatment response variability in LLD, mainly in the initial stages of treatment, through a gene-concentration interaction for SSRIs.[91] In addition, elderly subjects carrying the S allele may be at increased risk of adverse drug reactions and may require a higher initial SSRI plasma concentration to obtain a response.[91,92] Another recent candidate gene (OPRM1, the μ-opioid receptor) has been associated with citalopram response in the STAR*D sample.[93] However, a recent study of 72 candidate genes that also used a genome-wide associate study assessing more than 500,000 SNPs reported modest results.[94] None of the candidate genes provided evidence for association with response to antidepressants.[94]

Sequential treatment:

1. Pharmacotherapy followed by psychotherapy. A recent meta-analysis examined the efficacy of the sequential integration of psychotherapy and pharmacotherapy in reducing the risk of relapse and recurrence in MDD.[95] The pooled risk ratio (RR = 0.79) suggested a relative advantage in preventing relapse and recurrence for the sequential administration of psychotherapy after successful response to acute-phase pharmacotherapy compared with control conditions.[95]
2. ECT followed by pharmacotherapy. Relapse rates after ECT remain high, with virtually all remitted patients relapsing within 6 months of stopping ECT.[55] Most investigators have advocated the use of antidepressants or a combination of antidepressant and mood stabilizer (Li) after completion of ECT.[55] Some experts recommended using antidepressants during ECT to prevent early relapses.[96]
3. rTMS followed by pharmacotherapy. In a recent study, subjects received citalopram (20 mg/d) after either rTMS or sham treatment, with mixed results (of the 12 subjects who responded to rTMS, 9 maintained response and 4 had a relapse of depression).[97]

Various other lines of investigations are being developed. For example, homocysteine has been correlated with increased risk of depression (most likely through the link between the folate/methylation cycles and depression). Lowering homocysteine levels would reduce the incidence and severity of depressive symptoms; a meta-analysis found that older adults with high homocysteine plasma levels have increased risk of depression (odds ratio 1.7).[98]

Health Services Perspectives

The greatest limitation in treatment of LLD concerns treatment access and delivery. In primary care settings, the diagnosis of depression is frequently missed and treatment is often inadequate.[2] Studies such as Prevention of Suicide in Primary Care Elderly: Collaborative Trial (PROSPECT)[5,99] and Improving Mood Promoting Access to Collaborative Care Treatment (IMPACT)[100] have shown that collaborative care in primary care settings has better outcomes than usual care, and that downstream consequences of inadequately treated depression can be prevented. More importantly, a long-term, developmental perspective on depression across life span is needed.[3] Regarding prevention as protection (prolonging lifespan and healthspan), participation in studies such as PROSPECT[5] have been linked to lower rates of mortality from cancer at 4-year to 5-year follow-up.[3]

Many real-world challenges hinder implementing depression treatment recommendations, such as adequate funds, adequate management of various programs, overcoming barriers in training staff in intervention techniques, ensuring fidelity to established protocols, adequate support to evaluate outcomes, and ensuring accessibility.[101] Partnership among researchers, health care providers, and policy makers is necessary to implement successful treatment protocols for depression in late life.[101]

REFERENCES

1. Moussavi S, Chatterji S, Verdes E, et al. Depression, chronic diseases, and decrements in health: results from the World Health Surveys. Lancet 2007; 370:851–8.
2. Alexopoulos GS, Kelly RE Jr. Research advances in geriatric depression. World Psychiatry 2009;8:140–9.
3. Reynolds CF. The cutting edge: prevention of depressive disorders. Depress Anxiety 2009;26:1062–5.
4. Chapman DP, Perry GS. Depression as a major component of public health for older adults. Prev Chronic Dis 2008;5:A22.
5. Bruce ML, Ten Have TR, Reynolds CF, et al. Reducing suicidal ideation and depressive symptoms in depressed older primary care patients: a randomized controlled trial. J Am Med Assoc 2004;291:1081–91.
6. Charney DS, Reynolds CF, Lewis L, et al. Depression and bipolar support alliance consensus statement on the unmet needs in diagnosis and treatment of mood disorders in late life. Arch Gen Psychiatry 2003;60:664–72.
7. Stevens JA, Hasbrouck LM, Durant TM, et al. Surveillance for injuries and violence among older adults. MMWR CDC Surveill Summ 1999;48:27–50.
8. Mitchell AJ, Subramaniam H. Prognosis of depression in old age compared to middle age: a systematic review of comparative studies. Am J Psychiatry 2005;162:1588–601.
9. Mottram P, Wilson K, Strobl J. Antidepressants for depressed elderly. Cochrane Database Syst Rev 2006;1:CD003491.
10. Taylor WD, Doraiswamy PM. A systematic review of antidepressant placebo-controlled trials for geriatric depression: limitations of current data and directions for the future. Neuropsychopharmacology 2004;29:2285–99.
11. Nelson JC, Clary CM, Leon AC, et al. Symptoms of late-life depression: frequency and change during treatment. Am J Geriatr Psychiatry 2005;13:520–6.
12. Kozel FA, Trivedi MH, Wisniewski SR, et al. Treatment outcomes for older depressed patients with earlier versus late onset of first depressive episode: a Sequenced

Treatment Alternatives to Relieve Depression (STAR*D) report. Am J Geriatr Psychiatry 2008;16:58–64.

13. McGrath PJ, Khan AY, Trivedi MH, et al. Response to a selective serotonin reuptake inhibitor (citalopram) in major depressive disorder with melancholic features: a STAR*D report. J Clin Psychiatry 2008;69:1847–55.

14. Alexopoulos GS, Katz IR, Reynolds CF, et al. Pharmacotherapy of depression in older patients: a summary of the expert consensus guidelines. J Psychiatr Pract 2001;7:361–76.

15. Zis AP, Grof P, Webster M. Predictors of relapse in recurrent affective disorders. Psychopharmacol Bull 1980;16:47–9.

16. Reynolds CF, Dew MA, Pollock BG, et al. Maintenance treatment of major depression in old age. N Engl J Med 2006;354:1130–8.

17. Reynolds CF, Frank E, Perel JM, et al. Nortriptyline and interpersonal psychotherapy as maintenance therapies for recurrent major depression: a randomized controlled trial in patients older than 59 years. J Am Med Assoc 1999;281: 39–45.

18. Klysner R, Bent-Hansen J, Hansen HL, et al. Efficacy of citalopram in the prevention of recurrent depression in elderly patients: placebo-controlled study of maintenance therapy. Br J Psychiatry 2002;19:29–35.

19. Wilson KC, Mottram PG, Ashworth L, et al. Older community residents with depression: long-term treatment with sertraline. Randomised, double-blind, placebo-controlled study. Br J Psychiatry 2003;182:492–7.

20. Wilson KC, Mottram PG, Vassilas CA. Psychotherapeutic treatments for older depressed people. Cochrane Database Syst Rev 2008;1:CD004853.

21. Grant RW, Casey DA. Adapting cognitive behavioral therapy for the frail elderly. Int Psychogeriatr 1995;7:561–71.

22. Butters MA, Whyte EM, Nebes RD, et al. The nature and determinants of neuropsychological functioning in late-life depression. Arch Gen Psychiatry 2004;61: 587–95.

23. Alexopoulos GS, Raue P, Arean PA. Problem-solving therapy versus supportive therapy in geriatric major depression with executive dysfunction. Am J Geriatr Psychiatry 2003;11:46–52.

24. Alexopoulos GS, Raue PJ, Kanellopoulos D, et al. Problem-solving therapy for the depression-executive dysfunction syndrome of late life. Int J Geriatr Psychiatry 2008;23:782–8.

25. Arean PA, Perri MG, Nezu AM, et al. Comparative effectiveness of social problem-solving therapy and reminiscence therapy as treatments for depression in older adults. J Consult Clin Psychol 1993;61:1003–10.

26. Serfaty MA, Haworth D, Blanchard M, et al. Clinical effectiveness of individual cognitive behavioral therapy for depressed older people in primary care: a randomized controlled trial. Arch Gen Psychiatry 2009;66:1332–40.

27. Arean PA, Raue P, Mackin RS, et al. Problem-solving therapy and supportive therapy in older adults with major depression and executive dysfunction. Am J Psychiatry 2010;167:1391–8.

28. Pinquart M, Duberstein PR, Lyness JM. Treatments for later-life depressive conditions: a meta-analytic comparison of pharmacotherapy and psychotherapy. Am J Psychiatry 2006;163:1493–501.

29. Flint AJ, Rifat SL. The treatment of psychotic depression in later life: a comparison of pharmacotherapy and ECT. Int J Geriatr Psychiatry 1998;13:23–8.

30. Rice EH, Sombrotto LB, Markowitz JC, et al. Cardiovascular morbidity in high-risk patients during ECT. Am J Psychiatry 1994;151:1637–41.

31. van der Wurff FB, Stek ML, Hoogendijk WL, et al. Electroconvulsive therapy for the depressed elderly. Cochrane Database Syst Rev 2003;2:CD003593.

32. Driscoll HC, Karp JF, Dew MA, et al. Getting better, getting well: understanding and managing partial and non-response to pharmacological treatment of non-psychotic major depression in old age. Drugs Aging 2007;24:801–14.

33. Mulsant BH, Pollock B. Treatment-resistant depression in late-life. J Geriatr Psychiatry Neurol 1998;11:186–93.

34. Flint AJ. Treatment-resistant depression in late life. CNS Spectr 2002;7:733–8.

35. Shelton RC, Osuntokun O, Heinloth AN, et al. Therapeutic options for treatment-resistant depression. CNS Drugs 2010;24:131–61.

36. Kok RM, Nolen WA, Heeren TJ. Outcome of late-life depression after 3 years of sequential treatment. Acta Psychiatr Scand 2009;119:274–81.

37. Sheffrin M, Driscoll HC, Lenze EJ, et al. Pilot study of augmentation with aripiprazole for incomplete response in late-life depression: getting to remission. J Clin Psychiatry 2009;70:208–13.

38. Lavretsky H, Park S, Siddarth P, et al. Methylphenidate-enhanced antidepressant response to citalopram in the elderly: a double-blind placebo-controlled pilot trial. Am J Geriatr Psychiatry 2006;14:181–5.

39. Schmidt do Prado-Lima PA, Bacaltchuck J. Topiramate in treatment-resistant depression and binge-eating disorder. Bipolar Disord 2002;4:271–3.

40. Thomas SP, Nandhra HS, Jayaraman A. Systematic review of lamotrigine augmentation of treatment resistant unipolar depression (TRD). J Ment Health 2010;19:168–75.

41. Dew MA, Whyte EM, Lenze EJ, et al. Recovery from major depression in older adults receiving augmentation of antidepressant pharmacotherapy. Am J Psychiatry 2007;164:892–9.

42. Reynolds CF, Dew MA, Martire LM, et al. Treating depression to remission in older adults: a controlled evaluation of combined interpersonal psychotherapy versus escitalopram with depression care management. Int J Geriatr Psychiatry 2010;25:1134–41.

43. Lenze EJ. Comorbidity of depression and anxiety in the elderly. Curr Psychiatry Rep 2003;5:62–7.

44. Beekman AT, de Beurs E, van Balkom AJ, et al. Anxiety and depression in later life: co-occurrence and communality of risk factors. Am J Psychiatry 2000;157:89–95.

45. Andreescu C, Lenze EJ, Dew MA, et al. Effect of comorbid anxiety on treatment response and relapse risk in late-life depression: controlled study. Br J Psychiatry 2007;190:344–9.

46. Greenlee A, Karp JF, Dew MA, et al. Anxiety impairs depression remission in partial responders during extended treatment in late-life. Depress Anxiety 2010;27:451–6.

47. Andreescu C, Lenze E, Mulsant B, et al. High worry severity is associated with poorer acute and maintenance efficacy of antidepressants in late-life depression. Depress Anxiety 2009;26:266–72.

48. Coryell W, Leon A, Winokur G, et al. Importance of psychotic features to long-term course in major depressive disorder. Am J Psychiatry 1996;153:483–9.

49. Maj M, Pirozzi R, Magliano L, et al. Phenomenology and prognostic significance of delusions in major depressive disorder: a 10-year prospective follow-up study. J Clin Psychiatry 2007;68:1411–7.

50. Vythilingam M, Chen J, Bremner JD, et al. Psychotic depression and mortality. Am J Psychiatry 2003;160:574–6.

51. Mulsant BH, Pollock BG, Nebes R, et al. A twelve-week, double-blind, randomized comparison of nortriptyline and paroxetine in older depressed inpatients and outpatients. Am J Geriatr Psychiatry 2001;9:406–14.

52. Andreescu C, Mulsant BH, Rothschild AJ, et al. Pharmacotherapy of major depression with psychotic features: what is the evidence? Psychiatr Ann 2006;36:31–8.

53. Meyers BS, Flint AJ, Rothschild AJ, et al. A double-blind randomized controlled trial of olanzapine plus sertraline vs olanzapine plus placebo for psychotic depression: the study of pharmacotherapy of psychotic depression (STOP-PD). Arch Gen Psychiatry 2009;66:838–47.

54. Andreescu C, Mulsant BH, Peasley-Miklus C, et al. Persisting low use of antipsychotic in the treatment of major depression with psychotic features. J Clin Psychiatry 2007;68:194–200.

55. Sackeim HA, Haskett RF, Mulsant BH, et al. Continuation pharmacotherapy in the prevention of relapse following electroconvulsive therapy. J Am Med Assoc 2001;285:1299–307.

56. Sheline YI, Pieper CF, Barch DM, et al. Support for the vascular depression hypothesis in late-life depression: results of a 2-site, prospective, antidepressant treatment trial. Arch Gen Psychiatry 2010;67:277–85.

57. Hickie I, Scott E, Mitchell P, et al. Subcortical hyperintensities on magnetic resonance imaging: clinical correlates and prognostic significance in patients with severe depression. Biol Psychiatry 1995;37:151–60.

58. Simpson S, Baldwin RC, Jackson A, et al. Is subcortical disease associated with a poor response to antidepressants? Neurological, neuropsychological and neuroradiological findings in late-life depression. Psychol Med 1998;28:1015–26.

59. Salloway S, Boyle PA, Correia S, et al. The relationship of MRI subcortical hyperintensities to treatment response in a trial of sertraline in geriatric depressed outpatients. Am J Geriatr Psychiatry 2002;10:107–11.

60. Ramasubbu R, Goodyear BG. Methylphenidate modulates activity within cognitive neural networks of patients with post-stroke major depression: a placebo-controlled fMRI study. Neuropsychiatr Dis Treat 2008;4:1251–66.

61. Taragano FE, Allegri R, Vicario A, et al. A double blind, randomized clinical trial assessing the efficacy and safety of augmenting standard antidepressant therapy with nimodipine in the treatment of 'vascular depression'. Int J Geriatr Psychiatry 2001;16:254–60.

62. Taragano FE, Bagnatti P, Allegri RF. A double-blind, randomized clinical trial to assess the augmentation with nimodipine of antidepressant therapy in the treatment of "vascular depression". Int Psychogeriatr 2005;17:487–98.

63. Reynolds CF, Butters MA, Lopez O, et al. Maintenance treatment of depression in old age: a randomized, double-blind, placebo-controlled evaluation of the efficacy and safety of donepezil combined with antidepressant pharmacotherapy. Arch Gen Psychiatry 2011;68(1):51–60.

64. Lyketsos CG, DelCampo L, Steinberg M, et al. Treating depression in Alzheimer disease: efficacy and safety of sertraline therapy, and the benefits of depression reduction: the DIADS. Arch Gen Psychiatry 2003;60:737–46.

65. Roth M, Mountjoy CQ, Amrein R. Moclobemide in elderly patients with cognitive decline and depression: an international double-blind, placebo-controlled trial. Br J Psychiatry 1996;168:149–57.

66. Nyth AL, Gottfries CG, Lyby K, et al. A controlled multicenter clinical study of citalopram and placebo in elderly depressed patients with and without concomitant dementia. Acta Psychiatr Scand 1992;86:138–45.

67. Petracca G, Teson A, Chemerinski E, et al. A double-blind placebo-controlled study of clomipramine in depressed patients with Alzheimer's disease. J Neuropsychiatry Clin Neurosci 1996;8:270–5.

68. Weintraub D, Rosenberg PB, Drye LT, et al. Sertraline for the treatment of depression in Alzheimer disease: week-24 outcomes. Am J Geriatr Psychiatry 2010;18:332–40.

69. Karlsson I, Godderis J, Augusto De Mendonca Lima C, et al. A randomised, double-blind comparison of the efficacy and safety of citalopram compared to mianserin in elderly, depressed patients with or without mild to moderate dementia. Int J Geriatr Psychiatry 2000;15:295–305.

70. Young RC, Gyulai L, Mulsant BH, et al. Pharmacotherapy of bipolar disorder in old age: review and recommendations. Am J Geriatr Psychiatry 2004;12:342–57.

71. Sajatovic M, Gyulai L, Calabrese JR, et al. Maintenance treatment outcomes in older patients with bipolar I disorder. Am J Geriatr Psychiatry 2005;13:305–11.

72. Nemeroff CB. Advancing the treatment of mood and anxiety disorders: the first 10 years' experience with paroxetine. Psychopharmacol Bull 2003;37(Suppl 1): 6–7.

73. Smith RE, Helms PM. Adverse effects of lithium therapy in the acutely ill elderly patient. J Clin Psychiatry 1982;43:94–9.

74. Whyte EM, Dew MA, Gildengers A, et al. Time course of response to antidepressants in late-life major depression: therapeutic implications. Drugs Aging 2004; 21:531–54.

75. Andreescu C, Mulsant BH, Houck PR, et al. Empirically derived decision trees for the treatment of late-life depression. Am J Psychiatry 2008;165:855–62.

76. Kiernan M, Kraemer HC, Winkleby MA, et al. Do logistic regression and signal detection identify different subgroups at risk? Implications for the design of tailored interventions. Psychol Methods 2001;6:35–48.

77. Oquendo MA, Baca-Garcia E, Kartachov A, et al. A computer algorithm for calculating the adequacy of antidepressant treatment in unipolar and bipolar depression. J Clin Psychiatry 2003;64:825–33.

78. Dew MA, Reynolds CF, Houck PR, et al. Temporal profiles of the course of depression during treatment: predictors of pathways toward recovery in the elderly. Arch Gen Psychiatry 1997;54:1016–24.

79. Dew MA, Reynolds CF, Mulsant B, et al. Initial recovery patterns may predict which maintenance therapies for depression will keep older adults well. J Affect Disord 2001;65:155–66.

80. Jorge RE, Moser DJ, Acion L, et al. Treatment of vascular depression using repetitive transcranial magnetic stimulation. Arch Gen Psychiatry 2008;65: 268–76.

81. Narushima K, McCormick LM, Yamada T, et al. Subgenual cingulate theta activity predicts treatment response of repetitive transcranial magnetic stimulation in participants with vascular depression. J Neuropsychiatry Clin Neurosci 2010;22:75–84.

82. Mayberg HS, Lozano AM, Voon V, et al. Deep brain stimulation for treatment-resistant depression. Neuron 2005;45:651–60.

83. Malone DA Jr, Dougherty DD, Rezai AR, et al. Deep brain stimulation of the ventral capsule/ventral striatum for treatment-resistant depression. Biol Psychiatry 2009;65:267–75.

84. Nemeroff CB, Mayberg HS, Krahl SE, et al. VNS therapy in treatment-resistant depression: clinical evidence and putative neurobiological mechanisms. Neuropsychopharmacology 2006;31:1345–55.

85. MacQueen GM. Magnetic resonance imaging and prediction of outcome in patients with major depressive disorder. J Psychiatry Neurosci 2009;34:343–9.

86. Mayberg HS, Brannan SK, Tekell JL, et al. Regional metabolic effects of fluoxetine in major depression: serial changes and relationship to clinical response. Biol Psychiatry 2000;48:830–43.

87. Gunning-Dixon FM, Walton M, Cheng J, et al. MRI signal hyperintensities and treatment remission of geriatric depression. J Affect Disord 2010;126(3): 395–401.

88. Taylor WD, Kuchibhatla M, Payne ME, et al. Frontal white matter anisotropy and antidepressant remission in late-life depression. PLoS One 2008;3:e3267.

89. Malhotra AK. The pharmacogenetics of depression: enter the GWAS. Am J Psychiatry 2010;167:493–5.

90. Serretti A, Kato M, RonchiDe D, et al. Meta-analysis of serotonin transporter gene promoter polymorphism (5-HTTLPR) association with selective serotonin reuptake inhibitor efficacy in depressed patients. Mol Psychiatry 2007;12: 247–57.

91. Gerretsen P, Pollock BG. Pharmacogenetics and the serotonin transporter in late-life depression. Expert Opin Drug Metab Toxicol 2008;4:1465–78.

92. MacLeod C, Mathews A, Tata P. Attentional bias in emotional disorders. J Abnorm Psychol 1986;95:15–20.

93. Garriock HA, Tanowitz M, Kraft JB, et al. Association of mu-opioid receptor variants and response to citalopram treatment in major depressive disorder. Am J Psychiatry 2010;167:565–73.

94. Uher R, Perroud N, Ng MY, et al. Genome-wide pharmacogenetics of antidepressant response in the GENDEP project. Am J Psychiatry 2010;167:555–64.

95. Guidi J, Fava GA, Fava M, et al. Efficacy of the sequential integration of psychotherapy and pharmacotherapy in major depressive disorder: a preliminary meta-analysis. Psychol Med 2011;41(2):321–31.

96. Yildiz A, Mantar A, Simsek S, et al. Combination of pharmacotherapy with electroconvulsive therapy in prevention of depressive relapse: a pilot controlled trial. J ECT 2010;26:104–10.

97. Robinson RG, Tenev V, Jorge RE. Citalopram for continuation therapy after repetitive transcranial magnetic stimulation in vascular depression. Am J Geriatr Psychiatry 2009;17:682–7.

98. Almeida OP, McCaul K, Hankey GJ, et al. Homocysteine and depression in later life. Arch Gen Psychiatry 2008;65:1286–94.

99. Alexopoulos GS, Katz IR, Bruce ML, et al. Remission in depressed geriatric primary care patients: a report from the PROSPECT study. Am J Psychiatry 2005;162:718–24.

100. Unutzer J, Katon W, Callahan CM, et al. Collaborative care management of late-life depression in the primary care setting: a randomized controlled trial. J Am Med Assoc 2002;288:2836–45.

101. Snowden M, Steinman L, Frederick J. Treating depression in older adults: challenges to implementing the recommendations of an expert panel. Prev Chronic Dis 2008;5:A26.

102. Reynolds CF, Hoch CC, Buysse DJ, et al. Sleep in late-life recurrent depression: changes during early continuation therapy with nortriptyline. Neuropsychopharmacology 1991;5:85–96.

103. Smith GS, Reynolds CF, Pollock B, et al. Cerebral glucose metabolic response to combined total sleep deprivation and antidepressant treatment in geriatric depression. Am J Psychiatry 1999;156:683–9.

104. Mulsant BH, Houck PR, Gildengers AG, et al. What is the optimal duration of a short-term antidepressant trial when treating geriatric depression? J Clin Psychopharmacol 2006;26:113–20.

105. Gildengers AG, Houck PR, Mulsant BH, et al. Trajectories of treatment response in late-life depression: psychosocial and clinical correlates. J Clin Psychopharmacol 2005;25:S8–13.

106. Szanto K, Mulsant BH, Houck P, et al. Occurrence and course of suicidality during short-term treatment of late-life depression. Arch Gen Psychiatry 2003; 60:610–7.

107. Tew JD, Mulsant BH, Houck PR, et al. Impact of prior inadequate treatment exposure on response to antidepressant treatment in late life. Am J Geriatr Psychiatry 2006;14:957–65.

108. Martire LM, Schulz R, Reynolds CF, et al. Impact of close family members on older adults' early response to depression treatment. Psychol Aging 2008;23: 447–52.

109. Cohen A, Houck PR, Szanto K, et al. Social inequalities in response to antidepressant treatment in older adults. Arch Gen Psychiatry 2006;63:50–6.

110. Lotrich FE, Pollock BG, Kirshner M, et al. Serotonin transporter genotype interacts with paroxetine plasma levels to influence depression treatment response in geriatric patients. J Psychiatry Neurosci 2008;33(2):123–30.

Gene-Environment Interactions in Geriatric Depression

Francis E. Lotrich, MD, PhD

KEYWORDS

• Polymorphism • Stress • Elderly • Geriatric • Depression

Major depressive disorder (MDD) can be complicated to study—it has a heterogeneous manifestation and course. Even with respect to environmental precipitants, the onset of depressive episodes have been variously associated with the postpartum period,[1] the postmenopausal period,[2] thyroid disease,[3] circadian changes,[4] sleep impairment,[5] stimulant withdrawal,[6] cerebrovascular disease,[7–9] chronic illness,[10] inflammatory cytokines,[11] as well as psychosocial stresses[12] including interpersonal losses,[13,14] threats to safety, physical impairments,[15] pain,[16] and so forth. Because old age can be associated with deteriorating health, vascular disease, changing sleep patterns, bereavement, and so forth, many of these potential precipitants accumulate later in life.[17] However, only a minority of people exposed to a combination of these events actually develops depression. Stress does appear to have a causal influence on development of MDD in some people, sometimes[18]; but simple exposure to accumulating environmental stress is not enough to fully explain MDD.

Genetic influences on vulnerability and resilience to these precipitants likely play a role. But the heritability for MDD is estimated to be only about 37%.[19] Consistent with this, meta-analyses of case-control association studies suggest potential roles for polymorphisms in several genes,[20] with effect sizes that are typically very small. No single gene, acting alone, appears to play a major role. However, case-control genetic association studies generally face the limitation of not accounting for differences in exposure to the multitude of potential environmental influences. Thus, there remains the intriguing possibility that particular genes interact with particular environments to influence MDD. In examining this possibility, there are significant challenges to successfully completing gene × environment interaction (GxE) studies, although there recently has been encouraging progress. The field is nascent, but there are now multiple GxE studies examining the serotonin transporter (SERT), brain-derived

The author has nothing to disclose.
This work was supported by NIMH grant MH074012.
Department of Psychiatry, Western Psychiatric Institute and Clinics, University of Pittsburgh Medical Center, 3811 Ohara Street, Pittsburgh, PA 15213, USA
E-mail address: lotrichfe@upmc.edu

Psychiatr Clin N Am 34 (2011) 357–376
doi:10.1016/j.psc.2011.02.003
0193-953X/11/$ – see front matter © 2011 Elsevier Inc. All rights reserved.

psych.theclinics.com

neurotrophic factor (BDNF), the hypothalamic-pituitary-adrenal (HPA) axis, inflammatory cytokines, and other monoaminergic genes.

METHODOLOGICAL CONSIDERATIONS

Before reviewing these recent results, important methodological concerns should be noted.

How environment (E) is categorized likely matters. E can be (1) an acute precipitating trigger for the onset of an MDD episode, (2) an element of predispositional vulnerability to MDD, (3) a perpetuating factor once an MDD episode has occurred and preventing its remission, or (4) simply a secondary epiphenomenon statistically correlated with already having MDD. The question of whether MDD comorbidities (one type of E) are predispositions, precipitants, perpetuating factors, and/or epiphenomena can be a very complex question without a simple answer.[21] An example of a precipitating event that triggers the onset of an MDD episode could be a myocardial infarction.[22] A predisposition for MDD vulnerability could be lower childhood social class, resulting in decreased glucocorticoid and increased proinflammatory signaling later in life.[23] Perpetuating factors after MDD has developed could be social isolation and resultant inability to cope with stress.[24,25] Finally, having MDD may increase the likelihood of smoking, with secondary effects on pulmonary health.[26] It is conceivable that one set of genes interacts with environmentally influenced predisposition, another set interacts with environmental precipitants, and a third with perpetuating environments. Therefore, in determining the interaction of vulnerability genes with E, a longitudinal perspective is often necessary. Also, because environmental variables can obviously fluctuate over time, using a single period of time to assess E can sometimes be a misleading proxy for E.[27] Choosing what E to include in GxE studies should be guided by known science,[28] carefully defining the nature, extent, and timing of E.

Genetic correlations with E likely matter. Because each individual can shape the interpersonal interactions and environment around them, one's own genetic make-up appears to indirectly influence exposure to psychosocial stressors, social supports, and vascular disease. Statistically this means that there are often G-E correlations, situations in which G appears to "affect" E. Simply put, people can select and modify their own environments; and genetically similar people end up in similar environments. Examples of this abound. To illustrate, a Taq1A polymorphism in the dopamine receptor 2 gene has been associated with multiple illnesses that involve impulse dyscontrol, and children with the A1 allele are more likely to discontinue school. But this genetic risk can be mitigated by having a mentor, indicating an interaction between genetic vulnerability and mentorship.[29] However, children with A1 were also less likely to have a mentor in the first place, indicating the gene also adversely influenced access to this beneficial environment.[29] Thus, there is also a G-E correlation in addition to a GxE interaction.

In a similar fashion, genetic variability may be associated with almost two-thirds of the likelihood of experiencing personal stressful life events (ie, not all is simply bad luck).[30] Likewise, heritability may explain as much as 75% of differences in social support among people,[31] something that remains true later in life.[32] In fact, studies of older adult twins indicate that many environment stressors (eg, divorce, spouse in nursing home, change in residence) are under genetic influence, with as much as 43% heritability.[33] Thus in interpreting the results of GxE studies, one should recognize that the exposure to E itself can be partially "influenced" by G.

How MDD, E, and G are each measured likely matters.[34] Diagnoses of MDD by structured interview or by cut-off criteria on a self-report scale can be partially correlated, but these methods can also differ.[35] As just one example, brain injury, stroke, or Parkinson disease can affect the relationship between a self-reported score-based diagnosis and a diagnosis based on a structured interview.[36–38] Even in healthy old-old adults, self-reports may have limited correlation with interview-based diagnoses.[39] Taking a lesson from mice, different chromosomal areas are associated with different anxiety measures, depending on what behavioral test is used.[40] The differences could be associated with potentially different evolutionary constructs.[41] In humans, there are similarly unique heritabilities for specific depression symptoms,[42,43] and it is conceivable for some genes to better associate with MDD diagnosed using one methodology as compared with another.

Moreover, there may be etiologically different categories of MDD later in life,[44] depending on the concurrent development of cerebrovascular disease, recurrent lifetime history of episodes, new onset following the occurrence of a psychosocial stressor, prodromal symptoms of Alzheimer disease, and so forth. In confirming or replicating results across studies, the potential for nonreplication because of measurement "artifact" could be mitigated by studies using a variety of methods and instruments for assessing E and MDD.

In addition, both depression and environmental measures can also obviously be confounded by recall bias,[45] with this problem likely worsening with age.[46,47] It is possible that depressed mood as well as genes that affect memory could influence recall.[48] Thus, studies that rely on retrospective recall of E and/or MDD diagnosis face this limitation. For psychosocial "stressors," how E is perceived may be important. That is, the emotional valence or the controllability of major life events may both conceivably affect the relationship with depression. For example, a divorce could be a negative or a positive occasion, depending on the circumstances. Similarly, the extent to which one has control over the impact of the divorce may influence its impact on depression. Simply adding major life events together has the potential to be misleading, and there is vast heterogeneity among studies with respect to how life events are quantified, measured, and defined.

The information provided by genotyping can be affected by population stratification (particularly when cases and controls in association studies arise from different subpopulations); differing linkage between measured single nucleotide polymorphisms (SNPs) and potentially causal polymorphisms in populations of differing ancestry; effects on statistical power when testing multiple polymorphisms (particularly whole genome-wide studies); and laboratory reliability of different genotyping methods.[49,50]

Study design likely matters. A basic design is to examine two environments (eg, "stressed" and "not stressed") and to examine whether genotype interacts with E in predicting the presence of depression. A related design is to include quantitative gradations in level of E, and to assess for GxE interaction. A third design is to assume that E is probably influential, select only those subjects exposed to E, and test for a direct main effect of G. This latter design does not examine interaction per se, but is a powerful method for detecting G in the setting of known environmental stressors. Each of these designs can be employed in prospective, cross-sectional, or retrospective fashion, with varying degrees of attention to measurement, feasibility, assumptions, and statistical power.

Finally, the age of the population examined likely matters. The extent of potential predisposing factors (prior history of MDD episodes, poor sleep, chronic inflammation, frailty, pain, cognitive impairment, lack of social supports, and so forth) and potential precipitating factors (eg, major illness, sudden disability, loss of loved one, increased caregiver requirements) differ in the elderly. This difference could conceivably either mitigate or vitiate the effect size of GxE interactions.

These 5 general elements tremendously vary across the studies that have been done to date. Thus comparing results across studies is very difficult. Nonetheless, despite the interstudy variability, some tentative conclusions are possible.

POLYMORPHISMS IN THE SEROTONIN (5-HT) TRANSPORTER (SERT)

It has now been 7 years since the first report of an interaction between stress and an insertion/deletion polymorphism in the promoter region of the SERT gene (5-HTTLPR; with short [S] and long [L] alleles) in the development of depression in young adults.[51] This initial prospective study longitudinally assessed E as the cumulative number of stressful life events, including childhood maltreatment over a 5-year period.[51] Those with the S/S genotype were more sensitive to the adverse effects of stress on depression risk. This finding was soon "replicated" by another prospective study that assessed E as various threat levels within 1 month before depression assessment. In this second study, the difference between 5-HTTLPR genotypes was greatest at moderate threat levels,[52] suggesting a leftward shift in the "stress-depression" curve and greater sensitivity in the short term to moderate threats among those with the S/S genotype. This finding predicts minimal difference between genotypes when no stress exists or at very high levels of precipitating stress. There have now been almost 60 additional studies examining 5-HTTLPR for a potential GxE interaction, with mixed results.[53–55] A complete review of all these studies is not the intent of this article; rather, the authors attempt to highlight both inconsistencies and consistent findings.

Like the aforementioned prospective studies, several GxE studies are longitudinal. Most of these have replicated an interaction. In female twins, stressful life events in the 3 months before a diagnostic interview was more depressogenic in those with the S/S genotype,[56] an effect also seen in twins who reported childhood adversity,[57] and also 125 orphans with prior institutional deprivation.[58] A recent study specifically assessed bullying in 2017 children, and again reported evidence for the S/S subjects subsequently developing more depression.[59] Complicating this trend, some longitudinal studies have only replicated a GxE interaction for maltreatment and adolescent depression for females, but not males[60]; or the replication of GxE was evident later in life only when cumulative life events were tallied over 5 years and not just 1 year.[61] Conversely, another prospective study reported that S/S genotype increased risk for adult MDD in those with only one traumatic event, essentially shifting the stress-depression curve leftward.[62] In all of these studies, the S/S genotype was more prone to MDD than the L/L genotype; but whether there is an additive, recessive, or dominant effect for the S allele was not consistent between these studies.

There are some vitally important longitudinal studies that did not find a GxE interaction. A very large study of more than 4000 7-year-olds found no evidence for GxE, strongly arguing against a role for 5-HTTLPR as a risk factor for MDD in children at this very young age.[63] In another large study of subjects of various ages including older adult twins (total N = 3243), no role for 5-HTTLPR was again found.[64] In this study, depression symptoms in a telephone survey were assessed 1 to 10 years after a prior survey had queried about stressful events that initial year.

Also, one prospective study has found that the risk allele is actually the L allele.[65] Because of several negative and contradictory results, a recent meta-analysis examined a subset of these studies, along with several other cross-sectional studies, and concluded that there may be no GxE interaction for 5-HTTLPR.[55] Regardless, the clear conclusion is that the GxE interaction is definitely not universal. But what accounts for the differences between studies other than chance?[66]

One question is: does 5-HTTLPR interact with predispositional stress (eg, trauma in childhood influencing MDD risk in adulthood) or with adverse life events that are precipitants of depression (ie, stress immediately preceding an MDD episode)? Studies that assess childhood maltreatment or early trauma of some type and then MDD years later are often studies in which stress may result in some enduring change in predispositional vulnerability. Of these "predispositional" studies, most replicate the original finding of Caspi and colleagues.[60,67–69] Some other studies depend on how E was defined. For example, an interaction for 5-HTTLPR was found in adults when stressful traumatic events were assessed across 3 levels of diversity, but not when they were dichotomized.[70] In another, the GxE interaction was found only with child-hood sexual trauma but not with maltreatment more generally.[71] The few exceptions include a predispositional study in which no GxE was found in older adults when E was measured as father's education (a potential surrogate for childhood adversity).[72] Also, only a nonsignificant trend for greater depression symptoms in S/S carriers was noted in a study in which child adversity was measured as a continuous measure (with explicit items regarding sexual and physical abuse purposefully not asked).[57] Thus, most evidence implicates a role for the S/S genotype in augmenting the predisposition for MDD that results from severe childhood trauma, in particular sexual abuse. But the severity of the traumatic childhood experiences and how it is assessed and measured may be an important variable, and possibly account for the limited number of negative findings.

GxE studies examining cumulative stress as a potential precipitating event in the months or year preceding a depressive episode have been variable. Here, it is possible that the nature (eg, level of threat) and timing (eg, a few months preceding MDD) are crucial variables in determining whether GxE occurs. In a similar manner, 5-HTTLPR may affect the potency but not the efficacy of a selective serotonin reuptake inhibitor.[73] That is, 5-HTTLPR may shift the concentration-response curve, and thus at high or at very low concentrations there is no difference in antidepressant response. In the pharmacology case, E is readily quantified as a medication concentration in the blood. If G similarly shifts the stress-response curve (ie, it takes less stress to trigger an MDD episode in an S/S carrier), then a 5-HTTLPR influence on depression would be evident only at moderate levels of stress. Thus, assessing the magnitude, the duration, and the timing of stress becomes important for "precipitation studies," albeit more difficult than simply measuring a blood level. Whether this possibility may account for "negative" studies (eg, Coventry and colleagues[64]) is purely speculative at this point.

In older adults, medical illness is one specific type of precipitating environmental stressor. Here the results are fairly consistent. In 521 elderly subjects prospectively studied over 2 years, the S/S genotype increased the risk for MDD in those with 4 or more chronic medical disorders, supporting a GxE interaction.[74] Another study, interestingly, also reported that the S allele was associated with a leftward shift in the disease burden–depression relationship; however in this case those with 2 or 3 chronic medical illnesses were more at risk for depression symptoms if they had the S allele.[75] Examining more specific medical conditions, the S/S genotype has been associated with increased risk for depression in those with Parkinson disease,[76] with severe coronary disease,[22] following a myocardial infarction,[77,78] following a hip fracture,[15] and following a stroke.[79,80] The only two published exceptions to this trend that the authors have found to date include a large study of patients with existing cardiac illness where no role of 5-HTTLPR was found,[81] and a prospective examination of patients undergoing bypass graft surgery.[82] Of interest, this latter study found potential evidence for a complicating G-E correlation such that the L allele was associated with additional cardiac events following surgery. Therefore, studies examining cardiovascular disease may be confounded by the possibility that L allele increases the likelihood of being exposed to a cardiac event (potentially reversing its beneficial effect). This proposal is consistent with studies finding that the L allele is associated with increased platelet reactivity in depressed elderly.[83] Of note, the relationship between MDD and vascular disease is likely bidirectional.[84] Also, many of the potential genetic influences on depression may also influence coronary artery disease.[85] Thus with the potential exception of cardiac illness for which studies may be confounded by potential G-E correlation, there is fairly well-replicated support for the S/S genotype augmenting the detrimental effect of "medical illness burden" on depression risk.

There have also recently been a few prospective studies of patients who are treated with interferon-α, an inflammatory cytokine that can trigger MDD in about one-quarter of patients. Here, 2 studies have found that evidence for the S/S genotype increasing incidence for MDD during interferon-α therapy,[86,87] although there are 2 others (one in a Chinese population and one measuring depression symptoms using a questionnaire) that did not.[88,89] This finding raises the possibility that in older adults, the S/S genotype may sometimes be interacting with increased exposure to inflammatory cytokines (something associated with increasing medical burden). Elevated inflammatory cytokines may be important biomarkers for the development of geriatric depression during medical illnesses.[90] It is interesting that cytokines can affect expression of the serotonin transporter,[91] and this effect may be influenced by the 5-HTTLPR polymorphism.[92] As only a subset of patients with elevated cytokines develop MDD, this is an area of genetic vulnerability and resilience still awaiting further work.

Nonetheless, similar to findings in children and young adults, the interaction of 5-HTTLPR with psychosocial precipitating stressors later in life is less clear. In one study of adults aged 41 to 80, there was no GxE interaction either with total number of adverse life experiences recalled or with adverse events and long-term difficulties in the previous 5 years.[93] However, a study of Korean elders found a GxE interaction,[94] and the S/S genotype was also associated with increased risk in caregivers under this type of stress.[72] Another study of older adults found a GxE interaction only when the life event history was severe and traumatic, but not otherwise.[95] Again, differences in the severity stress among these studies may continue to play an important role.

To summarize, there are some tentative conclusions that can be made. (1) A universal interaction between "stress" and 5-HTTLPR is not likely, as evidenced by negative findings in several large studies. (2) Older adults with S/S genotypes have enhanced depression risk secondary to medical illness as a "precipitating" factor, and this appears to be mostly replicated. (3) In younger adults with S/S genotypes, enhanced "predispositional" risk from severe childhood trauma appears to be mostly replicated. The implication of this for the elderly is that the relative risk for late-life MDD episodes is 90-fold for people with a prior history of MDD episodes.[17] Thus, the 5-HTTLPR × early trauma interaction may affect recurrent MDD and extend into late-life. (4) Whether S/S also increases risk for the effect of cumulative precipitating stressors in late-life may depend on the severity of the stress. Findings among studies in this area are very variable, with notable heterogeneity in design as well as variability in E, G, and MDD assessment. At this point, therefore, this possibility is less conclusive.

The pathophysiology of how the S/S genotype could be influencing risk for MDD remains to be clarified, but plausible possibilities include effects on cerebral white matter disease,[96,97] effects on hippocampus volume,[98,99] effects on amygdala function,[100] effects on amygdala and frontal cortical connectivity,[101,102] effects on sleep quality,[86,103] effects on the cortisol stress axis,[104,105] among others.

POLYMORPHISMS IN THE HYPOTHALAMIC-PITUITARY-ADRENAL AXIS

Abnormal axis (HPA) feedback and hyperreactivity are often present in people with MDD,[106,107] and includes disrupted glucocorticoid receptor (GR) expression, translocation, and concomitant resistance to cortisol.[107] Chronic psychosocial stress may also impair appropriate regulation of the HPA axis.[108] One plausible hypothesis is that an imbalance between mineralocorticoid and glucocorticoid responses occurs in MDD.[109] Thus, polymorphisms in genes for GR, in corticotropin-releasing hormone (CRH), in both CRH receptors (CRHR1 and CRHR2), and in a GR chaperone (FKBP5), may all play roles in response to stress.[110] Over the past several years, a few GxE studies examining HPA genes have taken place. For example, in a longitudinal study of 906 aging subjects, child adversity affected both depression risk and cortisol levels; and polymorphisms in the GR gene increased the risk for depression.[111] The polymorphisms of interest for GR appear to influence acute corticosteroid response as well as HPA axis reactivity.[109]

CRHR1 gene polymorphisms also interact with childhood abuse to predict sensitivity to a dexamethasone/CRH challenge.[112] Consistent with this, several polymorphisms and a haplotype spanning intron 1 interact with childhood abuse to predict MDD in adulthood.[113] This haplotype finding was replicated in one longitudinal cohort but not in another (although the other cohort measured abuse differently).[114] Also, there appears to be a GxGxE interaction in which 5-HTTLPR and CRHR1 may interact with child abuse history to predict adult MDD.[70] Of note, these studies have specifically examined childhood trauma and not stressors more proximal to MDD episodes later in life. However, they are consistent with findings that serotonin transporter function can be influenced by glucocorticoids, and that this influence is moderated by 5-HTTLPR in creating a long-lasting predisposition to MDD.[115]

An immunophilin that is involved in translocation of GR from the cytosol to the nucleus, FKBP5, may likewise play an important role.[116,117] Alleles associated with enhanced expression of FKBP5 lead to an increased GR resistance and decreased efficiency of the negative feedback of the HPA axis. Polymorphisms for the FKBP5 gene have been primarily examined with respect to posttraumatic stress disorder, where they may be associated with prolonged HPA response to trauma, potentially resulting in long-lasting changes.[118] One hypothesis is that these HPA-related polymorphisms are primarily interactive with early-life trauma, leading to a lifelong predisposition or vulnerability to the effects of other types of stresses later in life.[118] Whether this is true for geriatric depression remains to be examined. Finally, it is biologically plausible that other polymorphisms in genes encoding for HPA-related proteins such as CRHR2 and CRH may also interact with stress.[119,120]

Although it is plausible that HPA genes may affect both vascular disease and MDD risk (including a plausible G-E correlation), any potentially interacting role for CRH1, CRH2, or FKBP5 in late-life MDD that remains awaits future study. Moreover, whether HPA axis genes may interact with more proximal "precipitating" factors or medical illness–related inflammatory changes is currently unknown.

BRAIN-DERIVED NEUROTROPHIC FACTOR

Impairment in growth factors such as BDNF may lead to MDD, and BDNF Met/Val variants have been associated with MDD.[121] Of interest, major traumas early in life can directly affect methylation and expression of BDNF.[122] Moreover, serotonin transporter function can be modulated by BDNF.[123] BDNF genetic variants may also influence GR sensitivity[124] and interact with stress to influence vulnerability.[68] Consequently, both the BDNF gene Val66Met polymorphism and polymorphisms in its receptor have been associated with late-life MDD,[125] along with increased suicidal ideation.[126]

Consistent with this, the BDNF Met/Val functional polymorphism has been found to interact with stress in a couple studies.[69,127] It is possible that the effect of early life stress on brain arousal pathways is influenced by this polymorphism, resulting in a predisposition to depression later in life.[128] The BDNF Val/Met polymorphism may also interact with both 5-HTTLPR and caregiving stress (as measured in parents of psychotic patients) to influence depression,[129] which is consistent with 2 BDNF × SERT × stress interactions found in younger patients.[57,68] There are a limited number of studies examining GxE for BDNF, and future work is clearly indicated. Nonetheless, the potential for GxGxE is enticing.

OTHER MONOAMINERGIC GENES

A very limited number of studies have started to explore the potential for other mono-aminergic genes and their interaction with E. There have not been enough published reports as yet to make any inferences regarding trends or consistencies among studies. However, there are some suggestive findings. A potentially functional polymorphism in catecholamine-O-methyltransferase (COMT) may interact with 5-HTTLPR and stress to influence depression risk.[130] It is interesting that the COMT polymorphism was also associated with depressive symptoms postpartum, both alone and in GxG interaction with monoamine oxidase A gene.[131] A polymorphism in the 5-HT1A gene interacted with recent stressful events in females aged either 20 to 24 or 60 to 64 years, associating with depression in select post hoc analyses, though no GxE interaction was noted in general for this gene.[132] Polymorphisms in 5-HT1A have been linked to depression, and 5-HT1A binding is reduced in depressed people.[133] A polymorphism in 5-HT1A has also been found to predict depressive symptoms in patients receiving interferon-α.[88] Using urban/rural residency to define E, the 5-HT2A gene may interact with residency to influence depression symptoms[134]; and a polymorphism in the 5-HT3A receptor gene may interact with early-life stress, resulting in differences in hippocampus and frontal gray matter.[135] Again using rural residency as a surrogate marker for stress in a recent study of Chinese citizens, a norepinephrine transporter polymorphism interacted to influence MDD risk.[136] Of note, these are all single studies with a variety of approaches, designs, and ways of defining E. Thus there are enticing leads, but further replication work is needed.

Two other monoaminergic genes of potential importance include tryptophan hydroxylases 1 and 2 (TPH1 and TPH2). In the peripheral systemic circulation, the relative action of TPH1 and indoleamine deoxygenase can influence whether tryptophan is metabolized to serotonin or to kynurenine and other glutamatergic compounds.[137] The kynurenine/tryptophan ratio is elevated in melancholic adolescents[138] and depressed subjects receiving interferon-α.[139] Elevated tryptophan may mitigate the effect of the S/S genotype on mood,[140] and 5-HTTLPR interacts with tryptophan depletion in acute studies of mood.[141,142] In adults, TPH1 polymorphisms may moderate the effect of social support on depression.[143] There is also some evidence that TPH1 polymorphisms interact with stressful childhood experiences to influence harm avoidance, which may increase risk for MDD.[144] Whether TPH1 polymorphisms interact with 5-HTTLPR in a GxGxE fashion remains to be determined. TPH2 also may interact with family structure to influence childhood depression symptoms.[145] Also, although the indoleamine deoxygenase gene has glucocorticoid response elements,[146] whether polymorphisms in this gene interact with stress in increasing MDD risk is not known to the authors' knowledge. Regardless, further work is required wlth respect to GxE studies.

OTHER GENES

There is preliminary evidence for other candidate genes. Although few of these studies have been replicated, there is the possibility that specific genes may interact with specific "precipitants." That is, there may be unique "subtypes" of depression in which different genes interact with different environmental precipitants; for example, risk genes for menopausal, for inflammatory cytokines, for circadian shift, and so forth. As noted in the introduction, there are many seemingly different and varied plausible "environmental" precipitants for MDD that have been described, and each may have its own unique genetic interactions.

As examples, a gene influencing metabolism of estrogen, coding for the enzyme CYP1A1, may double depression risk in perimenopausal women.[147] Polymorphisms affecting interleukin-6 may influence depression risk in the setting of increased inflammation, potentially in interaction with 5-HTTLPR.[87,148] In late-life, MDD has been associated with vascular disease as well as a prodromal condition to Alzheimer disease. Here, APOE4 may increase the risk of nonvascular late-life MDD, but not MDD associated with cerebrovascular disease.[149] A polymorphism in neuropeptide Y may protect against depression in the setting of stress,[150] and 2 studies have reported an interaction between the cannabinoid receptor gene polymorphism and stressful events in the risk for depression.[81,151] Thus ultimately there may be the potential for several cumulative GxE interactions in late-life, depending on which combinations of environmental precipitants are present. For the elderly, it is likely that future studies will need to increasingly attend multiple measures of E (in addition to childhood adversity or recent psychosocial stress).

POSSIBLE EPIGENETIC MECHANISMS

Early-life traumas appear to be the most studied and replicated risk for MDD in most of the GxE studies to date. So how does this affect risk later in life? Early-life trauma can manifest many years later as increased proinflammatory signaling,[23] and genomic studies of MDD have identified roles for genes such as TBX21 and PSMB4, which are influential in inflammation.[152] Therefore, changes in inflammatory and endocrine processes are implicated in the etiology of MDD. However, early-life stress has many additional potential long-lasting effects. Of particular note, epigenetic phenomena are increasingly being understood as mediating many of the lifelong effects of early environmental events.[153]

In other words, it is possible that environment can induce changes in the genome itself, either through modification of nucleotides or through packaging of the DNA in histones. In fact, chromatin remodeling may be one way in which early environmental conditions can have prolonged influences on vulnerability to MDD.[154] Alternatively, maternal effects on pups can influence HPA reactivity later in life via effects on DNA methylation of the GR gene.[155] This process is also possible in humans for whom early adversity may have prolonged influences on brain GR.[156] Thus, events in childhood could lead to enhanced sensitivity to "stress" later in life, as well as enhanced sensitivity of the inflammatory pathways.[23] Also, just as BDNF variants may interact with stress to influence MDD vulnerability, increased methylation of BDNF has also been found in the brains of suicidal subjects.[157] Furthermore, there appears to be a role for early traumas in increasing the level of BDNF methylation.[122]

In nonabused patients with MDD, no GR methylation differences from controls were found.[158] However, in this study production of NGFI-A, a transcription factor for GR, was decreased in the hippocampus of depressed subjects.[158] This finding is interesting because NGFI-A can mediate the effects of serotonergic signaling and BDNF. Thus, there may be alternative routes to MDD that converge on pathways such as this. That is, either GR methylation due to early-life trauma can occur or transcription factor changes in late-life can occur, and either of these paths could lead to decreased expression of GR.

To complicate the picture more, polymorphisms may affect epigenetic processes. For instance, 5-HT transporter levels are influenced by methylation of the SERT gene,[159] and this could interact with 5-HTTLPR in expression of the transporter.[160] One possibility is that both the 5-HTTLPR and increased methylation could additionally be necessary for decreased SERT expression.[161] However, research in this area is preliminary.

It is clear that there are many candidate pathways and interactions requiring explication. Epigenetic effects are just one of these. Future studies will need to (1) better delineate genetic influences on vulnerability to early-life trauma; (2) define which epigenetic effects of trauma are important for subsequent predisposition to depression; (3) assess how predisposition interacts with subsequent environmental precipitants; and (4) determine which genes interact with which precipitants, in the presence or absence of these other sources of vulnerability.

SUMMARY

After 7 years and almost 60 heterogeneous studies, it can probably safely be concluded that a 5-HTTLPR by "stress" interaction is not universal. However, the pattern of results suggests that the nature of "stress" that is measured, and how it is measured, matter. Based on the results of these studies, several intriguing hypotheses present themselves. Does S/S increase the maximal effect of childhood trauma, leading to recurrent MDD that recurs through old age? Does the S/S allele interact with elevated inflammatory cytokines, shifting the inflammation-MDD curve leftward? Does S/S shift the precipitating stress-MDD curve leftward, for psychosocial precipitants?

Only very tentative conclusions are possible. For 5-HTTLPR, there is some evidence that the long-lasting effects of severe early-life trauma is enhanced by the S/S genotype. Preliminary findings also support this for genes affecting the HPA axis and BDNF. In most of these studies, the interactive effects seem to be most evident for very severe stress, and often sexual trauma. This finding suggests that these genes may influence the maximal effect of early-life trauma (shifting the curve upward rather than leftward), a set of hypotheses that requires more definitive testing. In elderly adults, one would specifically predict that this type of GxE would result in an enhanced history of recurrent depression (ie, early-onset MDD) throughout life.

Whether 5-HTTLPR influences the potency of precipitating psychosocial stressors is debatable. One possibility is the "double-hit" hypothesis, whereby early trauma increases the risk for MDD by shifting the "precipitating stress–MDD" relationship in subsequent years.[162] In other words, traumatized children are more vulnerable to the effects of subsequent stresses as adults. Thus, 5-HTTLPR may influence the maximal effect of early trauma, and by this pathway indirectly influence the subsequent precipitating stress–MDD relationship later in life. Alternatively, 5-HTTLPR may shift leftward the precipitating stress–MDD relationship regardless of childhood trauma. There is some evidence for this.[52] Regardless, testing and replication of this hypothesis will require careful attention to measurement of E, including its timing, intensity, and chronicity.

In adults, the influence of medical illness on comorbid MDD does seem to be enhanced by the S/S genotype, with the preponderance of evidence suggesting that the "potency" of illness is affected (shifting the curve leftward). However, this effect on potency may conceivably be mitigated by concurrent effects on platelet reactivity and vascular risk. Nonetheless, one critical question is: what aspect of medical illness is in interaction with genetics? Is it psychosocial stress, increased inflammation, or something else? If it is increased inflammation, then this proffers the opportunity to have a blood-based measure of "environment." One speculative but tempting hypothesis is that the S/S genotype affects the "inflammation-MDD" relationship. To examine this, inflammatory cytokines such as interleukin-6 and interleukin-1b can be used as direct biomarkers of "medical stress." In other words, quantitatively measuring E using endocrine and inflammatory biomarkers may be one way of feasibly determining its interaction with 5-HTTLPR.

Polymorphisms in BDNF, the HPA axis, and other monoaminergic genes are also being examined as potential sources of vulnerability to adverse environments. This same set of questions will likely apply to them, but additional hypotheses arise. For example, do specific precipitants such as low-estrogen states interact with specific gene products such as CYP1A1? That is, should one be matching specific environments with specific polymorphisms? This question is particularly important for the elderly, for whom a variety of potential sources for depression can exist, sometimes simultaneously.

One might anticipate no progress for a complex, multifactorial disorder such as geriatric MDD, which can have a complicated recurring presentation, a new onset late in life, and/or comorbidity with either vascular disease or prodromal dementia. Nonetheless, progress has been made. As the potential nature of GxE interactions and the pathways that likely mediate these effects are better understood, further progress can be anticipated. With careful attention to robust measures of E, G, and MDD, it is likely that this trend will accelerate.

REFERENCES

1. Murphy-Eberenz K, Zandi PP, March D, et al. Is perinatal depression familial? J Affect Disord 2006;90(1):49–55.
2. Bromberger JT, Schott LL, Kravitz HM, et al. Longitudinal change in reproductive hormones and depressive symptoms across the menopausal transition: results from the Study of Women's Health Across the Nation (SWAN). Arch Gen Psychiatry 2010;67(6):598–607.
3. Panicker V, Evans J, Bjoro T, et al. A paradoxical difference in relationship between anxiety, depression and thyroid function in subjects on and not on T4: findings from the HUNT study. Clin Endocrinol 2009;71(4):574–80.
4. Mendlewicz J. Disruption of the circadian timing systems: molecular mechanisms in mood disorders. CNS Drugs 2009;23(Suppl 2):15–26.
5. Buysse DJ. Insomnia, depression and aging. Assessing sleep and mood interactions in older adults. Geriatrics 2004;59(2):47–51.
6. Kosten TR, Markou A, Koob GF. Depression and stimulant dependence: neurobiology and pharmacotherapy. J Nerv Ment Dis 1998;186(12):737–45.
7. Forster A, Young J. Specialist nurse support for patients with stroke in the community: a randomized controlled trial. BMJ 1996;312:1642–6.

8. Narushima K, Kosier TJ, Robinson RG. Preventing poststroke depression: a 12-week double blind randomized treatment trial and 21-month follow-up. J Nerv Ment Dis 2002;190:296–303.

9. Rasmussen BB, Lunde M, Loldrup PD, et al. A double-blind placebo-controlled study of sertraline in the prevention of depression in stroke patients. Psychosomatics 2003;44:216–21.

10. Smits F, Smits N, Schoevers R, et al. An epidemiological approach to depression prevention in old age. Am J Geriatr Psychiatry 2008;16(6):444–53.

11. Raison CL, Borisov AS, Majer M, et al. Activation of central nervous system inflammatory pathways by interferon-alpha: relationship to monoamines and depression. Biol Psychiatry 2009;65(4):296–303.

12. Brodaty H, Green AA, Koschera A. Meta-analysis of psychosocial interventions for caregivers of people with dementia. J Am Geriatr Soc 2003;51:657–64.

13. Vinkers DJ, Gussekloo J, Stek ML, et al. The 15-item geriatric depression scale (GDS-15) detects changes in depressive symptoms after a major negative life event. The Leiden 85-plus Study. Int J Geriatr Psychiatry 2004;19(1):80–4.

14. Cole MG. Evidence-based review of risk factors for geriatric depression and brief preventative interventions. Psychiatr Clin North Am 2005;28:785–803.

15. Lenze EJ, Munin MC, Ferrell RE, et al. Association of the serotonin transporter gene-linked polymorphic region (5-HTTLPR) genotype with depressive symptoms in elderly persons after hip fracture. Am J Geriatr Psychiatry 2004;13(5):428–31.

16. France RD, Krishnan KR, Trainor M. Chronic pain and depression. III. Family history study of depression and alcoholism in chronic low back pain patients. Pain 1986;24(2):185–90.

17. Beekman AT, Deeg DJ, van Tilberg T, et al. Major and minor depression in later life: a study of prevalence and risk factors. J Affect Disord 1995;36:65–75.

18. Kendler KS, Karkowski LM, Prescott CA. Causal relationship between stressful life events and the onset of major depression. Am J Psychiatry 1999;156:837–41.

19. Sullivan PF, Neale MC, Kendler KS. Genetic epidemiology of major depression: review and meta-analysis. Am J Psychiatry 2000;157:1552–62.

20. Lopez-Leon S, Janssens A, González-Zuloeta Ladd AM, et al. Meta-analyses of genetic studies on major depressive disorder. Mol Psychiatry 2008;13:772–85.

21. Alexopoulos GS, Buckwalter K, Olin J, et al. Comorbidity of late life depression: an opportunity for research on mechanisms and treatment. Biol Psychiatry 2002;52(6):543–58.

22. Otte C, McCaffery J, Ali S, et al. Association of a serotonin transporter polymorphism (5-HTTLPR) with depression, perceived stress, and norepinephrine in patients with coronary disease: the Heart and Soul Study. Am J Psychiatry 2007;164(9):1379–84.

23. Miller GE, Chen E, Fok AK, et al. Low early-life social class leaves a biological residue manifested by decreased glucocorticoid and increased proinflammatory signaling. Proc Natl Acad Sci U S A 2009;106(34):14716–21.

24. Checkley S. The neuroendocrinology of depression and chronic stress. Br Med Bull 1996;52(3):597–617.

25. Teasdale JD. Emotional processing, three modes of mind and the prevention of relapse in depression. Behav Res Ther 1999;37(Suppl 1):S53–77.

26. Husky MM, Mazure CM, Paliwal P, et al. Gender differences in the comorbidity of smoking behavior and major depression. Drug Alcohol Depend 2008;93(1–2):176–9.

27. Wolfe B, Havemen R, Ginther D, et al. The 'window problem' in studies of children's attainments. J Am Stat Assoc 1996;91:970–82.

28. Moffitt TE, Caspi A, Rutter M. Strategy for investigating interactions between measured genes and measured environments. Arch Gen Psychiatry 2005; 62(5):473–81.

29. Shanahan MJ, Erickson LD, Vaisey S, et al. Helping relationships and genetic propensities: a combinatoric study of DRD2, mentoring, and educational continuation. Twin Res Hum Genet 2007;10(2):285–98.

30. Foley DL, Kendler KS. A longitudinal study of stressful life events assessed at personal interview with an epidemiologic sample of adult twins: the basis of individual variation in event exposure. Psychol Med 1996;26:1239–52.

31. Kendler KS. Social support: a genetic epidemiologic analysis. Am J Psychiatry 1997;154:1309–404.

32. Bergemann CS, Neiderhiser JM, Pedersen NL, et al. Genetic and environmental influences on social support in later life: a longitudinal analysis. Int J Aging Hum Dev 2001;53:107–35.

33. Plomin R, Lichtenstein P, Pedersen NL, et al. Genetic influence on life events during the last half of the life span. Psychol Aging 1990;5:25–30.

34. Wermter AK, Laucht M, Schimmelmann BG, et al. From nature versus nurture, via nature and nurture, to gene x environment interaction in mental disorders. Eur Child Adolesc Psychiatry 2010;19(3):199–210.

35. Hedayati SS, Bosworth HB, Kuchibhatla M, et al. The predictive value of self-report scales compared with physician diagnosis of depression in hemodialysis patients. Kidney Int 2006;69(9):1662–8.

36. Homaifar BY, Brenner LA, Gutierrez PM, et al. Sensitivity and specificity of the Beck Depression Inventory-II in persons with traumatic brain injury. Arch Phys Med Rehabil 2009;90(4):652–6.

37. Healey AK, Kneebone II, Carroll M, et al. A preliminary investigation of the reliability and validity of the brief assessment schedule depression cards and the beck depression inventory-fast screen to screen for depression in older stroke survivors. Int J Geriatr Psychiatry 2008;23(5):531–6.

38. McDonald WM, Holtzheimer PE, Haber M, et al. Validity of the 30-item geriatric depression scale in patients with Parkinson's disease. Mov Disord 2006;21(10): 1618–22.

39. Watson LC, Lewis CL, Kistler CE, et al. Can we trust depression screening instruments in healthy 'old-old' adults? Int J Geriatr Psychiatry 2004;19(3): 278–85.

40. Henderson ND, Turri MG, DeFries JC, et al. QTL analysis of multiple behavioral measures of anxiety in mice. Behav Genet 2004;34:267–93.

41. Sturman ED, Mongrain M. Self-criticism and major depression: an evolutionary perspective. Br J Clin Psychol 2005;44(4):505–19.

42. Jang KL, Livesley WJ, Taylor S, et al. Heritability of individual depressive symptoms. J Affect Disord 2004;80(2–3):125–33.

43. Foley DL, Neale MC, Gardner CO, et al. Major depression and associated impairment: same or different genetic and environmental risk factors? Am J Psychiatry 2003;160:2128–33.

44. Brilman EI, Ormel J. Life events, difficulties and onset of depressive episodes in later life. Psychol Med 2001;31:859–69.

45. Moffitt TE, Caspi A, Taylor A, et al. How common are common mental disorders? Evidence that lifetime prevalence rates are doubled by prospective versus retrospective ascertainment. Psychol Med 2010;40(6):899–909.

46. Patten SB. Recall bias and major depression lifetime prevalence. Soc Psychiatry Psychiatr Epidemiol 2003;38(6):290–6.
47. Green JG, McLaughlin KA, Berglund PA, et al. Childhood adversities and adult psychiatric disorders in the national comorbidity survey replication I: associations with first onset of DSM-IV disorders. Arch Gen Psychiatry 2010;67(2): 113–23.
48. Drago A, Alboni S, Brunello N, et al. HTR1B as a risk profile maker in psychiatric disorders: a review through motivation and memory. Eur J Clin Pharmacol 2010; 66(1):5–27.
49. Yonan AL, Palmer AA, Gilliam TC. Hardy-Weinberg disequilibrium identified genotyping error of the serotonin transporter (SLC6A4) promoter polymorphism. Psychiatr Genet 2006;16(1):31–4.
50. van der Straaten T, van Schaik RH. Genetic techniques for pharmacogenetic analyses. Curr Pharm Des 2010;16(2):231–7.
51. Caspi A, Sugden K, Moffitt TE, et al. Influence of life stress on depression: moderation by a polymorphism in the 5-HTT gene. Science 2003;301(5631): 368–89.
52. Kendler KS, Kuhn JW, Vittum J, et al. The interaction of stressful life events and a serotonin transporter polymorphism in the prediction of episodes of major depression: a replication. Arch Gen Psychiatry 2005;62(5):529–35.
53. Uher R, McGuffin P. The moderation by the serotonin transporter gene of environmental adversity in the aetiology of mental illness: review and methodological analysis. Mol Psychiatry 2008;13(2):131–46.
54. Caspi A, Hariri AR, Holmes A, et al. Genetic sensitivity to the environment: the case of the serotonin transporter gene and its implications for studying complex diseases and traits. Am J Psychiatry 2010;167:509–27.
55. Risch N, Herrell R, Lehner T, et al. Interaction between the serotonin transporter gene (5-HTTLPR), stressful life events, and risk of depression. JAMA 2009; 301(23):2462–71.
56. Jacobs N, Kenis G, Peeters F, et al. Stress-related negative affectivity and genetically altered serotonin transporter function: evidence of synergism in shaping risk of depression. Arch Gen Psychiatry 2006;63:989–96.
57. Wichers M, Kenis G, Jacobs N, et al. The BDNF Val(66)Met x 5-HTTLPR x child adversity interaction and depressive symptoms: an attempt at replication. Am J Med Genet B Neuropsychiatr Genet 2008;147B:120–3.
58. Kumsta R, Stevens S, Brookes K, et al. HTT genotype moderates the influence of early institutional deprivation on emotional problems in adolescence: evidence from the English and Romanian Adoptee (ERA) study. J Child Psychol Psychiatry 2010;51(7):755–62.
59. Sugden K, Arseneault L, Harrington H, et al. Serotonin transporter gene moderates the development of emotional problems among children following bullying victimization. J Am Acad Child Adolesc Psychiatry 2010;49(8):830–40.
60. Aslund C, Leppert J, Comasco E, et al. Impact of the interaction between the 5HTTLPR polymorphism and maltreatment on adolescent depression. A population-based study. Behav Genet 2009;39(5):524–31.
61. Wilhelm K, Mitchell PB, Niven H, et al. Life events, first depression onset and the serotonin transporter gene. Br J Psychiatry 2006;188(3):210–5.
62. Cervilla JA, Rivera M, Molina E, et al. The 5-HTTLPR s/s genotype at the serotonin transporter gene (SLC6A4) increases the risk for depression in a large cohort of primary care attendees: the PREDICT-gene study. Am J Med Genet B Neuropsychiatr Genet 2007;141(8):912–7.

63. Araya R, Hu X, Heron J, et al. Effects of stressful life events, maternal depression and 5-HTTLPR genotype on emotional symptoms in pre-adolescent children. Am J Med Genet B Neuropsychiatr Genet 2009;150B(5):670–82.

64. Coventry WL, James MR, Eaves LJ, et al. Do 5HTTLPR and stress interact in risk for depression and suicidality? Item response analyses of a large sample. Am J Med Genet B Neuropsychiatr Genet 2010;153B(3):757–65.

65. Chorbov VM, Lobos EA, Todorov AA, et al. Relationship of 5-HTTLPR genotypes and depression risk in the presence of trauma in a female twin sample. Am J Med Genet B Neuropsychiatr Genet 2007;144B(6):830–3.

66. Munafo MR, Flint J. Replication and heterogeneity in gene x environment interaction studies. Int J Neuropsychopharmacol 2009;12(6):727–9.

67. Kaufman J, Yang BZ, Douglas-Palumberi H, et al. Social supports and serotonin transporter gene moderate depression in maltreated children. Proc Natl Acad Sci U S A 2004;101:17316–21.

68. Kaufman J, Yang BZ, Douglas-Palumberi H, et al. Brain-derived neurotrophic factor-5-HTTLPR gene interactions and environmental modifiers of depression in children. Biol Psychiatry 2006;59:673–80.

69. Aguilera M, Arias B, Wichers M, et al. Early adversity and 5-HT/BDNF genes: new evidence of gene-environment interactions on depressive symptoms in a general population. Psychol Med 2009;39(9):1425–32.

70. Ressler KJ, Bradley B, Mercer KB, et al. Polymorphisms in CRHR1 and the serotonin transporter loci: gene x gene x environment interactions on depressive symptoms. Am J Med Genet B Neuropsychiatr Genet 2010;153B(3): 812–24.

71. Cicchetti D, Rogosch FA, Sturge-Apple ML. Interactions of child maltreatment and serotonin transporter and monoamine oxidase A polymorphisms: depressive symptomatology among adolescents from low socioeconomic status backgrounds. Dev Psychopathol 2007;19(4):1161–80.

72. Brummett BH, Boyle SH, Siegler IC, et al. Effects of environmental stress and gender on associations among symptoms of depression and the serotonin transporter gene linked polymorphic region (5-HTTLPR). Behav Genet 2008; 38(1):34–43.

73. Lotrich FE, Pollock BG, Kirshner M, et al. Serotonin transporter genotype interacts with paroxetine plasma levels to influence depression treatment response. J Psychiatry Neurosci 2008;33(12):123–30.

74. Kim JM, Stewart R, Kim SW, et al. Modification by two genes of associations between general somatic health and incident depressive syndrome in older people. Psychosom Med 2009;71(3):286–91.

75. Grabe HJ, Lange M, Wolff B, et al. Mental and physical distress is modulated by a polymorphism in the 5-HT transporter gene interacting with social stressors and chronic disease burden. Mol Psychiatry 2005;10(2):220–4.

76. Mossner R, Henneberg A, Schmitt A, et al. Allelic variation of serotonin transporter expression is associated with depression in Parkinson's disease. Mol Psychiatry 2001;6(3):350–2.

77. Nakatani D, Sato H, Sakata Y, et al. Influence of serotonin transporter gene polymorphism on depressive symptoms and new cardiac events after acute myocardial infarction. Am Heart J 2005;150(4):652–8.

78. Leifheit-Limson EC, Reid KJ, Kasl SV, et al. The role of social support in health status and depressive symptoms after acute myocardial infarction: evidence for a stronger relationship among women. Circ Cardiovasc Qual Outcomes 2010; 3(2):143–50.

79. Ramasubbu R, Tobias R, Buchan A, et al. Serotonin transporter gene promoter region polymorphism associated with poststroke depression. J Neuropsychiatry Clin Neurosci 2006;18:96–9.

80. Kohen R, Cain KC, Mitchell PH, et al. Association of serotonin transporter gene polymorphisms with poststroke depression. Arch Gen Psychiatry 2008;65(11): 1296–302.

81. McCaffery JM, Duan QL, Frasure-Smith N, et al. Genetic predictors of depressive symptoms in cardiac patients. Am J Med Genet B Neuropsychiatr Genet 2009;150B(3):381–8.

82. Phillips-Bute B, Mathew JP, Blumenthal JA, et al. Relationship of genetic variability and depressive symptoms to adverse events after coronary artery bypass graft surgery. Psychosom Med 2008;70(9):953–9.

83. Whyte EM, Pollock BG, Wagner WR, et al. Influence of serotonin-transporter-linked promoter region polymorphism on platelet activation in geriatric depression. Am J Psychiatry 2001;158(12):2074–6.

84. Thomas AJ, Kalaria RN, O'Brien JT. Depression and vascular disease: what is the relationship? J Affect Disord 2004;79(1–3):81–95.

85. McCaffery JM, Frasure-Smith N, Dube M-P, et al. Common genetic vulnerability to depressive symptoms and coronary artery disease: a review and development of candidate genes related to inflammation and serotonin. Psychosom Med 2006;68(2):187–200.

86. Lotrich FE, Ferrell RE, Rabinovitz M, et al. Risk for depression during interferon-alpha treatment is affected by the serotonin transporter polymorphism. Biol Psychiatry 2009;65(4):344–8.

87. Bull SJ, Huezo-Diaz P, Binder EB, et al. Functional polymorphisms in the interleukin-6 and serotonin transporter genes, and depression and fatigue induced by interferon-a and ribavirin treatment. Mol Psychiatry 2008;14: 1095–104.

88. Kraus MR, Al-Taie O, Schefer A, et al. Serotonin-1A receptor gene (HTR1A) variation predicts interferon-induced depression chronic hepatitis C. Gastroenterology 2007;132(4):1279–86.

89. Su KP, Huang SY, Peng CY, et al. Phospholipase A2 and cyclooxygenase 2 genes influence the risk of interferon-a-induced depression by regulating polyunsaturated fatty acids levels. Biol Psychiatry 2010;67:550–7.

90. Musselman DL, Miller AH, Porter MR, et al. Higher than normal plasma interleukin-6 concentrations in cancer patients with depression: preliminary findings. Am J Psychiatry 2001;158(8):1252–7.

91. Morikawa O, Sakai N, Obara H, et al. Effects of interferon-alpha, interferon-gamma and cAMP on the transcriptional regulation of the serotonin transporter. Eur J Pharmacol 1998;349:317–24.

92. Mossner R, Daniel S, Schmitt A, et al. Modulation of serotonin transporter function by interleukin-4. Life Sci 2001;68:873–80.

93. Surtees PG, Wainwright NW, Willis-Owen SA, et al. Social adversity, the serotonin transporter (5-HTTLPR) polymorphism and major depressive disorder. Biol Psychiatry 2006;59:224–9.

94. Kim JM, Stewart R, Kim SW, et al. Interactions between life stressors and susceptibility genes (5-HTTLPR and BDNF) on depression in Korean elders. Biol Psychiatry 2007;62:423–8.

95. Goldman N, Glei DA, Lin YH, et al. The serotonin transporter polymorphism (5-HTTLPR): allelic variation and links with depressive symptoms. Depress Anxiety 2010;27(3):260–9.

96. Steffens DC, Taylor WD, McQuoid DR, et al. Short/long heterozygotes at 5HTTLPR and white matter lesions in geriatric depression. Int J Geriatr Psychiatry 2008;23(3):244–8.

97. Alexopoulos GS, Murphy CF, Gunning-Dixon FM, et al. Serotonin transporter polymorphisms, microstructural white matter abnormalities and remission of geriatric depression. J Affect Disord 2009;119(1–3):132–41.

98. Frodl T, Reinhold E, Koutsouleris N, et al. Childhood stress, serotonin transporter gene and brain structures in major depression. Neuropsychopharmacology 2010;35(6):1383–90.

99. Taylor WD, Steffens DC, Payne ME, et al. Influence of serotonin transporter promoter region polymorphisms on hippocampal volumes in late-life depression. Arch Gen Psychiatry 2005;62(5):537–44.

100. Hariri AR, Drabant EM, Munoz KE, et al. A susceptibility gene for affective disorders and the response of the human amygdala. Arch Gen Psychiatry 2005;62:146–52.

101. Friedel E, Schlagenhauf F, Sterzer P, et al. 5-HTT genotype effect on prefrontal-amygdala coupling differs between major depression and controls. Psychopharmacology 2009;205(2):261–71.

102. Pezawas L, Meyer-Lindenberg A, Drabant EM, et al. 5-HTTLPR polymorphism impacts human cingulate-amygdala interactions: a genetic susceptibility mechanism for depression. Nat Neurosci 2005;8:828–34.

103. Brummett BH, Krystal AD, Ashley-Koch A, et al. Sleep quality varies as a function of 5-HTTLPR genotype and stress. Psychosom Med 2008;69:621–4.

104. Alexander N, Kuepper Y, Schmitz A, et al. Gene-environment interactions predict cortisol responses after acute stress: implications for the etiology of depression. Psychoneuroendocrinology 2009;34(9):1294–303.

105. Mueller A, Brocke B, Fries E, et al. The role of the serotonin transporter polymorphism for the endocrine stress response in newborns. Psychoneuroendocrinology 2010;35(2):289–96.

106. Pariante CM, Miller AH. Glucocorticoid receptors in major depression: relevance to pathophysiology and treatment. Biol Psychiatry 2001;49(5):391–404.

107. Pace TW, Hu F, Miller AH. Cytokine-effects on glucocorticoid receptor function: relevance to glucocorticoid resistance and the pathophysiology and treatment of major depression. Brain Behav Immun 2007;21(1):9–19.

108. Miller GE, Cohen S, Ritchey AK. Chronic psychological stress and the regulation of pro-inflammatory cytokines: a glucocorticoid-resistance model. Health Psychol 2002;21:531–41.

109. de Kloet ER, Derijk RH, Meijer OC. Therapy insight: is there an imbalanced response of mineralocorticoid and glucocorticoid receptors in depression? Nat Clin Pract Endocrinol Metab 2007;3(2):168–79.

110. Derijk RH, de Kloet ER. Corticosteroid receptor polymorphisms: determinants of vulnerability and resilience. Eur J Pharmacol 2008;583(2–3):303–11.

111. Bet PM, Penninx BW, Bochdanovits Z, et al. Glucocorticoid receptor gene polymorphisms and childhood adversity are associated with depression: New evidence for a gene–environment interaction. Am J Med Genet B Neuropsychiatr Genet 2009;150B:660–9.

112. Tyrka AR, Price LH, Gelernter J, et al. Interaction of childhood maltreatment with the corticotropin-releasing hormone receptor gene: effects on hypothalamic-pituitary-adrenal axis reactivity. Biol Psychiatry 2009;66(7):681–5.

113. Bradley RG, Binder EB, Epstein MP, et al. Influence of child abuse on adult depression: moderation by the corticotropin-releasing hormone receptor gene. Arch Gen Psychiatry 2008;65(2):190–200.

114. Polanczyk G, Caspi A, Williams B, et al. Protective effect of CRHR1 gene variants on the development of adult depression following childhood maltreatment: replication and extension. Arch Gen Psychiatry 2009;66(9):978–85.

115. Glatz K, Mossner R, Heils A, et al. Glucocorticoid-regulated human serotonin transporter (5-HTT) expression is modulated by the 5-HTT gene-promoter-linked polymorphic region. J Neurochem 2003;86:1072–8.

116. Binder EB. The role of FKBP5, a co-chaperone of the glucocorticoid receptor in the pathogenesis and therapy of affective and anxiety disorders. Psychoneuroendocrinology 2009;34(Suppl 1):S186–95.

117. Binder EB, Salyakina D, Lichtner P, et al. Polymorphisms in FKBP5 are associated with increased recurrence of depressive episodes and rapid response to antidepressant treatment. Nat Genet 2004;36(12):1319–25.

118. Gillespie CF, Phifer J, Bradley K, et al. Risk and resilience: genetic and environmental influences on development of the stress response. Depress Anxiety 2009;26:984–92.

119. Claes S, Villafuerte S, Forsgren T, et al. The corticotropin-releasing hormone binding protein is associated with major depression in a population from Northern Sweden. Biol Psychiatry 2003;54(9):867–72.

120. Villafuerte SM, Del-Favero J, Adolfsson R, et al. Gene-based SNP genetic association study of the corticotropin-releasing hormone receptor-2 (CRHR2) in major depression. Am J Med Genet 2002;114(2):222–6.

121. Hwang JP, Tsai SJ, Hong CJ, et al. The Val66Met polymorphism of the brain-derived neurotrophic-factor gene is associated with geriatric depression. Neurobiol Aging 2005;27(12):1834–7.

122. Roth TL, Lubin FD, Funk AJ, et al. Lasting epigenetic influence of early-life adversity on the BDNF gene. Biol Psychiatry 2009;65(9):760–9.

123. Mossner R, Daniel S, Albert D, et al. Serotonin transporter function is modulated by brain-derived neurotrophic factor (BDNF) but not nerve growth factor (NGF). Neurochem Int 2000;36:197–202.

124. Schule C, Zill P, Baghai TC, et al. Brain-derived neurotrophic factor Val66Met polymorphism and dexamethasone/CRH test results in depressed patients. Psychoneuroendocrinology 2006;31(8):1019–25.

125. Lin E, Hong CJ, Hwang JP, et al. Gene-gene interactions of the brain-derived neurotrophic-factor and neurotrophic tyrosine kinase receptor 2 genes in geriatric depression. Rejuvenation Res 2009;12(6):387–93.

126. Perroud N, Aitchison KJ, Uher R, et al. Genetic predictors of increase in suicidal ideation during antidepressant treatment in the GENDEP project. Neuropsychopharmacology 2009;34(12):2517–28.

127. Drachmann BJ, Bock C, Vinberg M, et al. Interaction between genetic polymorphisms and stressful life events in first episode depression. J Affect Disord 2009;119(1–3):107–15.

128. Gatt JM, Nemeroff CB, Dobson-Stone C, et al. Interactions between BDNF Val66Met polymorphism and early life stress predict brain and arousal pathways to syndromal depression and anxiety. Mol Psychiatry 2009;14(7):681–95.

129. Golimbet V, Alfimova M, Korovaitseva G, et al. Emotional distress in parents of psychotic patients is modified by serotonin transporter gene (5-HTTLPR)–brain-derived neurotrophic factor gene interactions. Span J Psychol 2009;12(2):696–706.

130. Conway C, Hammen C, Brennan PA, et al. Interaction of chronic stress with serotonin transporter and catechol-O-methyltransferase polymorphisms in predicting youth depression. Depress Anxiety 2010;27(8):737–45.

131. Doornbos B, Dijck-Brouwer DA, Kema IP, et al. The development of peripartum depressive symptoms is associated with gene polymorphisms of MAOA, 5-HTT and COMT. Prog Neuropsychopharmacol Biol Psychiatry 2009;33(7): 1250–4.
132. Chipman P, Jorm AF, Tan XY, et al. No association between the serotonin-1A receptor gene single nucleotide polymorphism rs6295C/G and symptoms of anxiety or depression, and no interaction between the polymorphism and environmental stressors of childhood anxiety or recent stressful life events on anxiety or depression. Psychiatr Genet 2010;20(1):8–13.
133. Neumeister A, Young TL, Stastny J. Implications of genetic research on the role of the serotonin in depression: emphasis on the serotonin type 1A receptor and the serotonin transporter. Psychopharmacology (Berl) 2004;174:512–24.
134. Jokela M, Lehtimaki T, Keltikangas-Jarvinen L. The influence of urban/rural residency on depressive symptoms is moderated by the serotonin receptor 2A gene. Am J Med Genet B Neuropsychiatr Genet 2007;144B(7):918–22.
135. Gatt JM, Williams LM, Schofield PR, et al. Impact of the HTR3A gene with early life trauma on emotional brain networks and depressed mood. Depress Anxiety 2010;27(8):752–9.
136. Xu Y, Li F, Huang X, et al. The norepinephrine transporter gene modulates the relationship between urban/rural residency and major depressive disorder in a Chinese population. Psychiatry Res 2009;168(3):213–7.
137. Oxenkrug GF. Metabolic syndrome, age-associated neuroendocrine disorders, and dysregulation of tryptophan-kynurenine metabolism. Ann N Y Acad Sci 2010;1199:1–14.
138. Gabbay V, Klein RG, Katz Y, et al. The possible role of the kynurenine pathway in adolescent depression with melancholic features. J Child Psychol Psychiatry 2010;51(8):935–43.
139. Wichers MC, Maes M. The role of indoleamine 2,3-dioxygenase (IDO) in the pathophysiology of interferon-alpha-induced depression. J Psychiatry Neurosci 2004;29(1):11–7.
140. Markus CR, Firk C. Differential effects of tri-allelic 5-HTTLPR polymorphisms in healthy subjects on mood and stress performance after tryptophan challenge. Neuropsychopharmacology 2009;34(13):2667–74.
141. Walderhaug E, Magnusson A, Neumeister A, et al. Interactive effects of sex and 5-HTTLPR on mood and impulsivity during tryptophan depletion in healthy people. Biol Psychiatry 2007;62(6):593–9.
142. Neumeister A, Konstantinidis A, Stastny J, et al. Association between serotonin transporter gene promoter polymorphism (5HTTLPR) and behavioral responses to tryptophan depletion in healthy women with and without family history of depression. Arch Gen Psychiatry 2002;59(7):613–20.
143. Jokela M, Raikkonen K, Lehtimak IT, et al. Tryptophan hydroxylase 1 gene (TPH1) moderates the influence of social support on depressive symptoms in adults. J Affect Disord 2007;100(1–3):191–7.
144. Keltikangas-Jarvinen L, Puttonen S, Kivimaki ME, et al. Tryptophan hydroxylase 1 gene haplotypes modify the effect of a hostile childhood environment on adulthood harm avoidance. Genes Brain Behav 2007;6:305–13.
145. Nobile M, Ruscon IM, Bellina M, et al. The influence of family structure, the TPH2 G-703T and the 5-HTTLPR serotonergic genes upon affective problems in children aged 10–14 years. J Child Psychol Psychiatry 2009;50(3):317–25.
146. Comings DE, Muhleman D, Dietz G, et al. Sequence of human tryptophan 2,3-dioxygenase (TDO2): presence of a glucocorticoid response-like element

composed of a GTT repeat and an intronic CCCCT repeat. Genomics 1995;29: 390–6.
147. Kravitz M, Janssen I, Lotrich FE, et al. Sex steroid hormone gene polymorphisms and depressive symptoms. Am J Med 2006;119(Suppl 1):87–93.
148. Cole SW, Arevalo JM, Takahashi R, et al. Computational identification of gene-social environment interaction at the human IL6 locus. Proc Natl Acad Sci U S A 2010;107(12):5681–6.
149. Traykov L, Bayle A, Latour F, et al. Apolipoprotein E epsilon4 allele frequency in elderly depressed patients with and without cerebrovascular disease. J Neurol Sci 2007;257(1–2):280–3.
150. Sjoholm LK, Melas PA, Forsell Y, et al. PreproNPY Pro7 protects against depression despite exposure to environmental risk factors. J Affect Disord 2009; 118(1–3):124–30.
151. Juhasz G, Chase D, Pegg E, et al. CNR1 gene is associated with high neuroticism and low agreeableness and interacts with recent negative life events to predict current depressive symptoms. Neuropsychopharmacology 2009;34(8): 2019–27.
152. Wong ML, Dong C, Maestre-Mesa J, et al. Polymorphisms in inflammation-related genes are associated with susceptibility to major depression and antidepressant response. Mol Psychiatry 2008;13(8):800–12.
153. Chen P, Jiang T, Ouyang J, et al. Epigenetic programming of diverse glucocorticoid response and inflammatory/immune-mediated disease. Med Hypotheses 2009;73(5):657–8.
154. Tsankova NM, Berton O, Renthal W, et al. Sustained hippocampal chromatin regulation in a mouse model of depression and antidepressant action. Nat Neurosci 2006;9(4):519–25.
155. Weaver IC, Cervoni N, Champagne FA, et al. Epigenetic programming by maternal behavior. Nat Neurosci 2004;7:847–53.
156. McGowan PO, Sasaki A, D'Alessio AC, et al. Epigenetic regulation of the glucocorticoid receptor in human brain associates with childhood abuse. Nat Neurosci 2009;12(3):342–8.
157. Keller S, Sarchiapone M, Zarrilli F, et al. Increased BDNF promoter methylation in the Wernicke area of suicide subjects. Arch Gen Psychiatry 2010;67(3):258–67.
158. Alt SR, Turner JD, Klok MD, et al. Differential expression of glucocorticoid receptor transcripts in major depressive disorder is not epigenetically programmed. Psychoneuroendocrinology 2010;35(4):544–56.
159. Philibert R, Madan A, Andersen A, et al. Serotonin transporter mRNA levels are associated with the methylation of an upstream CpG island. Am J Med Genet B Neuropsychiatr Genet 2007;114B(1):101–5.
160. Philibert RA, Sandhu H, Hollenbeck N, et al. The relationship of 5HTT (SLC6A4) methylation and genotype on mRNA expression and liability to major depression and alcohol dependence in subjects from the Iowa Adoption Studies. Am J Med Genet B Neuropsychiatr Genet 2008;150B(1):153.
161. Olsson CA, Foley DL, Parkinson-Bates M, et al. Prospects for epigenetic research within cohort studies of psychological disorder: a pilot investigation of a peripheral cell marker of epigenetic risk for depression. Biol Psychol 2010;83(2):159–65.
162. Kendler KS, Kuhn J, Prescott CA. The interrelationship of neuroticism, sex, and stressful life events in the prediction of episodes of major depression. Am J Psychiatry 2004;161:631–6.

Psychosocial Interventions for Late-life Major Depression: Evidence-Based Treatments, Predictors of Treatment Outcomes, and Moderators of Treatment Effects

Dimitris N. Kiosses, PhD[a],*, Andrew C. Leon, PhD[b],
Patricia A. Areán, PhD[c]

KEYWORDS

- Psychosocial interventions • Evidence-based treatments
- Late-life depression • Moderators of treatment effects

The science of interventions is shifting from adapting current interventions for different populations and settings to investing in novel, potentially more effective, personalized interventions.[1] The recent *From Discovery to Cure* National Institute of Mental Health (NIMH) report on future directions for interventions research recommends that interventions researchers focus on understanding moderators of treatment response to better match patients to existing evidence-based practices and to develop new interventions for those who do not respond to any existing treatments.[2] This article reviews the efficacy of psychosocial interventions for the acute treatment of late-life major depression and identifies variables that predict treatment outcomes and moderate

[a] Department of Psychiatry, Weill-Cornell Medical College, 21 Bloomingdale Road, White Plains, NY 10605, USA
[b] Department of Psychiatry, Weill Cornell Medical College, 525 East 68th Street, Box 140, New York, NY 10065, USA
[c] Department of Psychiatry, University of California in San Francisco, 401 Parnassus Avenue, San Francisco, CA 94143, USA
* Corresponding author.
E-mail address: dkiosses@med.cornell.edu

Psychiatr Clin N Am 34 (2011) 377–401
doi:10.1016/j.psc.2011.03.001
0193-953X/11/$ – see front matter © 2011 Elsevier Inc. All rights reserved.

treatment effects. Based on the review of the literature as well as our scientific observations, we propose future directions that may advance the development of personalized treatments.

Our focus on major depressive disorder (MDD) in this population is important for the following reasons. First, major depression interacts with, and can exacerbate, cognitive impairment, disability, and medical illnesses, which often occur in older adults.[3] As a result, late-life MDD is associated with reduced quality of life, family disruption, high rates of use of medical services, and increased medical morbidity and mortality, including death from suicide.[4] Moreover, compared with milder forms of late-life depression, late-life MDD has more persistent and difficult to treat symptoms, greater disability, and higher rates of suicidal ideation.[5,6]

To our knowledge, this is the first systematic review of psychosocial interventions for late-life MDD that addresses questions related to personalized treatment development by examining predictors of treatment outcomes and moderators of treatment effects. Specifically, we answer the following questions: which treatments are efficacious in treating late-life MDD and which require more investigation? Which variables predict treatment outcomes and which variables moderate treatment effects of psychosocial interventions in late-life MDD? What are the necessary next steps to advance psychosocial interventions for older adults with MDD? The review may provide some guidance on the development of personalized interventions at the patient level.

METHODS

Studies were selected through searches of PUBMED (1966–2010), PsychINFO (1840–2010), Cochrane database, as well through previous reviews and meta-analyses.[7–22] Specifically, searches were conducted using combinations of the following keywords (the * denotes any combination of the word): random*, psychother*, psychosoc*, intervention, older, predict*, moderat*, mediat*,and elder*. The final selection of the publications was based on those American Psychological Association (APA) Division 12 criteria[23,24] that are pertinent to studies for the acute treatment of late-life MDD and additional statistical criteria regarding sample size and intent-to-treat analysis.

Selection of Studies

Inclusion of randomized controlled trials
The following are the criteria for the inclusion of studies: (a) a randomized controlled trial (RCT); (b) a psychosocial intervention (not including interventions at the organizational level or systems-level collaborative care models); (c) acute treatment of diagnosed unipolar MDD (based on a diagnosis by DSM-II, DSM-III-R, DSM-IV, RDC, ICD-9 or ICD-10, Primary Care Evaluation of Mental Disorders-PRIME-MD); (d) published in English; (e) with an average age of participants 60 years old or older. Consistent with the recent NIMH recommendation to broaden the focus of outcome measures,[25] we included RCTs that did not have a depression outcome, for example disability, quality of life, cost. We did not include articles that performed an interim analysis of an RCT because results of interim analyses are not conclusive about the efficacy of the interventions.

Initial selection Each study needed to meet the following APA Division 12[23] study design criteria:

1. study clearly stated inclusion and exclusion criteria
2. study determined clinical as well statistical significance

3. a treatment manual was used
4. treatment fidelity was assessed, or on-going supervision was provided, by experts in the psychosocial interventions
5. reliable and valid instruments were administered
6. research assessments were conducted by raters unaware of the participant's randomization status (**Table 1**).

Final selection Our final selection was based on the following statistical criteria:

1. The study had at least 30 participants per condition. The rationale for excluding studies with small sample sizes is that they do not provide a meaningful estimate of the between-group effect size because of the imprecision inherent in small samples, as embodied in wide confidence intervals.[26] Thirty participants per arm is the minimum number to detect a Cohen d of 0.74 effect size with 80% power.[27] Our choice of 30 participants per condition is arbitrary; ideally, we would have liked to use a much larger sample size that could detect smaller but clinically meaningful effects,[28] but these studies are rarely available in late-life MDD (see **Table 1**).
2. Intent-to-treat analyses were performed. We decided to include studies that have performed intent-to-treat analyses such that they adhere to the virtue of randomization for estimating treatment effects.[29]

Defining efficacy
Efficacy was assessed based on the RCTs that met both study design and statistical criteria. An intervention is considered efficacious, if there are at least 2 RCTs, conducted by independent investigators,[23,24] showing that the intervention is superior to a credible comparison group (ie, one that accounts for the passage of time, increased attention, expectation of therapeutic intervention, and the psychological consequences of legitimized sick role)[30] (Mental Health: A Report of the Surgeon General, 1999). An intervention is probably efficacious, pending replication (ie, the intervention has supportive evidence of efficacy but the results need to be replicated) if there is at least 1 RCT (or 2 or more RCTs conducted by the same investigative team) showing that the intervention is superior to a credible comparison group. An intervention has inconclusive evidence, if it does not fit into any of the 2 previous categories; for example, there has been only 1 RCT with negative results.

This review does not include interventions at the organizational level or systems-level collaborative care models, including IMPACT,[31] PROSPECT,[32] HOPE-D,[33] PRISM-E,[34] and RESPECT[35] because the relative effect of psychosocial interventions cannot be determined by the designs of these studies. The treatments were given in combination with other depression interventions, clouding the overall impact of psychosocial interventions[36]; for example, in IMPACT, patients who received problem-solving therapy (PST) were often also treated with antidepressant medication, and those who were not were provided with case management support and behavioral activation strategies.

During our search, we encountered RCTs of psychosocial interventions in mixed samples of participants with diagnosis of MDD and participants with diagnosis of minor depression and/or dysthymia. These studies were not included because they did not meet the study design and statistical criteria. Specifically, most of the studies did not have 30 or more MDD participants per arm, did not perform intent-to-treat between treatment groups statistical analyses in the MDD subgroup, or their randomization was not stratified by depression diagnosis (for example, see Refs.[37–48]).

Moderators of treatment effects in RCTs To design subsequent studies that focus on personalized treatment, we need to identify moderators of treatment effects.[49,50]

Table 1
Randomized clinical trials of psychosocial interventions for the acute treatment of late-life major depression that met study design criteria

Article	Comparison Groups	Total N	Mean Age (y)	≥30 Participants per Arm	Intent-to-treat Analysis	Outcomes	Summary of Results
Gallagher et al,[98] 1982	BT vs CT vs BIP	30	67.77	No	No	Depression	There were no significant differences between the 3 groups after treatment. However, there was reduction in depression in all 3 groups on HDRS, BDI, and Zung Self-rating Depression Scale, from an average of moderate depression severity (before treatment) to mild depression (after treatment)
Thompson et al,[83] 1987	BT vs CT vs BDT vs DEL	91	67.07	Yes	No	Depression/ anxiety/ coping skills	Combined treatment had significantly better scores than delayed treatment control on BDI, HDRS, BSI: depression, BSI: anxiety, BSI: global severity. There were no significant differences on any outcome among 3 treatments
Gallagher-Thompson et al,[84] 1990	BT vs CT vs BDT vs DEL	91	67.07	Yes	No	Depression	There were no significant differences among 3 treatments in diagnostic outcome (MDD, minor depression, not depressed based on SADS-change interview) after treatment
Areán et al,[77] 1993	PST vs RT vs WLC	75	66.5	No	Yes	Depression/well-being	Subjects in PST and RT had significantly less depression after treatment compared with their pretreatment scores according to all 3 depression measures (HDRS, GDS, BDI), whereas WLC subjects displayed no significant improvement. PST participants were also significantly less depressed than RT subjects according to their posttreatment HDRS and GDS scores but not according to their posttreatment BDI scores.
Klausner et al,[99] 1998	GFGP vs RT	13	66.8	No	No	Depression	Both groups had significant reduction in depression from before to after treatment, but participants in the GFGP group had more significant improvement than RT participants in HDRS

Study	Treatment	N	Age			Outcome	Results
Reynolds et al,[67] 1999	IPT+NT vs IPT+ PBO vs PBO vs NT	80	66.13	No	Yes	Depression/ bereavement severity	A significant positive NT effect was detected on remission vs no remission outcome; ie, remission: IPT+NT = 69%, IPT+PBO = 29%, NT = 56%, PBO = 45%. There was no main effect of IPT or an interaction effect of IPT by NT.
Rokke et al,[100] 2000	Self-Management Group vs Educational Group Therapy vs WLC	34	67.2	No	No	Depression/ pleasant events/self-management	Combined treatment vs no treatment: 56% of WLC participants had no diagnosis of depression after treatment vs 89% of participants in either self-management group or educational group. Participants in the combined treatment had significantly reduced depression scores after treatment compared with participants in the WLC condition on BDI but not on GDS or HDRS. Self-management vs educational group therapy: No significant differences between the 2 groups on percentage of participants without a diagnosis of depression after treatment and on reduction of depression on BDI, GDS, or HDRS
Thompson et al,[71] 2001	CBT vs desipramine vs CBT+ desipramine	100	66.85	Yes	Yes	Depression	There was a significant reduction in depressive symptoms as measured by the HDRS in all 3 conditions. The per-session rate of change for the combined condition was significantly greater than for the desipramine condition; however, the comparisons of the combined condition vs CBT-alone and of CBT vs desipramine were not significant
Alexopoulos et al,[78] 2003	PST vs ST	25	74.12	No	Yes	Depression/ disability	PST group had greater change in depression (HDRS) scores than the ST group. A significantly higher percentage of PST participants remitted than of ST participants. PST led to a more rapid improvement in disability (WHODAS-II) than ST

(continued on next page)

Table 1
(continued)

Article	Comparison Groups	Total N	Mean Age (y)	≥30 Participants per Arm	Intent-to-treat Analysis	Outcomes	Summary of Results
Sirey et al,[85] 2005	TIP vs TAU	52	73.2	No	Yes	Depression/antidepressant treatment adherence	TIP participants showed greater improvement in depression than the treatment as usual group. A significantly higher percentage of TIP participants remitted than of the control group participants. More intervention patients remained in treatment than patients in the nonintervention group
van Schaik et al,[72] 2006	IPT vs UC	143	67.93	Yes	Yes	Depression/physical functioning	There was a significantly higher percentage of participants in IPT without a depression diagnosis at 6 mo (1 mo after the end of treatment) compared with participants in UC. There was no significant difference between participants in IPT vs participants in UC in percentages of responders or remitters (MADRS<10). There was no significant difference in reduction of depression severity between the 2 groups at 6 mo
Bosmans et al,[73] 2007	IPT vs UC	143	67.93	Yes	Yes	Cost	There were no statistically significant differences in total costs between the 2 groups at 6 mo. IPT was not significantly more cost-effective than UC at 6 mo
Strachowski et al,[101] 2008	CBT vs WLC	48	62.24	No	No	Depression/positive affect/perceived stress/quality of life	CBT participants were significantly less depressed than WLC participants in post-treatment HDRS and BDI. Further, CBT participants, compared to WLC participants, had significantly greater improvement in positive affect and overall quality of life as well as reduction in perceived stress and negative affect
Laidlaw et al,[102] 2008	CBT vs TAU	40	74.03	No	Yes	Depression/worry/quality of life	Participants in both groups in this study benefited from treatment with significantly reduced scores on primary measures of mood (BDI, GDS, and HDRS) at end of treatment. However, there was no significant difference on depression outcomes between participants in CBT vs TAU

Study	Comparison	N	Age			Outcome	Results
Sirey et al,[76] 2010	TIP vs TAU	70	76	Yes	Yes	Depression/antidepressant treatment adherence	TIP participants had higher rates of adherence than TAU participants at 12 wk (end of intervention); specifically, 82% of TIP participants were adherent more than 80% of the time compared with 43% of participants in TAU. Participants in TIP had a greater reduction of depressive symptoms than participants in TAU at the end of intervention
Areán et al,[74] 2010	PST vs ST	221	73	Yes	Yes	Depression	Both PST and ST were associated with reduction of depression (HDRS) from baseline to 12 wk. However, participants in PST had greater reduction of depression (HDRS) than participants in the ST condition. There was no significant difference in response or remission rates between PST vs ST at 3 and 6 wk but there were significantly higher response and remission rates in PST vs ST at 9 and 12 wk
Alexopoulos et al,[75] 2011	PST vs ST	221	72.90	Yes	Yes	Disability	PST participants had significantly greater reduction in disability (total WHODAS scores) from baseline to 12 wk than ST participants
Kiosses et al,[103] 2010	PATH vs ST	30	79.41	No	Yes	Depression/disability	PATH participants had significantly greater reduction in depression and disability, from baseline to 12 wk, than ST participants. PATH and ST had comparable high rates of treatment satisfaction

Abbreviations: BDI, Beck Depression Inventory; BDT, brief dynamic therapy; BIP, brief relational/insight psychotherapy; BSI, brief symptom inventory; BT, behavior therapy; CBT, cognitive behavioral therapy; CT, cognitive therapy; DEL, delayed treatment condition; GDS, Geriatric Depression Scale; GFGP, goal-focused group psychotherapy; HDRS, Hamilton Depression Rating Scale; IPT, interpersonal psychotherapy; MADRS, Montgomery Asberg Depression Scale; NT, nortriptyline; PATH, problem adaptation therapy; PBO, placebo; PST, problem-solving therapy; RT, reminiscence therapy; ST, supportive therapy; TAU, treatment as usual; TIP, Treatment Initiation and Participation Program; UC, usual care; WHODAS, World Health Organization Disability Assessment Schedule; WLC, waiting-list condition.

Moderators are pretreatment variables that are associated with a between treatment groups effect size.[49] For instance, patients with baseline executive dysfunction may respond better to interventions that rely on compensatory cognitive strategies to improve mood than to interventions that do not use these strategies, whereas patients without cognitive impairment may have comparable responses with either intervention. Initial analyses of moderators are exploratory. Descriptive, not inferential, analyses are used; the focus is on the magnitude of the treatment effect, not on P values.[49]

Predictors of treatment outcomes To help identify potential moderators for future RCTs, we examined predictors of treatment outcomes in studies of psychosocial interventions for the acute treatment of late-life MDD. Predictors include baseline variables that have a main effect of, but not necessarily an interaction effect with, treatment (ie, if they had an interaction effect, they would be moderators) or postbaseline variables that are correlated with treatment outcome. To broaden the list of predictors, we used less stringent criteria than those evaluating efficacy and moderators of treatment effects, ie, including open acute trials in addition to RCTs (**Table 2**).

RESULTS AND DISCUSSION

We identified 404 articles, 78 of which were clinical trials of psychosocial interventions in older adults and were published in English. Thirty-nine of those focused on the acute treatment of elders with diagnosis of unipolar, nonpsychotic MDD. Eight articles were excluded because they performed interim analyses or did not fully randomize their participants.[51–58] Thirteen articles performed analyses only on predictors of treatment outcomes.[5,59–70] The remaining 18 RCT articles met the specified study design criteria and only 6 of those met the additional statistical criteria of 30 or more participants per arm and intent-to-treat analysis (see **Table 1**).

In the final selection of 6 studies, there were only 4 unique samples: (1) Thompson and colleagues,[71] 2001; (2) van Shaik and colleagues[72] and Bosmans and colleagues[73]; (3) Arean and colleagues[74] and Alexopoulos and colleagues[75]; and (4) Sirey and colleagues.[76] Specifically, van Shaik and colleagues,[72] and Bosmans and colleagues[73] conducted analyses of the same sample on depression and cost, respectively, while Arean and colleagues[74] and Alexopoulos and colleagues[75] performed analyses of the same sample using depression and disability outcomes respectively.

WHICH INTERVENTIONS ARE EFFICACIOUS?

This is the first important question whose answer can guide the efficient development of personalized approaches to psychosocial interventions. Our determination of efficacy was based on the 6 articles that met both study design and statistical criteria. No psychosocial interventions met the criteria of being efficacious for the acute treatment of late-life MDD. Three psychosocial interventions were probably efficacious, pending replication (problem solving therapy, cognitive behavioral therapy, treatment initiation and participation program), and 2 interventions showed inconclusive results (interpersonal psychotherapy, supportive therapy).

Psychosocial Interventions with Supportive Evidence of Efficacy, Pending Replication

Problem solving therapy
PST targets depression by systematically teaching patients skills for improving their ability to deal with specific everyday problems and life crises, rather than developing

generic skills. Patients identify problems, brainstorm different ways to solve their problems, create action plans, and evaluate their effectiveness in implementing the best possible solution.

Results Only 1 RCT met both study design and statistical criteria. Arean and colleagues[74] and Alexopoulos and colleagues[75] presented the study results on depression and disability outcomes respectively. The study tested PST versus supportive therapy in 221 older subjects with MDD and executive dysfunction.

Participants in PST had significantly greater reduction of depression on the Hamilton Depression Rating Scale (HDRS) than participants in the supportive therapy (ST) condition (at week 9, Cohen $d = 0.24$; at week 12, Cohen $d = 0.39$).[74] Further, PST participants had significantly greater reduction in disability (World Health Organization Disability Assessment Schedule [WHODAS]-II) than ST participants by approximately 0.18 points per week.[75]

Conclusion Based on this RCT, PST is probably efficacious in reducing depression and disability, pending replication. These results are consistent with 2 PST studies that met the study design but not the statistical criteria.[77,78]

Cognitive behavioral therapy

Studies followed the approach of Beck and colleagues,[79] which was modified by Emery[80] and Thompson and colleagues[81] for older adults. Patients were taught to monitor, evaluate, and modify negative dysfunctional thoughts and distorted perceptions and beliefs, and learn to use cognitive techniques such as reattribution, listing pros and cons, and examining the evidence. In addition to the cognitive techniques, patients were encouraged to increase their activity scheduling.

Results Only 1 RCT met both study design and statistical criteria (see **Table 1**).[70] In this study, cognitive behavioral therapy (CBT) plus desipramine was compared with CBT alone and desipramine alone. The patients were seen twice a week for the first 4 weeks and once for the following 8 to 12 weeks. Desipramine was started at a low dose of 10 mg and was gradually increased depending on the patient's tolerance to side effects, following a protocol developed by the NIMH Treatment of Depression Collaborative Research Program.[82] The mean stable daily dose of desipramine was 90 ($\pm$63) mg and the mean plasma level of desipramine was 123 ng/mL. In the CBT plus desipramine condition, the CBT therapist followed the same protocol as in the CBT-alone condition.

Patients in the CBT plus desipramine group had significantly greater reduction than participants in the desipramine-alone condition in both interviewer (HDRS) (rate of change per session, desipramine = -0.20; CBT plus desipramine = -0.41) and self-report depression (Beck Depression Inventory-Short Form [BDI-SF]) instruments (rate of change per session: desipramine = -0.10; CBT plus desipramine = -0.44). Participants in the CBT-alone condition had significantly greater reduction in depression compared with the desipramine-alone condition in BDI-SF and comparable reductions in depression in HDRS.

Conclusion Based on this RCT, CBT is a probably efficacious psychosocial intervention, pending replication. Additional RCTs that met the study design but not the statistical criteria have also shown that CBT participants had greater reduction in depression than those who were delayed treatment.[83,84] Further, in a large primary care study of participants diagnosed with major or minor depression (88% MDD, 12% minor), participants receiving CBT had significant greater reduction in

Table 2
Predictors of treatment outcomes in clinical trials of psychosocial interventions for the acute treatment of late-life major depression

Article	Comparison Groups	RCT	Predictors Examined	Results
Gallagher et al,[59] 1983	BT vs CT vs BIP	Yes	Endogenous vs nonendogenous depression at start of therapy	Participants with nonendogenous depression had significantly lower depression scores at the end of treatment compared with participants with endogenous depression on 2 out of 3 depression instruments (HDRS and BDI but not Zung Self-rating Depression Scale). The groups had comparable pretreatment depression scores. Similarly, a significantly higher percentage of participants with nonendogenous depression were responders at the end of treatment compared with participants with endogenous depression based on BDI≤10
Marmar et al,[60] 1989	BT vs CT vs BDT	Yes[a]	Patients' and therapists' ratings of treatment alliance at fifth session	Ratings of treatment alliance completed by therapists at fifth session were not significantly correlated with treatment outcome. However, ratings in a single domain of treatment alliance, patient commitment, when completed by patients at fifth session, were significantly correlated with treatment outcomes in the whole sample and in those patients in the CT arm
Gaston et al,[61] 1989	BT vs CT vs BDT	Yes[a]	Patients' expectations of 3 change processes (insight and support, behavioral and cognitive changes, and medication and environmental changes)	Levels of patient expectations of change processes were not significantly different among BT vs CT vs BDT. Patient expectations of change processes were not related to depression outcome (HDRS). However, greater expectation of gaining help through behavioral and cognitive changes was associated with less depressive symptoms at termination in CT; this association was not present in BT or BDT
Karp et al,[69] 1993	Open acute treatment of NT+IPT	No	Sociodemographic and clinical variables, including age, presence of a stress-provoking agent, PD, social support	Presence of a stress-provoking agent, eccentric cluster personality features (ie, paranoid, schizoid, and schizotypal) and earlier age at first episode were associated with prolonged time to remission. Two of the 4 variables, presence of a stress-provoking agent and perception of diminished social support, were also significant in the final model

Miller et al,[63] 1996	Open acute treatment of NT+IPT	No	Perception of illness, age, baseline depression severity, and medical burden	Age and baseline perception of illness, but not baseline medical burden or depression severity, predicted response in 75% of the participants
Dew et al,[64] 1997	Open acute treatment of NT+IPT	No	Baseline chronic stress, depression severity, anxiety level, social support, likelihood that a life stressor precipitated current episode, age at first lifetime episode, subjective sleep assessment, percentage of REM sleep, REM activity	Baseline low chronic stress, low likelihood that a life stressor precipitated current episode, older age at first lifetime episode, less severe depressive symptoms, lower anxiety level, less subjective sleep impairment, lower percentage of REM sleep, and less REM activity were the most important predictors of having a more rapid, sustained response. In contrast, poor social support, high likelihood that a major life stressor precipitated current episode, endogenous depression, and long sleep latency were associated with partial or mixed response
Reynolds et al,[88] 1999	Open acute treatment of NT+IPT	No	Two age groups (60–69 vs 70+ y old)	The two age groups (<70 and 70+ y) did not differ in absolute remission rates and in time to remission
Lenze et al,[65] 2001	Open acute treatment of NT+IPT	No	Age, gender, education, baseline depression severity, social adjustment, personality disorder, social adjustment, and disability	Lower self-rated health (perception of illness), greater personality disorder, and greater IADL disability were associated with greater likelihood of failure to remit in univariate analysis; however, only lower self-rated health was associated with greater likelihood of failure to remit in the multivariate model.
Gildengers et al,[5] 2005	Participants from open acute treatments with NT+IPT or paroxetine+IPT	No	Baseline depression severity, self-esteem, illness duration, age	Greater baseline depression severity was a significant risk factor for slower response in NT+IPT and in PX+IPT samples. Higher self-esteem was significantly associated with more rapid response in NT+IPT, whereas longer duration of illness was associated with a slower response trajectory in PX+IPT. Similarly, greater baseline depression severity was a significant risk factor for nonresponse in PX+IPT, but not in NT+IPT, whereas older age was associated with nonresponse in the NT+IPT sample

(continued on next page)

Table 2
(continued)

Article	Comparison Groups	RCT	Predictors Examined	Results
Oslin[62] 2005	Naltrexone+ sertraline+ psychosocial intervention vs sertraline+ psychosocial intervention	No	Heavy drinking, complete abstinence	Relapse to heavy drinking was associated with a reduction in treatment response as measured by remission of depression or by absolute improvement in symptoms. Complete abstinence was not associated with improvement in depression. Similar findings were found when considering the percentage of days of heavy drinking. More frequent bouts of heavy drinking during the trial were associated with lower rates of improvement in depression and reduction in HDRS scores
Karp et al,[66] 2005	Open acute treatment of paroxetine+IPT	No	Baseline depression severity, suicide ideation, body pain	Baseline severity of depressive symptoms, HDRS suicide probe, and pain were significantly lower in the subjects who responded vs in those who did not.
Morse et al,[70] 2005	Open acute treatment of NT+IPT	No	Cluster C PD	Cluster C PD was not associated with residual depressive symptom status or responder status at the end of acute treatment; however, cluster C PD predicted longer to response (median time to response: no PD = 9.86 wk; cluster C PD = 14.43 wk).
Andreescu et al,[68] 2007	Open acute treatment of paroxetine+IPT	No	Baseline anxiety level	A statistically lower percentage of patients with scores more than the median in the anxiety scale of BSI achieved response compared with the percentage of patients with scores less than the median who achieved response (52% vs 75% respectively). Patients with higher BSI scores had a significantly longer median time to response than those with lower BSI scores (11 vs 6.7 wk).

Abbreviations: BDI, Beck Depression Inventory; BIP, brief relational/insight psychotherapy; BT, behavior therapy; CBT, cognitive behavioral therapy; CT, cognitive therapy; GDS, Geriatric Depression Scale; HDRS, Hamilton Depression Rating Scale; IADL, instrumental activities of daily living; IPT, interpersonal psychotherapy; PD, personality disorder; PST, problem-solving therapy; REM, rapid eye movement; RT, reminiscence therapy; ST, supportive therapy; UC, usual care; WLC, waiting-list condition.

[a] Study was conducted on a subset of participants of the original RCT (Thompson and colleagues, 1987[83]; Gallagher-Thompson and colleagues, 1990[84]).

depression than participants in treatment as usual or participants in a talking control condition.[48]

Treatment Initiation and Participation Program

The Treatment Initiation and Participation (TIP) intervention is a brief, individualized intervention in primary care in conjunction with pharmacotherapy that identifies barriers to adherence in antidepressant medication treatment and uses cognitive behavior techniques to address these barriers and improve adherence to treatment.[76,85] TIP is based on the theory of reasoned actions and targets modifiable factors of adherence[86] including psychological barriers, stigma, concerns surrounding treatment, and fears of antidepressants.[76,85] TIP includes 3 in-person sessions (30 minutes each) during the first 6 weeks of pharmacotherapy and 2 short follow-up telephone sessions. The duration of intervention is 12 weeks.

Results Only 1 RCT[55] met both study design and statistical criteria (see **Table 1**). Participants in TIP had significantly greater reduction in depression at 12 weeks (end of intervention) than participants in the usual care (UC) group. Moreover, TIP participants achieved higher adherence rates to antidepressant treatment than participants in the control group. Specifically, at the 12-week follow-up, 82% of TIP participants were adherent (at the 80% level or more) compared with 43% of participants in the treatment as usual arm.

Conclusion TIP is a probably efficacious psychosocial intervention in conjunction with pharmacotherapy, pending replication. In another study that met the study design but did not meet the sample size criterion,[85] TIP participants had a significant reduction in depression at 12 weeks compared with UC participants.

Interventions with Inconclusive Evidence

Supportive therapy

ST is based on person-centered psychotherapy and consists of 12 individual sessions. The sessions focus on facilitating expression of affect, highlighting positive and successful experiences, offering empathy, and imparting therapeutic optimism. Therapists do not use main therapeutic strategies found in PST, CBT, interpersonal psychotherapy (IPT), or dynamic therapy but they engage in empathic listening, reflection, emotional processing, and encouragement.

Results and conclusion Only 1 RCT[74,75] met both criteria. In this study, PST was more efficacious than ST in reducing depression and disability (discussed earlier). However, ST reduced depression in 12 weeks and had a significant reduction in depression in the first 6 weeks of treatment.[74,75] Despite the encouraging results, ST has not yet shown greater efficacy than a credible comparison group in late-life MDD. Future studies may concentrate on comparing the efficacy of ST with psychological or pill placebo and on identifying subgroups of patients treated with ST (using moderators analysis) with a more beneficial course of illness.

Interpersonal psychotherapy

IPT focuses on complicated grief, role transition, role dispute/interpersonal conflicts, and interpersonal deficits.[87] The initial treatment phase includes exploration of depression symptoms and psychoeducation. In later phases, problems are identified and understood in the interpersonal context. Depending on each patient's problem, treatment focuses on facilitating grieving process, encouraging and facilitating role transition, exploring interpersonal disputes, and improving interpersonal skills. In the final phase, the therapist focuses on the gains and limitations of therapy and the prevention of relapses. Depending on the study, the duration of treatment and number of sessions ranged from 16 to 20 weeks and 12 to 16 sessions respectively.

Results One unique study met both study design and statistical criteria,[72,73] and 2 articles were published on depression[72] and cost[73] outcomes. IPT was compared with UC and participants were recruited through 12 primary care services in Amsterdam. The number of IPT sessions was reduced from 14 to 10 for use in primary care and the treatment was completed in 5 months.

Even though a significant higher percentage of IPT participants, compared with UC participants, did not have a depression diagnosis at 6 months (1 month after the end of treatment) (50.7% vs 33.8%), there were no significant differences in percentages of responders (50% reduction in Montgomery Asberg Depression Rating Scale [MADRS]) (IPT = 27.6% vs UC = 2 9%) or remitters (MADRS<10) (IPT = 32.8% vs UC = 32.3%) between the 2 groups. There were no significant differences between IPT and UC at 6 months on any subscale of SF-36. In another high-quality RCT of complicated grief[88] that did not meet the sample size criterion of 30 participants per arm, IPT did not show a significant main or interaction effect with nortriptyline (NT) on remission.

Conclusion Even though research has shown that IPT is an efficacious treatment of depression in young and middle-aged adults,[89] and clinical experience may suggest that IPT may reduce depression in older adults, there is no clear supportive evidence for the efficacy of IPT as an acute treatment of late-life MDD. Therefore, further research is recommended.

WHAT ARE THE KNOWN PREDICTORS OF TREATMENT OUTCOMES AND MODERATORS OF TREATMENT EFFECTS?

Few studies of psychosocial interventions in late-life MDD have included predictors of treatment outcomes and moderators of treatment effects. We identified 14 studies that investigated predictors of treatment outcomes (see **Table 2**); 4 of those were RCTs, 9 were open acute treatment trials using pharmacotherapy and IPT, and 1 study added a psychosocial intervention to randomized pharmacotherapy groups for the treatment of MDD with alcohol dependence.[62] Three RCTs examined moderators.[70,72,74,75] Two of these studies examined moderators of treatment effects in the same sample[74,75] but on different outcomes (depression and disability).

Predictors of Treatment Outcomes of Psychosocial Interventions in Late-life MDD

The most commonly examined predictors (ie, examined by at least 2 studies) are (1) baseline depression severity[5,63,64,66]; (2) age[6,63,65,88]; (3) baseline anxiety level[64,68]; (4) personality disorder[65,69,70]; (5) perception of illness or self-rated health[63,65]; (6) baseline stress level[64,69]; and (7) endogenous depression (see **Table 2**).[59,64]

Baseline depression severity

The results are inconsistent in predicting the effects of baseline depression severity to treatment outcomes. Dew and colleagues,[64] Gildengers and colleagues,[5] and Karp and colleagues,[66] found that more severe depressive symptoms at baseline predicted a slower response in acute trials of IPT plus NT and IPT plus paroxetine. However, Miller and colleagues,[63] and Lenze and colleagues,[65] showed that depression severity at baseline was not associated with response or remission status.

Age
The results are inconclusive on the effect of age on treatment outcomes. Older age was associated with worse response in the other 2 studies.[5,63]

Baseline anxiety level
Lower anxiety level predicted a more rapid, sustained response in a study of open acute treatment of NT plus IPT.[64] Similarly, in an open trial of paroxetine plus IPT, patients with high anxiety scores at baseline had a longer median time to response than those with low anxiety scores.[68]

Perception of illness (self-rated health)
Worse perception of illness and lower self-rated health at baseline were associated with lack of response and greater likelihood of failure to remit.[63,65]

Personality disorder
Greater personality pathology as measured by the Personality Assessment Form[90] was associated with greater likelihood of failure to remit in an open acute trial of NT plus IPT.[65,69] In a secondary analysis that focused on cluster C PDs,[70] cluster C PD was not associated with response status but predicted longer time to response (no PD = 9.86 weeks vs cluster C PD = 14.43 weeks).

Baseline stress
Low stress at baseline was associated with having a more rapid, sustained response[64] and shorter time to remission.[69]

Endogenous depression
Endogenous depression, a type of MDD that tends to have a higher genetic component and is related to poor affective control, anhedonia, and agitation, seems to have a negative effect on treatment outcomes. In their clinical trial comparing behavioral therapy, cognitive therapy, and brief relational/ insight therapy, Gallagher and Thompson[59] showed that patients with endogenous depression had worse depression outcomes than patients who had nonendogenous depression. Similarly, endogenous depression, in an open acute trial of NT and interpersonal psychotherapy, was associated with partial or mixed response.[64]

Moderators

Four articles investigated moderators of treatment outcomes in late-life MDD 3 with depression as the outcome and 1 with disability as the outcome (**Table 3**). Age, education, depression onset, number of depressive episodes, baseline depression and anxiety severity, social support, overall cognitive impairment, as well as executive dysfunction have been studied as potential moderators.

Thompson and colleagues[71] studied whether baseline depression severity would moderate treatment effects of CBT, desipramine, and the combination of the 2 treatments. The study found that in the high-severity group (HDRS 17 item $\geq$19) when an interviewer-administered instrument (HDRS) was used, participants in the combined group had -0.31 points in HDRS greater reduction in depression per session than participants in the desipramine group. However, in the low-severity group (HDRS 17 item <19), the between treatment difference was -0.11 in HDRS points. When a self-report measure (BDI-SF) was administered, participants in the combined condition had -0.48 points in the Beck depression inventory (BDI) greater reduction in depression per session than participants in the desipramine group in the high-severity group and -0.20 BDI points in the low-severity group. These results suggest

Table 3
Moderators of treatment effects in randomized clinical trials of psychosocial interventions for the acute treatment of late-life major depression

Article	Comparison Groups	Moderators: Examined	Moderators: Results
Thompson et al,[71] 2001	CBT vs desipramine vs CBT+desipramine	Baseline depression severity; high-severity group (HDRS>18) and low-severity group (HDRS≤18)	For BDI-short form: BDI improvement per session in CBT+desipramine participants between high-severity vs low-severity groups was significant (low severity = −0.29 vs high severity =0.58). However, BDI improvement per session in the other 2 treatment conditions was not significantly different between the high vs low initial severity groups
van Schaik et al,[72] 2006	IPT vs UC	Baseline depression severity: MADRS ≥21 (high) vs MADRS <21 (low)	In the subgroup of participants with high baseline depression severity, a significantly higher percentage of participants in the IPT group vs in UC had no diagnoses of depression (or lower depression score (measured by GDS-15) at 6 months. However, in the low baseline severity group, there was no significant difference in the percentage of participants in the IPT group vs those in UC with no diagnoses of depression or lower GDS-15 scores

Areán et al,[74] 2010[a]	PST vs ST	Examined moderators of treatment effects on depression. Baseline variables: age, education (years), depression severity, age at depression onset (years), total number depressive episodes, overall cognitive impairment, executive dysfunction, personality characteristics, disability, generalized anxiety disorder	None of these variables moderated the efficacy of treatment on depression
Alexopoulos et al,[75] 2010[a]	PST vs ST	Examined moderators of treatment effects on disability. Baseline variables: age, education (years), depression severity, age at depression onset (years), total number depressive episodes, overall cognitive impairment, executive dysfunction, personality characteristics, disability, generalized anxiety disorder	PST was associated with greater reduction of disability than ST in patients with higher number of depressive episodes and greater cognitive impairment (ie, lower MMSE scores). Specifically, for an increase of 1 additional depressive episode, the change in the difference between the WHODAS slopes of the PST and the ST groups was 4.15 points. When MMSE score was increased by 1 point, the change in the difference between the WHODAS slopes of the PST and the ST groups was 4.51 points

Abbreviations: CBT, cognitive behavioral therapy; HDRS, Hamilton Depression Rating Scale; IPT, interpersonal psychotherapy; MMSE, Mini Mental State Examination; PST, problem-solving therapy; ST, supportive therapy; UC, usual care; WHODAS, World Health Organization Disability Assessment Schedule.

[a] These 2 articles performed analyses on the same sample but with different outcomes: Arean and colleagues,[74] outcome = depression; Alexopoulos and colleagues,[75] outcome = disability.

that CBT plus desipramine compared with desipramine alone may have better depression outcomes in the high depression severity group than in the low depression severity group.

In another study, van Schaik and colleagues[72] investigated the moderating effect of depression severity on response to interpersonal therapy and care as usual, and found that the between-group treatment effect (interpersonal psychotherapy vs UC) was greater in those with high depression severity at baseline (MADRS score ≥ 21) than in those with low depression severity at baseline (MADRS<21). Specifically, in the high-severity group, there was a 1.1 score difference in Geriatric Depression Scale between interpersonal psychotherapy versus UC at 6 months, whereas in the low-severity group there was a -0.9 score difference between the 2 treatment groups. Despite a small difference (2 points), the results highlight that patients with high depression severity may respond better to interpersonal psychotherapy than patients with low depression severity.

Arean and colleagues[74] and Alexopoulos and colleagues[75] investigated a series of preplanned moderators in their comparison of PST with ST in older adults with comorbid MDD and executive dysfunction. The following moderators were investigated on depression and disability outcomes: baseline depression severity, age, education, gender, age of first onset, number of previous episodes, baseline severity of executive dysfunction, overall cognitive impairment, and anxiety. Although none of these variables moderated depression outcomes, patients with more cognitive impairment and higher number of depression episodes had better disability outcomes when treated with PST than with ST. Specifically, for an increase of 1 additional depressive episode, the change in the difference between the WHODAS slopes of the PST and the ST groups was 4.15 points at 12 weeks. Similarly, when Mini–Mental State Examination score was increased by 1 point, the change in the difference between the WHODAS slopes of the PST and the ST groups was 4.51 points.

Conclusion

The data on the predictors of treatment outcomes and moderators of treatment effects of psychosocial interventions for late-life MDD are still preliminary. It seems that increased baseline anxiety and stress level, personality disorder, endogenous depression, and reduced self-rated health are associated with worse depression outcomes. The review of moderators revealed that baseline depression severity may moderate the effects of CBT versus CBT plus medication or the effects of interpersonal psychotherapy versus UC. Further, problem-solving treatment may be a particularly good intervention in reducing disability for older adults who have mild cognitive deficits and high number of depression episodes. More work is needed to understand other predictors and moderators.

FUTURE DIRECTIONS

This article shows that PST, CBT, and TIP program are probably efficacious for the acute treatment of late-life MDD. Our findings are in agreement with findings from other reviews and meta-analyses that psychosocial interventions, including PST and CBT, are efficacious in the treatment of late-life depression (including diagnosable MDD, minor depression, dysthymia, or clinically significant depression).[7–9] In our review, 18 high-quality articles were initially identified, but only 6 met the statistical criteria of 30 or more participants per condition and intent-to-treat analyses. These 6 studies were published in the last 10 years, possibly reflecting the recent incorporation of statistical techniques to account for missing data (eg, mixed effects model analysis) and a better understanding of the limitations of small sample size pilot studies.[26] It is also likely that smaller sample sizes are a function of limited funding and the expense of conducting a psychotherapy trial. Most behavioral interventionists receive their funds from agencies such as the National Institutes for Health, and, as a result, only have limited budgets and a few years to recruit participants.

Our review highlights the need for novel research to identify moderators of treatment effects and guide the development of personalized approaches to psychosocial treatments. The National Advisory Mental Health Council report provides some direction for the focus of this research. One area that has been missing from the psychotherapy literature on late-life MDD is the role that cognitive impairments play on response to psychotherapy. As many as 30% of older adults with MDD have mild cognitive impairments and many more have cognitive complaints. The most common are memory, concentration, executive dysfunction, and language processing impairments, areas that have been earmarked for investigation by the NIMH Research Domain Criteria Project. These areas of function could be particularly important in determining differential treatment response in psychotherapy. Given that psychotherapies tend to rely on these cognitive processes, and some provide a compensatory framework for certain disabilities (eg, PST for executive dysfunction), exploring the role that cognitive impairment plays in response to psychotherapy could prove to be paradigm shifting for the psychotherapy field overall. Other areas that deserve attention are early life stress, emotional control, and biomarkers associated with poor response to treatment.

Some qualifiers require mention, because the samples of the efficacy studies are highly selective. Most studies of psychosocial interventions have selected relatively healthy, cognitively intact, white, "young-old," and educated samples. Specifically, the average age of participants in the 14 unique samples that met our study design criteria was 69.78 years, the average number of years of education (of the studies that reported years of education) was 13.11 years, and the average percentage of white participants (of those studies that reported percentages) was 86%. Therefore, there has been little focus on participants older than 80 years, ethnic minorities, and those with cognitive impairment and low education. Future research may investigate the effect of these demographic variables on treatment outcomes.

As older adults become more cognitively and physically impaired, novel psychosocial interventions for MDD may be designed to address their needs. Application of psychosocial interventions in nontraditional settings (patients' residence, assisted living facilities, nursing homes, home care), and focus on the patient's ecosystem (including the patient, the living environment, and the caregiver) may be necessary. Despite the advances in the diagnosis and treatment of depression in nontraditional settings, most of the studies of psychosocial interventions in these settings have been conducted with older adults without MDD diagnosis or in patients with milder forms of depression.[11,45,91,92] As cognitive impairment and disability increases, patients may benefit from the involvement of an available and willing caregiver, as well as from modifications in their immediate living environment that may help improve their functioning. Therefore, future studies with cognitively and functionally compromised older adults with MDD may focus on the patient's ecosystem, including the patient, their living environment, and their caregiver.[93]

Despite the abundance of studies on dementia, the literature on psychosocial interventions for the treatment of MDD in dementia is sparse.[15,20] Most psychosocial interventions have been tested in demented patients with either milder forms of depression, a wide range of neuropsychiatric symptoms, but not depression per se, or in samples without MDD diagnosis.[15,20] Teri and colleagues investigated a promising intervention for depression in dementia in a mixed sample of demented elders with major and minor depression.[43] The study showed that a behavioral treatment of depression significantly reduced depression in this population. In another high-quality study in patients suffering from dementia of the Alzheimer type but without any depression diagnosis, exercise training combined with teaching caregivers behavioral management techniques reduced depressive symptoms compared with routine UC.[94] Finally, a recent pilot study testing a modified version of Dr Teri's treatment in nursing homes has shown encouraging feasibility data[45] in a small, mixed sample of patients with major and minor depression.

The dearth of studies on psychosocial interventions for patients with MDD and dementia may reflect limited funding as well as diagnostic considerations of MDD in dementia.[95,96] Nevertheless, MDD has detrimental consequences for demented patients and their caregivers, including increased medical morbidity, mortality, and death from suicide (see article by Nowrangi and colleagues elsewhere in this issue for further exploration of this topic). Because antidepressant medications have limited efficacy in this population (see article by Nowrangi and colleagues elsewhere in this issue for further exploration of this topic),[97] psychosocial interventions for MDD in dementia may help provide relief to a large number of demented patients and their caregivers.

The task of intervention developers and scientists is to now focus on fine-tuning treatment choices by determining which treatments are effective for the different ways that late-life MDD presents. Cognitive impairments, physical disability, socioeconomic and biologic factors may all influence response to psychotherapy overall and by type of treatment. The next steps are to better study moderators and then to guide the matching of treatments to late-life MDD presentation, as well as to develop novel interventions that address comorbidities for which no treatments have been developed.

REFERENCES

1. Chambers DA, Wang PS, Insel TR. Maximizing efficiency and impact in effectiveness and services research. Gen Hosp Psychiatry 2010;32(5):453–5.
2. From discovery to cure: accelerating the development of new and personalized interventions for mental illnesses. Report from the National Advisory Mental Health Council's Workgroup. National Institute of Mental Health, 2010. Available at: http://www.nimh.nih.gov/about/advisory-boards-and-groups/namhc/reports/fromdiscoverytocure.pdf. Accessed March 14, 2011.
3. Lebowitz BD, Pearson JL, Schneider LS, et al. Diagnosis and treatment of depression in late life. Consensus statement update. JAMA 1997;278(14):1186–90.
4. Alexopoulos GS, Buckwalter K, Olin J, et al. Comorbidity of late life depression: an opportunity for research on mechanisms and treatment. Biol Psychiatry 2002;52(6):543–58.
5. Gildengers AG, Houck PR, Mulsant BH, et al. Trajectories of treatment response in late-life depression: psychosocial and clinical correlates. J Clin Psychopharmacol 2005;25(Suppl 1):S8–13.
6. Raue PJ, Morales KH, Post EP, et al. The wish to die and 5-year mortality in elderly primary care patients. Am J Geriatr Psychiatry 2010;18:341–50.
7. Cuijpers P, van Straten A, Smit F. Psychological treatment of late-life depression: a meta-analysis of randomized controlled trials. Int J Geriatr Psychiatry 2006;21:1139–49.

8. Mackin RS, Areán PA. Evidence-based psychotherapeutic interventions for geriatric depression. Psychiatr Clin North Am 2005;28:805–20, vii–viii.

9. Pinquart M, Duberstein PR, Lyness JM. Effects of psychotherapy and other behavioral interventions on clinically depressed older adults: a meta-analysis. Aging Ment Health 2007;11(6):645–57.

10. Bartels SJ, Dums AR, Oxman TE, et al. Evidence-based practices in geriatric mental health care. Psychiatr Serv 2002;53(11):1419–31.

11. Bharucha AJ, Dew MA, Miller MD, et al. Psychotherapy in long-term care: a review. J Am Med Dir Assoc 2006;7(9):568–80.

12. Bohlmeijer E, Roemer M, Cuijpers P, et al. The effects of reminiscence on psychological well-being in older adults: a meta-analysis. Aging Ment Health 2007;11:291–300.

13. Bohlmeijer E, Smit F, Cuijpers P. Effects of reminiscence and life review on late-life depression: a meta-analysis. Int J Geriatr Psychiatry 2003;18: 1088–94.

14. Cuijpers P. Psychological outreach programmes for the depressed elderly: a meta-analysis of effects and dropout. Int J Geriatr Psychiatry 1998;13:41–8.

15. Livingston G, Johnston K, Katona C, et al, Old Age Task Force of the World Federation of Biological Psychiatry. Systematic review of psychological approaches to the management of neuropsychiatric symptoms of dementia. Am J Psychiatry 2005;162(11):1996–2021.

16. O'Connor DW, Ames D, Gardner B, et al. Psychosocial treatments of psychological symptoms in dementia: a systematic review of reports meeting quality standards. Int Psychogeriatr 2009;21(2):241–51.

17. Pinquart M, Duberstein PR, Lyness JM. Treatments for later-life depressive conditions: a meta-analytic comparison of pharmacotherapy and psychotherapy. Am J Psychiatry 2006;163(9):1493–501.

18. Scogin F, McElreath L. Efficacy of psychosocial treatments for geriatric depression: a quantitative review. J Consult Clin Psychol 1994;62(1):69–74.

19. Scogin F, Welsh D, Hanson D, et al. Evidence-based psychotherapies for depression in older adults. Clin Psychol Sci Pract 2005;12:222–37.

20. Teri L, McKenzie G, LaFazia D. Psychosocial treatment of depression in older adults with dementia. Clin Psychol Sci Pract 2005;12:303–16.

21. Wilson KC, Mottram PG, Vassilas CA. Psychotherapeutic treatments for older depressed people. Cochrane Database Syst Rev 2008;1:CD004853.

22. Niederehe G, Schneider LS. Treatments for depression and anxiety in the aged. In: Nathan PE, Gorman JM, editors. A guide to treatments that work. New York: Oxford University Press; 1998.

23. Chambless DL, Hollon SD. Defining empirically supported therapies. J Consult Clin Psychol 1998;66(1):7–18.

24. Chambless DL, Ollendick TH. Empirically supported psychological interventions: controversies and evidence. Annu Rev Psychol 2001;52:685–716.

25. National Institute of Mental Health: strategic plan, 2008. Available at: http://www.nimh.nih.gov/about/strategic-planning-reports/nimh-strategic-plan-2008.pdf. Accessed March 14, 2011.

26. Leon AC, Davis LL, Kraemer HC. The role and interpretation of pilot studies in clinical research. J Psychiatr Research 2010. [Epub ahead of print].

27. Cohen J. Statistical power analysis for the behavioral sciences. 2nd edition. Hillsdale (NJ): Erlbaum; 1988.

28. Leon AC, Davis LL. Enhancing clinical trial design of interventions for posttraumatic stress disorder. J Trauma Stress 2009;22(6):603–11.

29. Lachin JM. Statistical considerations in the intent-to-treat principle. Control Clin Trials 2000;21(3):167–89.
30. Klerman GL. Scientific and ethical considerations in the use of placebo controls in clinical trials in psychopharmacology. Psychopharmacol Bull 1986;22(1):25–9.
31. Unutzer J, Katon W, Callahan CM, et al. Collaborative care management of late-life depression in the primary care setting: a randomized controlled trial. JAMA 2002;288(22):2836–45.
32. Bruce ML, Ten Have TR, Reynolds CF 3rd, et al. Reducing suicidal ideation and depressive symptoms in depressed older primary care patients: a randomized controlled trial. JAMA 2004;291(9):1081–91.
33. Ell K, Katon W, Xie B, et al. Collaborative care management of major depression among low-income, predominantly Hispanic subjects with diabetes: a random-ized controlled trial. Diabetes Care 2010;33(4):706–13.
34. Bartels SJ, Coakley EH, Zubritsky C, et al. Improving access to geriatric mental health services: a randomized trial comparing treatment engagement with inte-grated versus enhanced referral care for depression, anxiety, and at-risk alcohol use. Am J Psychiatry 2004;161(8):1455–62.
35. Dietrich AJ, Oxman TE, Williams JW Jr, et al. Re-engineering systems for the treatment of depression in primary care: cluster randomised controlled trial. BMJ 2004;329(7466):602.
36. van Marwijk HW, Ader H, de Haan M, et al. Primary care management of major depression in patients aged > or =55 years: outcome of a randomised clinical trial. Br J Gen Pract 2008;58(555):680–6.
37. Lichtenberg PA, Kimbarow ML, Morris P, et al. Behavioral treatment of depres-sion in predominantly African-American medical patients. Clin Gerontol 1996; 17:15–33.
38. Floyd M, Scogin F, McKendree-Smith NL, et al. Cognitive therapy for depres-sion: a comparison of individual psychotherapy and bibliotherapy for depressed older adults. Behav Modif 2004;28(2):297–318.
39. Haringsma R, Engels GI, Cuijpers P, et al. Effectiveness of the Coping with Depression (CWD) course for older adults provided by the community-based mental health care system in the Netherlands: a randomized controlled field trial. Int Psychogeriatr 2006;18(2):307–25.
40. Singh NA, Clements KM, Singh MA. The efficacy of exercise as a long-term anti-depressant in elderly subjects: a randomized, controlled trial. J Gerontol A Biol Sci Med Sci 2001;56(8):M497–504.
41. Rosen J, Rogers JC, Marin RS, et al. Control-relevant intervention in the treat-ment of minor and major depression in a long-term care facility. Am J Geriatr Psychiatry 1997;5(3):247–57.
42. Teri L. Behavioral treatment of depression in patients with dementia. Alzheimer Dis Assoc Disord 1994;8(Suppl 3):66–74.
43. Teri L, Logsdon RG, Uomoto J, et al. Behavioral treatment of depression in dementia patients: a controlled clinical trial. J Gerontol B Psychol Sci Soc Sci 1997;52(4):P159–66.
44. Gum AM, Areán PA, Bostrom A. Low-income depressed older adults with psychiatric comorbidity: secondary analyses of response to psychotherapy and case management. Int J Geriatr Psychiatry 2007;22(2):124–30.
45. Meeks S, Looney SW, Van Haitsma K, et al. BE-ACTIV: a staff-assisted behavioral intervention for depression in nursing homes. Gerontologist 2008;48(1):105–14.
46. Areán PA, Gum A, McCulloch CE, et al. Treatment of depression in low-income older adults. Psychol Aging 2005;20(4):601–9.

47. Gallagher-Thompson D, Steffen AM. Comparative effects of cognitive-behavioral and brief psychodynamic psychotherapies for depressed family caregivers. J Consult Clin Psychol 1994;62(3):543–9.
48. Serfaty MA, Haworth D, Blanchard M, et al. Clinical effectiveness of individual cognitive behavioral therapy for depressed older people in primary care: a randomized controlled trial. Arch Gen Psychiatry 2009;66(12):1332–40.
49. Kraemer HC, Wilson GT, Fairburn CG, et al. Mediators and moderators of treatment effects in randomized clinical trials. Arch Gen Psychiatry 2002;59(10): 877–83.
50. Leon AC. Two clinical trial designs to examine personalized treatments for psychiatric disorders. J Clin Psychiatry 2010. [Epub ahead of print].
51. Sloane RB, Staples FR, Schneider LS. Interpersonal therapy versus nortriptyline for depression in the elderly. In: Burrows GD, Norman TR, Dennerstein L, editors. Clinical and pharmacological studies in psychiatric disorders. London: Libbey; 1985. p. 344–6.
52. Thompson LW, Gallagher D. Efficacy of psychotherapy in the treatment of late-life depression. Adv Behav Res Ther 1984;6:127–39.
53. Jarvik LF, Mintz J, Steuer JL. Treating geriatric depression: a 26-week interim analysis. J Am Geriatr Soc 1982;30:713–7.
54. Wilson KC, Scott M, Abou-Saleh M, et al. Long-term effects of cognitive-behavioural therapy and lithium therapy on depression in the elderly. Br J Psychiatry 1995;167(5):653–8.
55. Brand E, Clingempeel WG. Group behavioral therapy with depressed geriatric inpatients: an assessment of incremental efficacy. Behav Ther 1992;23:475–82.
56. Steuer JL, Mintz J, Hammen CL, et al. Cognitive-behavioral and psychodynamic group psychotherapy in treatment of geriatric depression. J Consult Clin Psychol 1984;52(2):180–9.
57. Lynch TR. Dialectical behavior therapy for depressed older adults: a randomized pilot study. Am J Geriatr Psychiatry 2003;11:33–45.
58. Beutler LE, Scogin F, Kirish P, et al. Group cognitive therapy and alprazolam in the treatment of depression in older adults. J Consult Clin Psychol 1987;55:550–6.
59. Gallagher DE, Thompson LW. Effectiveness of psychotherapy for both endogenous and nonendogenous depression in older adult outpatients. J Gerontol 1983;38:707–12.
60. Marmar CR, Gaston L, Gallagher D, et al. Alliance and outcome in late-life depression. J Nerv Ment Dis 1989;177:464–72.
61. Gaston L, Gallagher D, Thompson L. Impact of confirming patient expectations of change processes in behavioral, cognitive, and brief dynamic psychotherapy. Psychotherapy 1989;26:296–302.
62. Oslin DW. Treatment of late-life depression complicated by alcohol dependence. Am J Geriatr Psychiatry 2005;13(6):491–500.
63. Miller MD, Schulz R, Paradis C, et al. Changes in perceived health status of depressed elderly patients treated until remission. Am J Psychiatry 1996;153: 1350–2.
64. Dew MA, Reynolds CF 3rd, Houck PR, et al. Temporal profiles of the course of depression during treatment. Predictors of pathways toward recovery in the elderly. Arch Gen Psychiatry 1997;54:1016–24.
65. Lenze EJ, Miller MD, Dew MA, et al. Subjective health measures and acute treatment outcomes in geriatric depression. Int J Geriatr Psychiatry 2001;16:1149–55.
66. Karp JF, Weiner D, Seligman K, et al. Body pain and treatment response in late-life depression. Am J Geriatr Psychiatry 2005;13(3):188–94.

67. Reynolds CF, Miller MD, Pasternak RE, et al. Treatment of bereavement-related major depressive episodes in later life: a controlled study of acute and continuation treatment with nortriptyline and interpersonal psychotherapy. Am J Psychiatry 1999;156:202–8.

68. Andreescu C, Lenze EJ, Dew MA, et al. Effect of comorbid anxiety on treatment response and relapse risk in late-life depression: controlled study. Br J Psychiatry 2007;190:344–9.

69. Karp JF, Frank E, Anderson B, et al. Time to remission in late-life depression: analysis of effects of demographic, treatment, and life-events measures. Depression 1993;1:250–6.

70. Morse JQ, Pilkonis PA, Houck PR, et al. Impact of cluster C personality disorders on outcomes of acute and maintenance treatment in late-life depression. Am J Geriatr Psychiatry 2005;13(9):808–14.

71. Thompson LW, Coon DW, Gallagher-Thompson D, et al. Comparison of desipramine and cognitive/behavioral therapy in the treatment of elderly outpatients with mild-to-moderate depression. Am J Geriatr Psychiatry 2001;9:225–40.

72. van Schaik A, van Marwijk H, Adèr H, et al. Interpersonal psychotherapy for elderly patients in primary care. Am J Geriatr Psychiatry 2006;14(9):777–86.

73. Bosmans JE, van Schaik DJF, Heymans MW, et al. Cost-effectiveness of interpersonal psychotherapy for elderly primary care patients with major depression. Int J Technol Assess Health Care 2007;23(4):480–7.

74. Areán PA, Raue P, Mackin RS, et al. Problem-solving therapy and supportive therapy in older adults with major depression and executive dysfunction. Am J Psychiatry 2010;167(11):1391–8.

75. Alexopoulos GS, Raue PJ, Kiosses DN, et al. Problem solving therapy and supportive therapy in older adults with major depression and executive dysfunction: effect on disability. Arch Gen Psychiatry 2011;68(1):33–41.

76. Sirey JA, Bruce ML, Kales HC. Improving antidepressant adherence and depression outcomes in primary care: the Treatment Initiation and Participation (TIP) program. Am J Geriatr Psychiatry 2010;18(6):554–62.

77. Arean PA, Perri MG, Nezu AM, et al. Comparative effectiveness of social problem-solving therapy and reminiscence therapy as treatments for depression in older adults. J Consult Clin Psychol 1993;61:1003–10.

78. Alexopoulos GS, Raue PJ, Arean P. Problem-solving therapy versus supportive therapy in geriatric major depression with executive dysfunction. Am J Geriatr Psychiatry 2003;11:46–52.

79. Beck AT, Rush AJ, Shaw BF, et al. Cognitive therapy of depression. New York: Guilford Press; 1979.

80. Emery G. Cognitive therapy with the elderly. In: Emery G, Hollon S, Bedrosian R, editors. New directions in cognitive therapy. New York: Guilford Press; 1981.

81. Thompson LW, Gallagher-Thompson D, Laidlaw K, et al. Cognitive-behavioural therapy for late life depression: a therapist manual. UK version. Edinburgh (UK): University of Edinburgh, Department of Psychiatry; 2000.

82. Fawcett J, Epstein P, Fiester SJ, et al. Clinical management: imipramine/placebo administration manual: NIMH Treatment of Depression Collaborative Research Program. Psychopharmacol Bull 1987;23:309–24.

83. Thompson LW, Gallagher D, Breckenridge JS. Comparative effectiveness of psychotherapies for depressed elders. J Consult Clin Psychol 1987;55:385–90.

84. Gallagher-Thompson D, Hanley-Peterson P, Thompson LW. Maintenance of gains versus relapse following brief psychotherapy for depression. J Consult Clin Psychol 1990;58:371–4.

85. Sirey JA, Bruce ML, Alexopoulos GS. The treatment initiation program: an intervention to improve depression outcomes in older adults. Am J Psychiatry 2005; 162:184–6.

86. Zivin K, Kales HC. Adherence to depression treatment in older adults. Drugs Aging 2008;25:559–71.

87. Klerman GL, Weissman MM, Rounsaville BJ, et al. Interpersonal psychotherapy of depression. New York: Academic Press; 1984.

88. Reynolds CF III, Frank E, Dew MA, et al. Treatment of 70∼-year-olds with recurrent major depression. Excellent short-term but brittle long-term response. Am J Geriatr Psychiatry 1999;7:64–9.

89. Holon SD, Ponniah K. A review of empirically supported psychological therapies for mood disorders in adults. Depress Anxiety 2010;27:891–932.

90. Pilkonis PA, Frank E. Personality pathology in recurrent depression: nature, prevalence, and relationship to treatment response. Am J Psychiatry 1988; 145:435–41.

91. Gellis ZD, McGinty J, Horowitz A, et al. Problem-solving therapy for late-life depression in home care: a randomized field trial. Am J Geriatr Psychiatry 2007;15(11):968–78.

92. Gellis ZD, Bruce ML. Problem solving therapy for subthreshold depression in home healthcare patients with cardiovascular disease. Am J Geriatr Psychiatry 2010;18(6):464–74.

93. Alexopoulos GS, Bruce ML. A model for intervention research in late-life depression. Int J Geriatr Psychiatry 2009;24(12):1325–34.

94. Teri L, Gibbons LE, McCurry SM, et al. Exercise plus behavioral management in patients with Alzheimer disease: a randomized controlled trial. JAMA 2003; 290(15):2015–22.

95. Olin JT, Katz IR, Meyers BS, et al. Provisional diagnostic criteria for depression of Alzheimer disease: rationale and background. Am J Geriatr Psychiatry 2002; 10(2):129–41 Review. Erratum appears in Am J Geriatr Psychiatry 2002;10(3): 264.

96. Olin JT, Schneider LS, Katz IR, et al. Provisional diagnostic criteria for depression of Alzheimer disease. Am J Geriatr Psychiatry 2002;10(2):125–8.

97. Bains J, Birks JS, Dening TR. The efficacy of antidepressants in the treatment of depression in dementia. Cochrane Database Syst Rev 2002;4:CD003944.

98. Gallagher DE, Thompson LW. Treatment of major depressive disorder in older adult outpatients with brief psychotherapies. Psychother Theor Res Pract 1982;19:482–90.

99. Klausner EJ, Clarkin JF, Spielman L, et al. Late-life depression and functional disability: the role of goal-focused group psychotherapy. Int J Geriatr Psychiatry 1998;13:707–16.

100. Rokke PD, Tomhave JA, Jocic Z. Self-management therapy and educational group therapy for depressed elders. Cognit Ther Res 2000;24:99–119.

101. Strachowski D, Khaylis A, Conrad A, et al. The effects of cognitive behavior therapy on depression in older patients with cardiovascular risk. Depress Anxiety 2008;25(8):E1–10.

102. Laidlaw K, Davidson K, Toner H, et al. A randomised controlled trial of cognitive behaviour therapy vs treatment as usual in the treatment of mild to moderate late life depression. Int J Geriatr Psychiatry 2008;23(8):843–50.

103. Kiosses DN, Arean PA, Teri L, et al. Home-delivered problem adaptation therapy (PATH) for depressed, cognitively impaired, disabled elders: a preliminary study. Am J Geriatr Psychiatry 2010;18(11):988–98.

Functional Neuroimaging in Geriatric Depression

Faith M. Gunning, PhD[a],*, Gwenn S. Smith, PhD[b]

KEYWORDS

• Geriatric depression • PET • fMRI • Spectroscopy

OVERVIEW

Geriatric depression is a complex syndrome that is associated with a high degree of interindividual variability and determined by multiple biological and environmental factors. Among these factors, abnormalities in specific cerebral functions likely confer vulnerability that increases the susceptibility for development of geriatric depression and affect the course of symptoms. Functional neuroimaging makes possible the identification of alterations in cerebral function that not only characterize disease vulnerability but also may be responsible for variability in mood and cognitive responses to treatment. Thus, thoughtful use of functional neuroimaging approaches can inform conceptual models of late-life depression and guide treatment developments.

This article reviews several techniques, such as regional cerebral blood flow (rCBF) and cerebral metabolism studies, molecular imaging, blood oxygenation level–dependent (BOLD) imaging, and magnetic resonance spectroscopy (MRS), that have been used to examine abnormalities in brain function, with a focus on the pattern of results obtained by each method as well as recommendations for future research.

THE FUNCTIONAL NEUROANATOMY OF GERIATRIC DEPRESSION AND TREATMENT

Positron Emission Tomographic Cerebral Glucose Metabolism Studies

The major focus of positron emission tomographic (PET) neuroimaging studies in affective disorders has been the characterization of rCBF and glucose metabolic

This work was supported in part by National Institute of Mental Health grants K23MH74818 (F.M.G.), MH01621(G.S.S.), MH 64823(G.S.S.) and MH 86881(G.S.S.).
The authors have nothing to disclose.
[a] Department of Psychiatry, Institute of Geriatric Psychiatry, Weill Cornell Medical College, 21 Bloomingdale Road, White Plains, NY 10605, USA
[b] Department of Psychiatry and Behavioral Sciences, Johns Hopkins Bayview Medical Center, Alpha Commons Building, 4th floor, 5300 Alpha Commons Drive, Baltimore, MD 21224, USA
* Corresponding author.
E-mail address: fgd2002@med.cornell.edu

Psychiatr Clin N Am 34 (2011) 403–422
doi:10.1016/j.psc.2011.02.010
0193-953X/11/$ – see front matter © 2011 Published by Elsevier Inc.

psych.theclinics.com

alterations in midlife patients with primary unipolar depression and secondary depression caused by stroke or movement disorders (Huntington and Parkinson diseases) as well as the effects of antidepressant interventions.[1–3] Fewer studies comparing geriatric depressed patients with controls or evaluating treatment effects have been performed.[2,4–8] Because cerebral glucose metabolism is the final common pathway of neurochemical activity, these studies identify the neural circuitry of pathophysiology and treatment response to inform the design of mechanistic studies within the pathways identified.

These rCBF and cerebral metabolism studies, in addition to preclinical and postmortem data, have been integrated to develop a functional neuroanatomic model of depression and of antidepressant effects in midlife depressed patients. This model involves increased metabolism in dorsal structures and decreased metabolism in ventral structures.[1] Many of the brain regions that comprise this model have been implicated in a recent meta-analysis of neuroimaging studies in major depression.[3] The regions that are hypoactive at rest show a lack of activation during negative mood states and that increase with selective serotonin reuptake inhibitor (SSRI) treatment include the dorsal pregenual cingulate gyrus, middle and dorsolateral prefrontal cortex (DLPFC), insula, and superior temporal gyrus. A second network identified was a cortical-limbic network including the medial and inferior frontal cortex and basal ganglia, structures that were overactive at rest and during induction of negative mood states and reduced in activity with antidepressant treatment. The amygdala and thalamus were also implicated in the network in some studies. Other regions highlighted in the meta-analysis included the cerebellum (which showed increased activity at rest), posterior cingulate, and medial temporal lobe (including the parahippocampal gyrus [PHG]), all of which show abnormal activation in mood induction paradigms. The applicability of this model to geriatric patients can be tested, given that such data have become available recently.[9–11]

Comparison of the Neural Circuitry of Depression Across the Life Span

Differences between the functional neuroanatomic alterations in older depressed patients and younger patients have been observed.[10] Relative to younger patients, geriatric depressed patient demonstrate increased glucose metabolism in a more extensive network of both anterior and posterior cortical regions.[10] In younger depressed patients, antidepressant treatment increased anterior cortical metabolism and decreased limbic metabolism. Within the cingulate gyrus, effects are observed in rostral areas (Brodmann areas [BAs] 24, 25) in midlife depressed patients.[1] In contrast, in studies in older depressed patients,[8,9,11,12] decreased anterior cortical and limbic metabolisms and increases in posterior cortical regions and cerebellum with antidepressant treatment (including SSRIs and total sleep deprivation) have been observed. With respect to the cingulate gyrus, effects are observed in caudal subregions of the cingulate gyrus (BA 32) with acute treatment and in rostral subregions (BA 24) with chronic treatment in geriatric depression. The regional differences in metabolic response to antidepressant medications between younger and older depressed patients may be attributable to differences in depression phenomenology as well as differential compensatory processes in the aging brain.

Mood and Cognitive Networks of Treatment Response in Geriatric Depression

Functional connectivity (FC) methods have identified neural networks associated with improvement of affective and cognitive symptoms in geriatric depressed patients who underwent PET glucose metabolism studies before and during a course of treatment with the antidepressant citalopram.[9] The partial least squares method identified that a subcortical-limbic-frontal network was associated with improvement in affect (mood and anxiety), whereas a medial temporal-parieto-frontal network was associated with improvement in cognition (immediate verbal learning/memory and verbal fluency). The network of regions that correlated with the left anterior cingulate cortex (ACC; BA 24) seed and with improved affect was composed of the left amygdala, frontal regions (right orbitofrontal cortex [BA 11], bilateral medial frontal gyrus [BA 10], bilateral middle frontal gyrus [BA 46], bilateral superior frontal gyrus [BA 6], right inferior frontal gyrus [BA 45]), right ACC (BA 24), the bilateral insula (BA 13), and left midbrain. The network of regions that correlated with the right PHG seed and with improved scores in the California Verbal Learning Test (CVLT; sum of the first 5 trials) and the Controlled Oral Word Association Test (COWAT) included the left hippocampus, frontal regions (bilateral middle frontal gyrus [BA 46], bilateral orbitofrontal cortex [BA 11], and left inferior frontal gyrus [BA 47]), temporal regions (left inferior temporal gyrus [BA 20], bilateral middle temporal gyrus [BA 21], and right superior temporal gyrus [BA 22]), parietal regions (left inferior parietal lobule [BA 40] and right postcentral gyrus [BA 2]), and the bilateral cerebellum. In contrast, the bilateral insula and occipital areas (bilateral lateral occipital gyrus [BA 19], right superior occipital gyrus [BA 39], and right fusiform gyrus [BA 37]) showed increased metabolism and also correlated with improvements in the two cognitive measures. The underlying mechanisms of the midbrain-limbic-frontal affective network may involve interactions between monoaminergic and glutamatergic systems. The regions involved in the medial temporal-parietal-frontal cognitive network overlap with the regions affected in Alzheimer dementia (AD) and may reflect neuronal vulnerability to a neurodegenerative processes (such as β amyloid deposition[13]). Thus, an understanding of the cerebral metabolic networks associated with the affective and cognitive responses to antidepressant treatment is critical to the design of future mechanistic studies.

PET cerebral glucose metabolism measures have provided a fundamental understanding of the functional neuroanatomic pathways underlying depressive symptoms and treatment response. This information is critical for designing studies to evaluate specific neurochemical substrates with molecular imaging methods.

MOLECULAR IMAGING IN DEPRESSION

The initial application of neurochemical imaging methods was to test the hypothesis of decreased monoaminergic function (norepinephrine; dopamine; and, in particular, serotonin)[14–16] in depression. Most studies have been performed in midlife depressed patients. Advances in radiotracer chemistry over the last decade have made possible the ability to image neuropathologic processes that may be relevant to understanding neurodegenerative and cerebrovascular mechanisms involved in geriatric depression. The monoamine imaging data in depression are reviewed in this section with a focus on the serotonin and dopamine systems, the major areas of investigation. The amyloid imaging data are reviewed next, followed by a discussion of future directions that is based on new developments in radiotracer chemistry and recent data that implicate the role of therapeutic mechanisms beyond the monoamine systems.

The Serotonin System

The evidence supporting serotonin hypofunction in major depression includes (1) alterations in serotonin transporter (SERT) binding, 5-hydroxytryptamine (5-HT) receptor 1A and 5-HT$_{2A}$ binding in postmortem and in vivo studies; (2) a blunted neuroendocrine response to acute pharmacologic interventions of the serotonin system; and (3) alterations in mood in depressed patients by pharmacologic manipulations of serotonin system (improvement in mood with increased serotonin concentrations and worsening of mood with reduced serotonin concentrations).[17–19] Neurochemical imaging studies have evaluated serotonin synthesis, SERT binding, the initial target site of action of the SSRIs, as well as 5-HT$_{1A}$ and 5-HT$_{2A}$ binding. Radiotracers for other relevant serotonin receptor sites are being evaluated, such as for 5-HT$_{1B}$,[20] 5-HT$_4$,[21] 5-HT$_6$.[22]

Reduced serotonin synthesis in depression has been observed in several studies. Agren and colleagues[23] reported lower uptake of [11C]-5-hydroxytryptophan, a radio-labeled precursor for serotonin synthesis, in depressed patients. Serotonin synthesis as measured by trapping of the radiotracer α-[11C]-methyl-L-tryptophan was shown to be reduced in the ACC (bilaterally in women, left hemisphere in men) and left medial temporal cortex in unmedicated depressed patients.[24]

Several studies have evaluated SERT binding in midlife unipolar and bipolar depressed patients. The results include increased SERT,[25,26] decreased SERT,[27–31] or no difference in unmedicated recovered patients or unmedicated patients.[32,33] Although the direction of the results across studies is different, the regions implicated are remarkably consistent (eg, cingulate gyrus, frontal cortex, insula, thalamus, and striatum). The factors that may contribute to differences across studies include differences in the radiotracers used ([11C]-DASB vs [11C]-McN5652) and sample characteristics. At this time, there do not seem to be any published studies of SERT in geriatric depression. Preliminary studies in 2 samples of geriatric depression patients suggest decreased SERT relative to controls in the ACC (BA 24), middle temporal gyrus, PHG, amygdala, caudate, and thalamus (Smith and colleagues, unpublished data, 2011). Two studies have reported that higher baseline SERT binding predicted remission to acute fluoxetine treatment, as well as remission at 1 year.[34,35]

SERT occupancy by SSRIs has been evaluated in midlife depressed patients. Studies in midlife depressed patients treated for 4 weeks with either paroxetine or citalopram have reported significant SERT occupancy in the caudate, putamen, and thalamus, in addition to prefrontal and anterior cingulate cortices. The magnitude occupancy for both compounds was similar (ranging from 65% 87% across regions).[36] The magnitude of occupancy and the relationship between brain occupancy and plasma concentrations is consistent with that observed in elderly depressed patients treated with the citalopram at steady state doses.[2] There was a remarkable degree of similarity between regions of SERT occupancy that were correlated with improvement in depressive symptoms and regions of cerebral metabolic alterations by citalopram (eg, ACC, middle frontal gyrus, precuneus, inferior parietal lobule, cuneus).[2,9] These data suggest that a serotonergic mechanism (decreased serotonin function in corticolimbic pathways) may underlie observations of altered cerebral blood flow and metabolism associated with the antidepressant response and that voxelwise analyses of the neurochemical imaging data may be informative to detecting changes in brain regions relevant to the antidepressant response that have lower concentrations of the transporters/receptors of interest. Although the data concerning SERT binding in the baseline unmedicated state in unipolar depressed patients are controversial, there is consistency between studies to show the predictive value of baseline SERT binding with respect to treatment outcome and remission, as well as occupancy by antidepressant medications. The available data suggest that striatal and thalamic occupancy (70% or greater) is necessary to observe an antidepressant response; however, less occupancy of cortical and limbic SERT may be associated with treatment resistance.

Studies of the 5-HT$_{1A}$ receptor have either shown decreased[37,38] or increased[39] binding. In a study by Parsey and colleagues,[39] antidepressant naive subjects and subjects homozygous for the functional 5-HT$_{1A}$ G (-1019) allele of the promoter poly-morphism demonstrated higher 5-HT$_{1A}$ binding. A correlation between higher baseline 5-HT$_{1A}$ binding and poorer treatment response has been reported.[40,41] The one study of geriatric depressed patients observed decreased 5-HT$_{1A}$ binding in the dorsal raphe as well as in the middle temporal cortex and hippocampus.[42] A similar selective reduction in 5-HT$_{1A}$ binding in temporal cortex has also been observed in patients with AD,[43] which might suggest that decreased serotonin modulation of temporal cortical regions may be associated with affective or cognitive deficits similar to depression and AD.

Alterations in 5-HT$_{1A}$ binding after SSRI treatment has not been observed in human neuroimaging studies,[38,41] a finding that is not expected based on animal studies showing 5-HT$_{1A}$ desensitization induced by SSRI treatment.[44] One of the explanations for the lack of an observed effect is that the 5-HT$_{1A}$ antagonist radiotracers bind to low-affinity sites, whereas the changes with treatment may be observed in high-affinity sites. To test this hypothesis, a promising 5-HT$_{1A}$ agonist radiotracer has been developed.[45]

5-HT$_{2A}$ receptor binding has reported to be unchanged in both midlife and late-life depressed patients,[36,46,47] decreased in orbitofrontal cortex in one report,[48] or increased.[49] Treatment studies have shown either a decrease[50,51] or an increase in 5-HT$_{2A}$ binding.[52,53] The discrepancy between studies may be that in the study by Yatham and colleagues,[51] desipramine was administered, which binds directly to the 5-HT$_{2A}$ receptors, whereas SSRIs were used in the other studies. In addition, different radiotracers were used across studies, [18F]-setoperone versus the spiper-one derivative radiotracer [18F]-FESP.

Studies of SERT and the 5-HT$_{1A}$ and 5-HT$_{2A}$ receptors have been performed in mainly in midlife unipolar depressed patients. The within-group variability obtained in transporter or receptor binding has been explained in some studies by correlations with affective or cognitive symptoms or particular genetic polymorphisms related to the transporters or receptors of interest.[33,39]

The Dopamine System

The role of the dopamine system in depression has been reviewed in detail.[54,55] There are several lines of evidence to support dopamine dysfunction in depression, including improvement in depressive symptoms with dopamine agonists, the induction of a depressive relapse by pharmacologic depletion of dopamine, and low cerebrospinal fluid homovanillic acid levels in depressed patients compared with controls. The avail-able imaging data suggest modest decreases or no change in dopamine metabolism, dopamine transporter, and D$_1$ and D$_2$ receptor binding.[56–58] Dopamine transporter binding was reduced in major depression disorder (MDD) relative to controls.[57] Several studies of striatal and extrastriatal D$_2$ receptor availability have not shown differences between patients and controls, including studies in medication-naive patients.[59–61] Greater psychomotor slowing has been associated with increased stria-tal D$_2$ receptor binding, indicating that perhaps differences may be observed in subgroups of depressed patients.[62] With respect to the D$_1$ receptor, decreased binding was observed in the left middle caudate in one report.[63] In addition, no differ-ences in amphetamine-induced striatal dopamine release have been observed in either euthymic bipolar patients or patients with unipolar depression.[60,64]

The available dopamine neuroimaging data suggest a presynaptic deficit in the dopamine system because the postsynaptic receptors are not significantly altered, except in patients with psychomotor slowing. Several lines of evidence suggest that dopamine dysfunction may play a more prominent role in geriatric depression, including the substantial age-related decline in dopamine transporters and receptors as well as the evidence for the augmentation of the antidepressant response by psychostimulants (such as methylphenidate).[65,66] A better understanding of the nature of the dopaminergic deficits in geriatric depression leads to targeted treatments that would potentially be more effective.

β Amyloid Imaging

The development of radiotracers to image β amyloid deposition, one of the pathologic hallmarks of AD (in addition to hyperphosphorylated tau), represents a significant advance in neuroimaging studies of neurodegenerative disease. Several PET radiotracers for β amyloid have been evaluated in human subjects and show good diagnostic sensitivity between normal controls, individuals with mild cognitive impairment (MCI), and those with AD ([18F]-FDDNP, [11C]-SB13, [11C]-PIB).[67-72] [11C]-PIB is the best-characterized and most commonly used radiotracer and has a high binding affinity and specificity to amyloid in the brain of those with AD.[69,73,74]

Several lines of evidence suggest that [11C]-PIB measures are sensitive to subtle cognitive impairment and may predict subsequent cognitive decline. Higher cortical PIB concentrations are associated with cognitive impairment in healthy controls, as well as cognitive impairment and cognitive decline in subjects with MCI.[72,75-77]

The initial study of [11C]-PIB in geriatric depression was recently published.[78] Nine remitted depressed patients underwent cognitive testing, magnetic resonance imaging, and [11C]-PIB scanning. Individuals who met criteria for amnestic MCI demonstrated greater binding than those with nonamnestic MCI and those who were cognitively normal. These results are consistent with that of nondepressed subjects with cognitive impairment. In a recent study of geriatric depressed patients who do not meet criteria for MCI, greater β amyloid deposition relative to that in controls was observed in the ACC, superior and middle frontal gyrus, left orbitofrontal gyrus, precuneus bilateral insula, and left PHG.[79] In patients with MCI and cognitively normal controls, greater depression and anxiety symptoms were associated with higher [18F]-FDDNP binding.[80] These studies suggest that depressive symptoms in normal control subjects and depressed patients without cognitive impairment are associated with AD neuropathology. β Amyloid deposition may underlie the cognitive impairment that persists after mood symptom remission.

FUTURE DIRECTIONS FOR MOLECULAR IMAGING STUDIES

As reviewed in the previous sections, the serotonin and dopamine systems have been the major focus of neurochemical imaging studies in depression, and most studies have been performed in younger patients. Recent studies have focused on imaging β amyloid deposition in geriatric depression as a mechanism underlying cognitive impairment that might be related to the increased risk of AD in depressed patients. There are several other potentially relevant molecular targets for which radiotracers are in development and/or promising new radiotracers are available. These important future directions for molecular imaging studies, of particular relevance to geriatric patients, are reviewed.

Radiotracer development for the noradrenergic system (including the norepinephrine transporter and β-adrenergic receptors) has been challenging because of the lack of pharmacologically selective agents and the low signal-to-noise levels of binding in the brain.[81,82] Given the role of the norepinephrine transporter in the mechanism of action of antidepressant agents, a suitable radiotracer permits drug occupancy studies as well as studies of pathophysiology. Such studies are especially critical in older patients, given the side effects associated with noradrenergic agents.[83]

The recent evidence for the antidepressant effects of N-methyl-D-aspartate (NMDA) antagonist, ketamine, and the genetic data implicating glutamate receptor polymorphisms in response to SSRIs has stimulated research to evaluate the role of glutamate in depression.[84] Several radiotracers have been evaluated for the NMDA receptor[85–87] and do not have suitable imaging properties for human studies. The recent emphasis and greatest success for glutamate radiotracer development has been the metabotropic glutamate subtype 5 receptor.[88] Given the role of glutamate in neurotoxicity as shown in preclinical studies,[89] glutamatergic dysfunction in geriatric depression may be associated with subsequent neurodegenerative processes and cognitive decline.

The antidepressant effects of cholinergic agents, such as muscarinic antagonists and nicotinic agonists, highlight a possible primary or secondary role of the cholinergic system in depression.[90,91] For the cholinergic system, radiotracers have been developed for the vesicular acetylcholine transporter, acetylcholinesterase, and nicotinic and muscarinic receptors. These radiotracers have not been studied extensively in mood disorders. One study using a muscarinic receptor (M2 subtype selective) radiotracer, [18F]FP-TZTP, observed reduced muscarinic receptor binding in the ACC in bipolar depressed patients relative to that in patients with MDD and controls.[92] The reduction in receptor binding was negatively correlated with depressive symptoms. The further investigation of muscarinic and nicotinic mechanisms in geriatric depression is of potential mechanistic and therapeutic relevance for mood symptoms and cognitive deficits.

Inflammation may be a common underlying mechanism for depression, as well as cardiovascular disease, diabetes, and cancer and may be more relevant to geriatric depression, given the increasing medical comorbidity in late-life.[93] A recent focus in radiotracer chemistry is the development of peripheral benzodiazepine radiotracers that bind with high affinity to translocator protein (TSPO). TSPO is upregulated in activated microglia and represents a marker of neuroinflammation. Several radiotracers have been developed and evaluated in human subjects[94–96] and offer promise for the evaluation of the role of inflammation in the pathophysiology of geriatric depression.

MRS

MRS is a noninvasive imaging tool that can provide a quantitative measure of the biochemical concentration in the brains of elderly depressed patients. Different molecules have unique magnetic resonance spectra that can be quantified by taking the area under the signal curve. In most cases, the values are not absolute, so it is customary to take ratios of the measure of interest to some standard metabolite, for example, choline. MRS measures complement PET imaging methods and permit the noninvasive evaluation of concentrations of amino acids (γ-aminobutyric acid, glutamate) and membrane lipids in the brain that are found in high concentrations that are difficult to image with PET because of high nonspecific binding of radiotracers.

Kumar and colleagues[97] used MRS to examine biochemical abnormalities in the left frontal white matter and bilateral anterior cingulate gray matter of elderly depressed patients. The investigators observed higher choline to creatine as well as myo-inositol to creatine ratios in the white matter of patents relative to age-matched controls. In a follow-up study using 2-dimensional MRS, the investigators detected a significant difference in the overall pattern of associations between the measured metabolites (choline, myo-inositol, creatine, phosphoethanolamine, phosphocholine) and verbal learning and processing speed in elderly depressed patients compared with elderly controls.[98] The investigators interpreted the weaker relationship between metabolites and specific cognitive domains in patients with late-life depression because of evidence that cognitive decline in geriatric depression may be associated with biochemical changes in frontolimbic circuitry. Further, in a recent study of elderly depressed patients and age-matched control subjects, MRS spectra were acquired from voxels that were placed in the left frontal white matter, left periventricular white matter, and left basal ganglia. Elderly depressed patients had significantly lower N-acetyl aspartate (NAA) to creatine ratio in the left frontal white matter and higher choline to creatine and myo-inositol to creatine ratios in the left basal ganglia when compared with the control subjects. Furthermore, the myo-inositol concentration correlated with global cognitive function among the patients.[99] Taken together, these findings suggest that biochemical abnormalities are not only present in geriatric depression but also associated with the cognitive deficits that characterize the illness.

MRS and course of illness

Single-voxel ^{1}H-MRS was used to examine biochemical abnormalities related to late-life depression in the medial prefrontal cortex and medial temporal lobe. Elderly previously depressed individuals had significantly reduced concentrations of total NAA, choline, and creatine in the medial prefrontal cortex, suggesting that reduced neuronal, phospholipid, and energy metabolisms are present even in clinically improved depression.[100] Furthermore, using a 3-dimensional chemical shift imaging sequence, tissue-specific differences in markers of energy metabolism, including high-energy phosphate compounds (β and total nucleoside triphospates [NTP], PCr) and pH, were examined in 13 older adults with major depression before and after 12 weeks of treatment with sertraline and 10 age-matched controls. Relative to controls, total NTP was reduced in the white matter, but not in the gray matter, in the depressed group before treatment. In addition, intracellular pH was higher in the gray matter of subjects with pretreatment depression but similar to levels of controls after treatment.[101]

Most spectroscopic studies thus far have used single-voxel acquisitions, with a high number of repetitions to get adequate signal-to-noise ratio. Other studies use chemical shift imaging to obtain spectroscopic data on an image slice or set of slices. The key limitation for chemical shift imaging is that the signal-to-noise ratio increases in magnitude as more voxels are acquired. Although there are only a handful of published reports that have used MRS to examine the neurochemical environment in geriatric depression, MRS seems to be a promising technique that, especially if used in combination with other measures of biochemistry, is likely to be a quite powerful tool to advance the understanding of the neurobiological underpinnings of late-life depression.

FUNCTIONAL MAGNETIC RESONANCE IMAGING STUDIES

The most commonly used functional magnetic resonance imaging (fMRI) technique, BOLD, is a noninvasive indirect measure of cerebral activity that enables functional imaging with a temporal resolution in the order of 100 milliseconds and a spatial resolution of 1 to 2 mm. Thus, BOLD fMRI is ideal for localizing activity in response to transient cognitive events, even in relatively small brain structures that have been implicated in late-life depression (eg, the amygdala and brain stem nuclei). This section begins with a brief overview of the initial task-based findings and then focuses on fMRI studies of 2 networks that seem to be critical to the pathophysiology of geriatric depression (ie, the cognitive control network, the affective network) followed by some recommendations regarding 2 additional networks that the authors believe should be examined in late-life depression.

Functional neuroimaging studies in late-life depression reveal a pattern of abnormal activation of frontolimbic regions, generally characterized by hypoactivation of specific dorsal cortical regions, including the DLPFC and the dorsal ACC. One of the first published reports of task-related activation in geriatric depression was a PET study that compared cerebral blood flow during a word activation task between elderly patients with severe depression and normal elderly individuals. During the word activation task, hypoactivation of the dorsal ACC and the hippocampus was detected.[102] This finding of attenuated activation of the dorsal ACC during a verbal fluency task was later replicated by another group in an fMRI study of older depressed individuals in remission who had experienced multiple previous episodes of depression.[103] Furthermore, in depressed elderly patients, relative to age-matched controls, Aizenstein and colleagues[104] reported decreased DLPFC in addition to increased caudate activation in response to an explicit sequence-learning task.

These initial task-based activation studies of late-life depression converge with emerging evidence from other clinical and cognitive neuroscience techniques that cognitive control systems are disrupted in late-life depression (see the earlier sections on PET and MRS).[105,106] The cognitive control system of interest is composed of the dorsal ACC, DLPFC, and select parietal regions and enables efficient information processing by facilitating the adaptation to changing environmental demands and personal goals.[107,108] Several previous studies of midlife depression have reported activation abnormalities during cognitive control tasks, mostly involving hypoactivation of the dorsal ACC and the DLPFC,[109–111] with some evidence for abnormal FC within this network.[112,113]

Cognitive control is of particular interest in geriatric depression because of the vulnerability of cognitive control structures to aging[114–116] and the potential of specific cognitive control dysfunctions to explain several salient cognitive and other behavioral features of the illness, including the inability to ignore irrelevant, especially negative, stimuli. In elderly depressed patients, the DLPFC was observed to be hypoactive during the depressed state in response to a cognitive control paradigm along with reduced FC between the DLPFC and dorsal ACC.[117] An fMRI study of elderly depressed patients that used an emotional oddball task reported that relative to healthy comparison subjects, the elderly depressed patients demonstrated attenuated activation in select frontolimbic regions, including the right middle frontal gyrus and the cingulate, as well as the inferior parietal cortex.[118] In this sample, activation in the middle frontal gyrus seemed depressive state related, whereas attenuated activation in the posterior cingulate and inferior parietal regions persisted in the remitted subjects, suggesting a state-related alteration in cognitive control systems.

Functional abnormalities in the affective network in depression, which includes the ventral ACC, the amygdala, and portions of the orbitofrontal cortex, were first observed using PET (see the earlier section on PET).[1] Structures involved in the affective network typically demonstrate increased resting-state metabolism during depressed states in mixed-age–depressed people.[1,7,119–121] Subsequent fMRI studies in young and middle-aged adults with major depression have shown hyperactivation of ventral limbic regions most consistently, including the perigenual cingulate and amygdala, in response to emotional stimuli.[110,111,122–126] In contrast to the pattern of hyperactivity in the affective network in midlife depression, in an fMRI study that used an affective paradigm in elderly acutely depressed patients, relative to elderly control subjects, depressed patients exhibited hypoactivation of the ventromedial prefrontal cortex in response to the emotional evaluation of negatively valenced relative to positively valenced words.[127]

Activation and Antidepressant Treatment in Midlife Depression

fMRI studies in midlife depression on change in activation from baseline to posttreatment suggest that hyperactivity of the perigenual ACC[128–130] and amygdala[120,128,130] and hypoactivity of DLPFC[131,132] occurring during depressed states tend to resolve with antidepressant treatment. For example, fMRI studies conducted by Fales and colleagues[110,131] reported hypoactivity of the DLPFC and hyperactivity of the amygdala in depressed patients during a cognitive control task involving emotional interference. Hypoactivity of the DLPFC resolved after SSRI treatment.[131] Furthermore, the studies in midlife depression of the relationship of pretreatment fMRI activation to antidepressant response suggest that in response to affective stimuli, greater activity in the rostral ACC[133,134] and amygdala[133–136] before treatment may be associated with better clinical outcomes.

Activation, Antidepressant Treatment, and Geriatric Depression

There are only 2 published studies that report the relationship between fMRI activation and antidepressant response. In a study of the affective network that examined the relationship of cerebral activation to course of illness, acutely depressed patients exhibited hypoactivation of the ventromedial prefrontal cortex in response to the emotional evaluation of negatively valenced relative to positively valenced words. However, this hypoactivation normalized after several months of uncontrolled antidepressant treatment.[127] Furthermore, in a controlled antidepressant treatment trial, during a cognitive control task elderly depressed patients demonstrated hypoactivation in the DLPFC and diminished FC between the DLPFC and dorsal ACC before treatment.[117] Although the hypoactivity in the right DLPFC subsided after successful antidepressant treatment, the reduced FC between the dorsal ACC and the DLPFC persisted.

Future Directions

Taken together, the functional neuroimaging results indicate that abnormal frontolimbic activation is present in elderly depressed patients during the depressed state and some of these abnormalities may normalize (eg, hypoactivation of the DLPFC and hyperactivation of the amygdala), at least in part, in response to antidepressant treatment, whereas other abnormalities (ie, reduced FC, abnormal activity in the posterior cingulate) may persist despite antidepressant treatment.[117,118] However, the bulk of the existent fMRI data are from midlife depression, and it is quite likely that as more data become available, a different pattern of results may emerge in late-life that can clarify conceptual models of the pathophysiology of geriatric depression.

Reward Systems

To date, the task-based activation studies in geriatric depression have concentrated on cognitive control and affective regions. However, there are other systems that have been shown to be central to the behavioral disturbances observed in geriatric depression. For example, reward functions are disrupted in depression,[54] and these disruptions may be fundamental to the presentation of core symptoms of geriatric depression, including anhedonia.[136,137] fMRI studies of midlife depression indicate hypoactivation of the brain's reward structures, including dopaminergically mediated ascending mesolimbic projections areas such as the dorsal and ventral striata as well as the medial prefrontal cortex.[136,138,139] However, despite the vulnerability of reward systems to aging (see the section "The Dopamine System"),[140] to the authors' knowledge, there are no published reports that have examined task-related activation of reward systems in late-life depression, a syndrome for which anhedonia is especially problematic.[141]

The Default Mode Network

Traditionally, fMRI studies have focused on regional activation and, more recently, network activation related to task performance. However, there is a growing body of evidence that the resting brain is organized in a way that reflects interrelationships among structures with related functions and, therefore, resting-state FC analysis can identify functionally integrated, biologically meaningful networks.[142–144] These relationships can be examined using resting-state FC, which refers to the temporal correlation of brain activity across disparate regions.

The default mode network is one of several functionally connected networks that have been identified under resting-state conditions. The default mode network overlaps with the affective network and is composed of a set of regions (posterior cingulate/precuneus, medial prefrontal cortex, ventral ACC, inferior lateral parietal lobes, and parts of the temporal lobe) that consistently decrease their activity during cognitive task performance.[142,144] The default mode network is important in self-referential activities, including evaluating salience of internal and external cues, remembering the past, and planning the future.[144,145] Resting-state studies of midlife depression suggest that the default network may demonstrate higher FC in depression than in controls.[146,147] Furthermore, there is preliminary evidence that resting-state FC in the subgenual ACC is correlated with the length of major depressive episode with higher FC found during longer episodes of depression.[146] Given the influence of age on the FC of the default mode network[148] and the putative role of the default mode network in depression-related cognitive biases,[149] future studies should focus on the characterization of the default mode network in geriatric depression and how this network may interact with other cerebral systems to produce the depressive syndrome in late-life.

SUMMARY

Thus far, most of the functional neuroimaging data in late-life depression have focused on patterns of cerebral abnormalities that characterize the illness. As with many areas of study of psychiatric illnesses, functional neuroimaging observations are notable for the variability of findings between studies. However, when considering evidence from multiple functional neuroimaging modalities, a general pattern of findings has emerged. For example, studies that examine cerebral activity using either cerebral glucose metabolism or BOLD fMRI, generally yield a pattern of functional abnormalities in select aspects of corticolimbic networks, as well as elements of the default network, although the direction of the activation abnormalities (hypo vs hyper) tends to vary across imaging modalities and across the life span. Furthermore, abnormal activation in these systems seems to normalize, at least in part, in response to antidepressant treatment, but we are beginning to be able to dissociate networks associated with changes in cognitive symptoms from those associated with changes in affective symptoms.[150] To date, few molecular imaging studies have been performed in elderly depressed patients. However, based on the data in midlife depressed patients and age-related neurochemical changes, studies of monoaminergic and glutamatergic systems are a logical focus of future molecular imaging studies. In addition, studies of β amyloid and neuroinflammation may advance our understanding of the neurobiological basis of the cognitive and affective symptoms of the illness, including the increased risk of dementia associated with depression.

The authors believe that a critical next step in geriatric depression research is to use functional neuroimaging techniques to focus on dysfunctions in the networks that have been implicated in the pathophysiology of depression and relate these specific network dysfunctions to salient features of the illness, including the response of both cognitive and affective symptoms to treatments. In July 2010, the National Institute of Mental Health (NIMH) published the NIMH Research Domain Criteria (RDoC) Project,[151] which called for a search for "clinically relevant models of circuitry-behavior relationships." The RDoC mandates that investigators focus "on neural circuitry, with a level of analysis progressing…upwards from measures of circuitry function to clinically relevant variation." Because of the age-related vulnerability of some of the brain systems that have been implicated in mood disorders (eg, dopamine system, cognitive control system), geriatric depression is likely to be associated with more severe cerebral abnormalities than in midlife depression. Thus, consistent with the RDoC mandate, geriatric depression provides a logical context within which to study the role of specific functional abnormalities in both antidepressant response and key behavioral and cognitive abnormalities of mood disorders.

REFERENCES

1. Mayberg HS. Modulating dysfunctional limbic-cortical circuits in depression: towards development of brain-based algorithms for diagnosis and optimised treatment. Br Med Bull 2003;65:193–207.
2. Smith G, Kahn A, Hanratty K, et al. Serotonin transporter occupancy by citalopram treatment in geriatric depression. Neuroimage 2008;41:T168.
3. Fitzgerald PB, Laird AR, Maller J, et al. A meta-analytic study of changes in brain activation in depression. Hum Brain Mapp 2008;29:736.
4. Kumar A, Newberg A, Alavi A, et al. Regional cerebral glucose metabolism in late-life depression and Alzheimer disease: a preliminary positron emission tomography study. Proc Natl Acad Sci U S A 1993;90:7019–23.
5. Sackeim HA, Prohovnik I, Moeller JR, et al. Regional cerebral blood flow in mood disorders. I. Comparison of major depressives and normal controls at rest. Arch Gen Psychiatry 1990;47:60–70.
6. Nobler MS, Roose SP, Prohovnik I, et al. Regional cerebral blood flow in mood disorders, V: effects of antidepressant medication in late-life depression. Am J Geriatr Psychiatry 2000;8:289–96.
7. Smith G, Reynolds C, Pollock B, et al. Acceleration of the cerebral glucose metabolic response to antidepressant treatment by total sleep deprivation in geriatric depression. Am J Psychiatry 1999;156:683–9.
8. Smith G, Reynolds C, Houck P, et al. The glucose metabolic response to total sleep deprivation, recovery sleep and acute antidepressant treatment as functional neuroanatomic correlates of treatment outcome in geriatric depression. Am J Geriatr Psychiatry 2002;10:561–7.
9. Diaconescu AO, Kramer E, Hermann C, et al. Distinct functional networks associated with improvement of affective symptoms and cognitive function during citalopram treatment in geriatric depression. Hum Brain Mapp 2010 Sep 30. [Epub ahead of print].
10. Smith G, Kramer E, Hermann C, et al. The functional neuroanatomy of geriatric depression. Int J Geriatr Psychiatry 2009;24:798–808.
11. Smith G, Kramer E, Hermann C, et al. Serotonin modulation of cerebral glucose metabolism in depressed older adults. Biol Psychiatry 2009;66:259–66.

12. Smith G, Kramer E, Hermann C, et al. Serotonin modulation of cerebral glucose metabolism in geriatric depression. Am J Geriatr Psychiatry 2002;45:105–12.

13. Buckner RL, Snyder AZ, Shannon BJ, et al. Molecular, structural, and functional characterization of Alzheimer's disease: evidence for a relationship between default activity, amyloid, and memory. J Neurosci 2005;25:7709–17.

14. Schildkraut JJ. The catecholamine hypothesis of affective disorders: a review of supporting evidence. Am J Psychiatry 1965;122:509–22.

15. Lapin IP, Oxenkrug GF. Intensification of the central serotonergic processes as a possible determinant of the thymoleptic effect. Lancet 1969;1:132–6.

16. Ressler KJ, Nemeroff CB. Role of serotonergic and noradrenergic systems in the pathophysiology of depression and anxiety disorders. Depress Anxiety 2000; 12(Suppl 1):2–19.

17. Mann JJ. Role of the serotonergic system in the pathogenesis of major depression and suicidal behavior. Neuropsychopharmacology 1999;21(Suppl 2): 99S–105S.

18. Nobler MS, Mann JJ, Sackeim HA. Serotonin, cerebral blood flow, and cerebral metabolic rate in geriatric major depression and normal aging. Brain Res 1999; 30:250–63.

19. Nobler MS, Pelton GH, Sackeim HA. Cerebral blood flow and metabolism in late-life depression and dementia. J Geriatr Psychiatry Neurol 1999;12:118–27.

20. Pierson ME, Andersson J, Nyberg S, et al. [11C]AZ10419369: a selective 5-HT1B receptor radioligand suitable for positron emission tomography (PET): characterization in the primate brain. Neuroimage 2008;41:1075–85.

21. Comley R, Parker C, Wishart M, et al. In vivo evaluation and quantification of the 5-HT4 receptor PET ligand [11C]SB-207145. Neuroimage 2006;31:T23.

22. Parker CA, Cunningham VJ, Martarello L, et al. Evaluation of the novel 5-HT6 receptor radioligand, [11C] GSK-215083 in human. Neuroimage 2008;41:T20.

23. Agren H, Reibring L, Hartvig P, et al. Low brain uptake of L-[11C]5-hydroxytryptophan in major depression: a positron emission tomography study on patients and healthy volunteers. Acta Psychiatr Scand 1991;83:449–55.

24. Rosa-Neto P, Diksic M, Okazawa H, et al. Measurement of brain regional alpha-[11C]methyl-L-tryptophan trapping as a measure of serotonin synthesis in medication-free patients with major depression. Arch Gen Psychiatry 2004;61: 556–63.

25. Cannon DM, Ichise M, Fromm SJ, et al. Serotonin transporter binding in bipolar disorder assessed using [11C]DASB and positron emission tomography. Biol Psychiatry 2006;60:207–17.

26. Cannon DM, Ichise M, Rollis D, et al. Elevated serotonin transporter binding in major depressive disorder assessed using positron emission tomography and [11C]DASB; comparison with bipolar disorder. Biol Psychiatry 2007;62:870–7.

27. Reimold M, Batra A, Knobel A, et al. Anxiety is associated with reduced central serotonin transporter availability in unmedicated patients with unipolar major depression: a [11C]DASB PET study. Mol Psychiatry 2008;13:606–13, 557.

28. Oquendo MA, Hastings RS, Huang YY, et al. Brain serotonin transporter binding in depressed patients with bipolar disorder using positron emission tomography. Arch Gen Psychiatry 2007;64:201–8.

29. Parsey RV, Hastings RS, Oquendo MA, et al. Lower serotonin transporter binding potential in the human brain during major depressive episodes. Am J Psychiatry 2006;163:52–8.

30. Malison RT, Price LH, Berman R, et al. Reduced brain SERT availability in major depression as measured by [123I]-2 beta-carbomethoxy-3 beta–(4-iodophenyl)

tropane and single photon emission computed tomography. Biol Psychiatry 1998;44:1090–8.

31. Newberg AB, Amsterdam JD, Wintering N, et al. 123I-ADAM binding to serotonin transporters in patients with major depression and healthy controls: a preliminary study. J Nucl Med 2005;46:973–7.

32. Bhagwagar Z, Murthy N, Selvaraj S, et al. 5-HTT binding in recovered depressed patients and healthy volunteers: a positron emission tomography study with [11C]DASB. Am J Psychiatry 2007;164:1858–65.

33. Meyer JH, Houle S, Sagrati S, et al. Brain serotonin transporter binding potential measured with carbon 11-labeled DASB positron emission tomography: effects of major depressive episodes and severity of dysfunctional attitudes. Arch Gen Psychiatry 2004;61:1271–9.

34. Kugaya A, Sanacora G, Staley JK, et al. Brain serotonin transporter availability predicts treatment response to selective serotonin reuptake inhibitors. Biol Psychiatry 2004;56:497–502.

35. Miller JM, Oquendo MA, Ogden RT, et al. Serotonin transporter binding as a possible predictor of one-year remission in major depressive disorder. J Psychiatr Res 2008;42:1137–44.

36. Meyer JH, Wilson AA, Ginovart N, et al. Occupancy of SERTs by paroxetine and citalopram during treatment of depression: a [(11)C]DASB PET imaging study. Am J Psychiatry 2001;158(11):1843–9.

37. Drevets WC, Frank E, Price JC, et al. PET imaging of serotonin 1A receptor binding in depression. Biol Psychiatry 1999;46:1375–87.

38. Sargent PA, Kjaer KH, Bench CJ, et al. Brain serotonin 1A receptor binding measured by positron emission tomography with [11C]WAY-100635: effects of depression and antidepressant treatment. Arch Gen Psychiatry 2000;57: 174–80.

39. Parsey RV, Oquendo MA, Ogden RT, et al. Altered serotonin 1A binding in major depression: a [carbonyl-C-11] WAY100635 positron emission tomography study. Biol Psychiatry 2006;59:106–13.

40. Parsey RV, Olvet DM, Oquendo MA, et al. Higher 5-HT1A receptor binding potential during a major depressive episode predicts poor treatment response: preliminary data from a naturalistic study. Neuropsychopharmacology 2006;31: 1745–9.

41. Moses-Kolko EL, Price JC, Thase ME, et al. Measurement of 5-HT1A receptor binding in depressed adults before and after antidepressant drug treatment using positron emission tomography and [11C]WAY-100635. Synapse 2007; 61:523–30.

42. Meltzer CC, Price JC, Mathis CA, et al. Serotonin 1A receptor binding and treatment response in late-life depression. Neuropsychopharmacology 2004;29: 2258–65.

43. Lanctot KL, Hussey DF, Herrmann N, et al. A positron emission tomography study of 5-hydroxytryptamine-1A receptors in Alzheimer disease. Am J Geriatr Psychiatry 2007;15:888–98.

44. Blier P, De Montigny C, Azzaro AJ. Modification of serotonergic and noradrenergic neurotransmissions by repeated administration of monoamine oxidase inhibitors: electrophysiological studies in the rat central nervous system. J Pharmacol Exp Ther 1986;237:987–94.

45. Milak MS, Severance AJ, Ogden RT, et al. Modeling considerations for 11C-CUMI-101, an agonist radiotracer for imaging serotonin 1A receptor in vivo with PET. J Nucl Med 2008;49:587–96.

46. Meltzer CC, Price JC, Mathis CA, et al. PET imaging of serotonin type 2A receptors in late-life neuropsychiatric disorders. Am J Psychiatry 1999;156:1871–8.
47. Meyer JH, Kapur S, Houle S, et al. Prefrontal cortex 5-HT2 receptors in depression: an [18Γ] setoperone PET imaging study. Am J Psychiatry 1999;156:1029–34.
48. Biver F, Wikler D, Lotstra F, et al. Serotonin 5-HT2 receptor imaging in major depression: focal changes in orbito-insular cortex. Br J Psychiatry 1997;171:444–8.
49. Bhagwagar Z, Hinz R, Taylor M, et al. Increased 5-HT(2A) receptor binding in euthymic, medication-free patients recovered from depression: a positron emission study with [(11)C]MDL 100,907. Am J Psychiatry 2006;163:1580–7.
50. Meyer JH, Kapur S, Eisfeld B, et al. The effect of paroxetine on 5-HT2A receptors in depression: an [18F] setoperone PET imaging study. Am J Psychiatry 2001;158:78–85.
51. Yatham LN, Liddle PF, Dennie J, et al. Decrease in brain serotonin 2 receptor binding in patients with major depression following desipramine treatment: a positron emission tomography study with fluorine-18-labeled setoperone. Arch Gen Psychiatry 1999;56:705–11.
52. Moresco RM, Colombo C, Fazio F, et al. Effects of fluvoxamine treatment on the in vivo binding of [F-18]FESP in drug naive depressed patients: a PET study. Neuroimage 2000;12:452–65.
53. Massou JM, Trichard C, Attar-Levy D, et al. Frontal 5-HT2A receptors studied in depressive patients during chronic treatment by selective serotonin reuptake inhibitors. Psychopharmacology 1997;133:99–101.
54. Brown AS, Gershon S. Dopamine and depression. J Neural Transm 1993;91:75–109.
55. Nestler EJ, Carlezon WA Jr. The mesolimbic dopamine reward circuit in depression. Biol Psychiatry 2006;59:1151–9.
56. Agren H, Reibring L. PET studies of presynaptic monoamine metabolism in depressed patients and healthy volunteers. Pharmacopsychiatry 1994;27:2–6.
57. Meyer JH, Krüeger S, Wilson AA, et al. Lower dopamine transporters binding potential in striatum during depression. Neuroreport 2001;12:4121–5.
58. Suhara T, Nakayama K, Inoue O, et al. D1 dopamine receptor binding in mood disorders measured by positron emission tomography. Psychopharmacology 1992;106:14–8.
59. Klimke A, Larisch R, Janz A, et al. Dopamine D2 receptor binding before and after treatment of major depression measured by [123I]IBZM SPECT. Psychiatry Res 1999;90:90–101.
60. Parsey RV, Oquendo MA, Zea-Ponce Y, et al. Dopamine D(2) receptor availability and amphetamine-induced dopamine release in unipolar depression. Biol Psychiatry 2001;50:313–22.
61. Hirvonen J, Karlsson H, Kajander J, et al. Striatal dopamine D2 receptors in medication-naïve patients with major depressive disorder as assessed with [11C]raclopride PET. Psychopharmacology (Berl) 2008;197:581–90.
62. Meyer JH, McNeely HE, Sagrati S, et al. Elevated putamen D(2) receptor binding potential in major depression with motor retardation: an [11C]raclopride positron emission tomography study. Am J Psychiatry 2006;163:1594–602.
63. Cannon DM, Klaver JM, Peck SA, et al. Dopamine type-1 receptor binding in major depressive disorder assessed using positron emission tomography and [11C]NNC-112. Neuropsychopharmacology 2009;34:1277–87.
64. Anand A, Verhoeff P, Seneca N, et al. Brain SPECT imaging of amphetamine-induced dopamine release in euthymic bipolar disorder patients. Am J Psychiatry 2000;157:1108–14.

65. Volkow ND, Wang GJ, Fowler JS, et al. Parallel loss of presynaptic and postsynaptic dopamine markers in normal aging. Ann Neurol 1998;44:143–7.
66. Lavretsky H, Kumar A. Methylphenidate augmentation of citalopram in elderly depressed patients. Am J Geriatr Psychiatry 2001;9:298–303.
67. Shoghi-Jadid K, Small GW, Agdeppa ED, et al. Localization of neurofibrillary tangles and beta-amyloid plaques in the brains of living patients with Alzheimer disease. Am J Geriatr Psychiatry 2002;10:24–35.
68. Verhoeff NP, Wilson AA, Takeshita S, et al. In-vivo imaging of Alzheimer disease beta-amyloid with [11C]SB-13 PET. Am J Geriatr Psychiatry 2004;12:584–95.
69. Klunk WE, Engler H, Nordberg A, et al. Imaging brain amyloid in Alzheimer's disease with Pittsburgh compound-B. Ann Neurol 2004;55:306–19.
70. Small GW, Kepe V, Ercoli LM, et al. PET of brain amyloid and tau in mild cognitive impairment. N Engl J Med 2006;355:2652–63.
71. Rowe CC, Ng S, Ackermann U, et al. Imaging beta-amyloid burden in aging and dementia. Neurology 2007;68:1718–25.
72. Forsberg A, Engler H, Almkvist O, et al. PET imaging of amyloid deposition in patients with mild cognitive impairment. Neurobiol Aging 2008;29:1456–65.
73. Mathis CA, Wang Y, Holt DP, et al. Synthesis and evaluation of 11C-labeled 6-substituted 2-arylbenzothiazoles as amyloid imaging agents. J Med Chem 2003;46:2740–54.
74. Ikonomovic MD, Klunk WE, Abrahamson EE, et al. Post-mortem correlates of in vivo PIB-PET amyloid imaging in a typical case of Alzheimer's disease. Brain 2008;131:1630–4.
75. Villemagne VL, Pike KE, Darby D, et al. A beta deposits in older non-demented individuals with cognitive decline are indicative of preclinical Alzheimer's disease. Neuropsychologia 2008;46:1688–97.
76. Pike KE, Savage G, Villemagne VL, et al. Beta-amyloid imaging and memory in non-demented individuals: evidence for preclinical Alzheimer's disease. Brain 2007;130:2837–44.
77. Kemppainen NM, Aalto S, Wilson IA, et al. PET amyloid ligand [11C]PIB uptake is increased in mild cognitive impairment. Neurology 2007;68:1603–6.
78. Butters MA, Klunk WE, Mathis CA, et al. Imaging Alzheimer pathology in late-life depression with PET and Pittsburgh compound-B. Alzheimer Dis Assoc Disord 2008;22:261–8.
79. Marano C, Workman C, Zhou Y, et al. Cortical beta-amyloid deposition in late-life depression. Abstract presented at the American College of Neuropsychopharmacology 49th Annual Meeting. Miami (FL), 2010.
80. Lavretsky H, Siddarth P, Kepe V, et al. Depression and anxiety symptoms are associated with cerebral FDDNP-PET binding in middle-aged and older nondemented adults. Am J Geriatr Psychiatry 2009;17:493–502.
81. Schou M, Pike VW, Halldin C. Development of radioligands for imaging of brain norepinephrine transporters in vivo with positron emission tomography. Curr Top Med Chem 2007;7:1806–16.
82. Ding YS, Lin KS, Logan J. PET imaging of norepinephrine transporters. Curr Pharm Des 2006;12:3831–45.
83. Wu E, Greenberg P, Yang E, et al. Comparison of treatment persistence, hospital utilization and costs among major depressive disorder geriatric patients treated with escitalopram versus other SSRI/SNRI antidepressants. Curr Med Res Opin 2008;24:2805–13.
84. Mathew SJ, Manji HK, Charney DS. Novel drugs and therapeutic targets for severe mood disorders. Neuropsychopharmacology 2008;33:2080–92.

85. Blin J, Denis A, Yamaguchi T, et al. PET studies of [18F]methyl-MK-801, a potential NMDA receptor complex radioligand. Neurosci Lett 1991;121:183–6.

86. Ferrarese C, Guidotti A, Costa E, et al. In vivo study of NMDA-sensitive glutamate receptor by fluorothienylcyclohexylpiperidine, a possible ligand for positron emission tomography. Neuropharmacology 1991;30:899–905.

87. Shiue CY, Shiue GG, Mozley PD, et al. P-[18F]- MPPF: a potential radioligand for PET studies of 5-HT1A receptors in humans. Synapse 1997;25:147–54.

88. Brown AK, Kimura Y, Zoghbi SS, et al. Metabotropic glutamate subtype 5 receptors are quantified in the human brain with a novel radioligand for PET. J Nucl Med 2008;49:2042–8.

89. Olney JW, Wozniak DF, Farber NB. Excitotoxic neurodegeneration in Alzheimer disease. New hypothesis and new therapeutic strategies. Arch Neurol 1997;54:1234–40.

90. Furey ML, Drevets WC. Antidepressant efficacy of the antimuscarinic drug scopolamine: a randomized, placebo-controlled clinical trial. Arch Gen Psychiatry 2006;63:1121–9.

91. George TP, Sacco KA, Vessicchio JC, et al. Nicotinic antagonist augmentation of selective serotonin reuptake inhibitor-refractory major depressive disorder: a preliminary study. J Clin Psychopharmacol 2008;28:340–4.

92. Cannon DM, Carson RE, Nugent AC, et al. Reduced muscarinic type 2 receptor binding in subjects with bipolar disorder. Arch Gen Psychiatry 2006;63:741–7.

93. Smith G, Gunning-Dixon F, Lotrich F, et al. Translational research in late-life mood disorders: implications for future intervention and prevention research. Neuropsychopharmacology 2007;32:1857–75.

94. Chauveau F, Boutin H, Van Camp N, et al. Nuclear imaging of neuroinflammation: a comprehensive review of [(11)C]PK11195 challengers. Eur J Nucl Med Mol Imaging 2008;35:2304–19.

95. Fujita M, Imaizumi M, Zoghbi SS, et al. Kinetic analysis in healthy humans of a novel positron emission tomography radioligand to image the peripheral benzodiazepine receptor, a potential biomarker for inflammation. Neuroimage 2008;40:43–52.

96. Endres CJ, Pomper MG, James M, et al. Initial evaluation of 11C-DPA-713, a novel TSPO PET ligand, in humans. J Nucl Med 2009;50:1276–82.

97. Kumar A, Thomas A, Lavretsky H, et al. Frontal white matter biochemical abnormalities in late-life major depression detected with proton magnetic resonance spectroscopy. Am J Psychiatry 2002;15:630–6.

98. Elderkin-Thompson V, Thomas MA, Binesh N, et al. Brain metabolites and cognitive function among older depressed and healthy individuals using 2D MR spectroscopy. Neuropsychopharmacology 2004;29:2251–7.

99. Chen CS, Chiang IC, Li CW, et al. Proton magnetic resonance spectroscopy of late-life major depressive disorder. Psychiatry Res 2009;172:210–4.

100. Venkatraman TN, Krishnan RR, Steffens DC, et al. Biochemical abnormalities of the medial temporal lobe and medial prefrontal cortex in late-life depression. Psychiatry Res 2009;172:49–54.

101. Forester BP, Harper DG, Jensen JE, et al. 31Phosphorus magnetic resonance spectroscopy study of tissue specific changes in high energy phosphates before and after sertraline treatment of geriatric depression. Int J Geriatr Psychiatry 2009;24:788–97.

102. de Asis JM, Stern E, Alexopoulos GS, et al. Hippocampal and anterior cingulate activation deficits in patients with geriatric depression. Am J Psychiatry 2001;158:1321–3.

103. Takami H, Okamoto Y, Yamashita H, et al. Attenuated anterior cingulate activation during a verbal fluency task in elderly patients with a history of multiple-episode depression. Am J Geriatr Psychiatry 2007;15:594–603.

104. Aizenstein HJ, Butters MA, Figurski JL, et al. Prefrontal and striatal activation during sequence learning in geriatric depression. Biol Psychiatry 2005;58:290–6.

105. Alexopoulos GS, Kiosses DN, Heo M, et al. Executive dysfunction and the course of geriatric depression. Biol Psychiatry 2005;58:204–10.

106. Murphy CF, Gunning-Dixon FM, Hoptman MJ, et al. White-matter integrity predicts stroop performance in patients with geriatric depression. Biol Psychiatry 2007;61:1007–10.

107. Carter CS, van Veen V. Anterior cingulate cortex and conflict detection: an update of theory and data. Cogn Affect Behav Neurosci 2007;7:367–79.

108. Egner T, Etkin A, Gale S, et al. Dissociable neural systems resolve conflict from emotional versus nonemotional distracters. Cereb Cortex 2008;18:1475–84.

109. Fitzgerald PB, Oxley TJ, Laird AR, et al. An analysis of functional neuroimaging studies of dorsolateral prefrontal cortical activity in depression. Psychiatry Res 2006;148:33–45.

110. Fales CL, Barch DM, Rundle MM, et al. Altered emotional interference processing in affective and cognitive-control brain circuitry in major depression. Biol Psychiatry 2008;63:377–84.

111. Siegle GJ, Thompson W, Carter CS, et al. Increased amygdala and decreased dorsolateral prefrontal BOLD responses in unipolar depression: related and independent features. Biol Psychiatry 2006;612:198–209.

112. Schlosser RG, Wagner G, Koch K, et al. Fronto-cingulate effective connectivity in major depression: a study with fMRI and dynamic causal modeling. Neuroimage 2008;43:645–55.

113. Vasic N, Walter H, Sambataro F, et al. Aberrant functional connectivity of dorsolateral prefrontal and cingulate networks in patients with major depression during working memory processing. Psychol Med 2009;39:977–87.

114. Gunning-Dixon FM, Raz N. Neuroanatomical correlates of selected executive functions in middle-aged and older adults: a prospective MRI study. Neuropsychologia 2003;41:1929–41.

115. Gunning-Dixon FM, Brickman AM, Cheng JC, et al. Aging of cerebral white matter: a review of MRI findings. Int J Geriatr Psychiatry 2009;24:109–17.

116. Raz N, Gunning-Dixon FM, Head D, et al. Neuroanatomical correlates of cognitive aging: evidence from structural magnetic resonance imaging. Neuropsychology 1998;12:95–114.

117. Aizenstein HJ, Butters MA, Wu M, et al. Altered functioning of the executive control circuit in late-life depression: episodic and persistent phenomena. Am J Geriatr Psychiatry 2009;17:30–42.

118. Wang L, Krishnan KR, Steffens DC, et al. Depressive state- and disease-related alterations in neural responses to affective and executive challenges in geriatric depression. Am J Psychiatry 2008;165:863–71.

119. Drevets WC, Bogers W, Raichle ME. Functional anatomical correlates of antidepressant drug treatment assessed using PET measures of regional glucose metabolism. Eur Neuropsychopharmacol 2002;12:527–44.

120. Kennedy SH, Evans KR, Kruger S, et al. Changes in regional brain glucose metabolism measured with positron emission tomography after paroxetine treatment of major depression. Am J Psychiatry 2001;158:899–905.

121. Mayberg HS, Liotti M, Brannan SK, et al. Reciprocal limbic-cortical function and negative mood: converging PET findings in depression and normal sadness. Am J Psychiatry 1999;156:675–82.
122. Anand A, Li Y, Wang Y, et al. Activity and connectivity of brain mood regulating circuit in depression: a functional magnetic resonance study. Biol Psychiatry 2005;57:1079–88.
123. Canli T, Sivers H, Thomason ME, et al. Brain activation to emotional words in depressed vs healthy subjects. Neuroreport 2004;15:2585–8.
124. Elliott R, Rubinsztein JS, Sahakian BJ, et al. The neural basis of mood-congruent processing biases in depression. Arch Gen Psychiatry 2002;59:597–604.
125. Sheline YI, Barch DM, Donnelly JM, et al. Increased amygdala response to masked emotional faces in depressed subjects resolves with antidepressant treatment: an fMRI study. Biol Psychiatry 2001;50:651–8.
126. Surguladze S, Brammer MJ, Keedwell P, et al. A differential pattern of neural response toward sad versus happy facial expressions in major depressive disorder. Biol Psychiatry 2005;57:201–9.
127. Brassen S, Kalisch R, Weber-Fahr W, et al. Ventromedial prefrontal cortex processing during emotional evaluation in late-life depression: a longitudinal functional Magnetic resonance imaging study. Biol Psychiatry 2008;64:349–55.
128. Anand A, Li Y, Wang Y, et al. Reciprocal effects of antidepressant treatment on activity and connectivity of the mood regulating circuit: an fMRI study. J Neuropsychiatry Clin Neurosci 2007;19:274–82.
129. Fu CH, Williams SC, Cleare AJ, et al. Attenuation of the neural response to sad faces in major depression by antidepressant treatment: a prospective, event-related functional magnetic resonance imaging study. Arch Gen Psychiatry 2004;61:877–89.
130. Robertson B, Wang L, Diaz MT, et al. Effect of bupropion extended release on negative emotional processing in major depressive disorder: a pilot functional magnetic resonance imaging study. J Clin Psychiatry 2007;68:261–7.
131. Fales C, Barch D, Rundle M, et al. Antidepressant treatment normalizes hypoactivity in dorsolateral prefrontal cortex during emotional interference processing in major depression. J Affect Disord 2009;112:206–11.
132. Davidson RJ, Irwin W, Anderle MJ, et al. The neural substrates of affective processing in depressed patients treated with venlafaxine. Am J Psychiatry 2003; 160:64–75.
133. Langenecker S, Kennedy S, Guidotti L, et al. Frontal and limbic activation during inhibitory control predicts treatment response in major depressive disorder. Biol Psychiatry 2007;62:1272–80.
134. Canli T, Cooney R, Goldin P, et al. Amygdala reactivity to emotional faces predicts improvement in major depression. Neuroreport 2005;16:1267–70.
135. Siegle GJ, Carter CS, Thase ME. Use of fMRI to predict recovery from unipolar depression with cognitive behavior therapy. Am J Psychiatry 2006;163:735–8.
136. Pizzagalli DA, Holmes AJ, Dillon DG, et al. Reduced caudate and nucleus accumbens response to rewards in unmedicated individuals with major depressive disorder. Am J Psychiatry 2009;166:702–10.
137. Wacker J, Dillon DG, Pizzagalli DA. The role of the nucleus accumbens and rostral anterior cingulate cortex in anhedonia: integration of resting EEG, fMRI, and volumetric techniques. Neuroimage 2009;46:327–37.
138. Epstein J, Pan H, Kocsis JH, et al. Lack of ventral striatal response to positive stimuli in depressed versus normal subjects. Am J Psychiatry 2006;163: 1784–90.

139. Mitterschiffthaler MT, Kumari V, Malhi GS, et al. Neural response to pleasant stimuli in anhedonia: an fMRI study. Neuroreport 2003;14:177–82.
140. Volkow ND, Logan J, Fowler JS, et al. Association between age-related decline in brain dopamine activity and impairment in frontal and cingulate metabolism. Am J Psychiatry 2000;157:75–80.
141. Krishnan KR, Hays JC, Tupler LA, et al. Clinical and phenomenological comparisons of late-onset and early-onset depression. Am J Psychiatry 1995;152: 785–8.
142. Fox MD, Snyder AZ, Vincent JL, et al. The human brain is intrinsically organized into dynamic, anticorrelated functional networks. Proc Natl Acad Sci U S A 2005; 102:9673–8.
143. Fox MD, Raichle ME. Spontaneous fluctuations in brain activity observed with functional magnetic resonance imaging. Nat Rev Neurosci 2007;8:700–11.
144. Raichle ME, Snyder AZ. A default mode of brain function: a brief history of an evolving idea. Neuroimage 2007;37:1083–90.
145. Raichle ME, MacLeod AM, Snyder AZ, et al. A default mode of brain function. Proc Natl Acad Sci U S A 2001;98:676–82.
146. Greicius MD, Flores BH, Menon V, et al. Resting-state functional connectivity in major depression: abnormally increased contributions from subgenual cingulate cortex and thalamus. Biol Psychiatry 2007;62:429–37.
147. Sheline YI, Price JL, Yan Z, et al. Resting-state functional MRI in depression unmasks increased connectivity between networks via the dorsal nexus. Proc Natl Acad Sci U S A 2010;107:11020–5.
148. Damoiseaux JS, Beckmann CF, Arigita EJ, et al. Reduced resting-state brain activity in the "default network" in normal aging. Cereb Cortex 2008;18:1856–64.
149. Sheline YI, Barch DM, Price JL, et al. The default mode network and self-referential processes in depression. Proc Natl Acad Sci U S A 2009;106:1942–7.
150. Smith GS, Workman CI, Kramer E, et al. The relationship between the acute cerebral metabolic response to citalopram and chronic citalopram treatment outcome. Am J Geriatr Psychiatry 2011;19:53–63.
151. Insel T, Cuthbert B, Garvey M, et al. Research domain criteria (RDoC): toward a new classification framework for research on mental disorders. Am J Psychiatry 2010;167:748–51.

Structural Neuroimaging of Geriatric Depression

Sophiya Benjamin, MD[a], David C. Steffens, MD, MHS[b],*

KEYWORDS

- Geriatric depression • Late-life depression • Neuroimaging
- MRI • White matter hyperintensities
- Magnetic resonance spectroscopy

Neuroimaging has been a powerful tool in our search to identify neuroanatomic markers that provide information about the diagnostic and prognostic status of elderly patients with depressive symptoms. After decades of research, we now know several regions in the brain that are implicated in depression such as the anterior cingulate, orbitofrontal cortex (OFC), and the hippocampus. Successes in delineating the neural circuits in depression have closely paralleled progress in neuroimaging techniques and advances in image analysis. Such noninvasive methods are critical as access to the tissue of interest, the brain, is otherwise impossible except in postmortem samples.

Magnetic resonance (MR) or nuclear MR occurs when protons in the nuclei of certain atoms (usually hydrogen) are subjected to a static magnetic field, then exposed to a second oscillating magnetic field (pulse). During the application of the pulse, the alignment of the protons within the static magnetic field is disturbed. Following the application of the pulse, the misaligned protons relax and return to their original alignment emitting energy signals in the process. The relaxation times of different tissues vary, forming the basis of MRI.[1] MR-based methods such as MR morphometry, diffusion tensor imaging (DTI), and MR spectroscopy (MRS), among others, are used to detect differences between the brains of depressed and nondepressed elderly. Readers interested in further details about individual methods, their strengths and weaknesses in the context of geriatric depression, are referred to the excellent review by Hoptman and colleagues.[1]

Financial Disclosures: The authors have nothing to disclose.
[a] Department of Psychiatry, Duke University Medical Center, DHSP, Box 3837, Durham 27710, NC, USA
[b] Division of Geriatric Psychiatry, Department of Psychiatry and Behavioral Sciences, Duke University Medical Center, DHSP, Box 3903, Durham, NC 27710, USA
* Corresponding author.
E-mail address: david.steffens@duke.edu

Psychiatr Clin N Am 34 (2011) 423–435
doi:10.1016/j.psc.2011.02.001
0193-953X/11/$ – see front matter © 2011 Elsevier Inc. All rights reserved.

Several differences in the structure of the brain between depressed and nondepressed elderly have been found and replicated. In this article, the authors summarize some of the salient structural imaging findings in geriatric depression and their implications to the neurobiology of late-life depression. First, morphometric studies focusing on volumetric differences are discussed; followed by findings from studies that examine white matter pathology using different imaging techniques. Finally, the biochemical correlates of depression found by MRS are summarized.

VOLUMETRIC DIFFERENCES IN SPECIFIC BRAIN STRUCTURES

Volumetric studies examine differences in the volumes of different brain structures among patients with depression compared with those who are not depressed. This can be accomplished either by traditional morphometric studies that focus on a predetermined, specific structure, based on previous knowledge about pathophysiology, or by voxel-based morphometry (VBM) that is not biased toward any one structure and assesses anatomical differences throughout the brain.

Morphometric Studies

Most morphometric studies use T1-weighted images to compare the volumes of specific structures such as the hippocampus or a particular region in the frontal cortex. These areas are called regions of interest (ROI). This hypothesis-driven approach has identified several volumetric differences between depressed and nondepressed elderly.

The hippocampus

The hippocampus is one of the most commonly studied structures in depression. Studies in late-life depression have repeatedly demonstrated a reduction in hippocampal volume among the depressed.[2–7] Though some studies did find negative results,[8,9] two recent meta-analyses of MRI studies have confirmed that there is indeed an association between depression and decreased hippocampal volume.[10,11] It has been suggested that earlier negative findings may be due either to the inclusion of the amygdala along with the hippocampus[12] or lower resolution of images.[13] Further exploration of this association has revealed that age of onset of depression correlates negatively with hippocampal volume as patients with late-onset depression had smaller hippocampal volumes when compared with those with early onset depression and controls.[4] In a younger cohort of patients followed over 3 years, depressed participants exhibited greater decline in bilateral hippocampal volume.[14]

Evidence from animal studies indicates that the mechanism underlying decreased hippocampal volumes is stress-induced decrease in cell proliferation in the hippocampal region.[15,16] Further, administration of antidepressants has been shown to prevent such stress-induced suppression of neurogenisis.[17] Hippocampal volume reduction has also been shown to correlate with serotonin transporter promoter region polymorphism (5-HTTLPR) in which individuals who were homozygous for the L allele exhibited smaller hippocampal volumes.[18] A similar correlation with the val66met polymorphism of the brain-derived neurotrophic factor gene has been found to be positive in younger adults,[19] but was not replicated in an elderly sample.[20] Though decrease in hippocampal volume has been proposed as an endophenotype for depression, it is by no means specific as similar decreases occur in mild cognitive impairment and Alzheimer's dementia, which are common comorbidities in older adults with depression.[21,22]

The amygdala

The amygdala is an important structure in emotion regulation as it identifies and integrates the emotional salience with perception. Functional studies have demonstrated that patients with depression have increased reactivity of the amygdala to negative stimuli that can be reversed by antidepressant treatment.[23] However, findings from structural studies have been conflicting as studies in younger cohorts have shown an increase in volume during the first episode of depression but not in those with recurrent episodes; further, it did not correlate with age of onset, illness duration, or severity of symptoms.[24] Earlier studies included the amygdala and hippocampus together, making the results hard to interpret.[8] A meta-analysis combining amygdala volumes in depression from 14 studies found that there was a significant heterogeneity among the studies and that there was no significant association between amygdala volume and depression.[10] There is some evidence that the differences in volume might be heritable, thereby making it harder to detect differences between depressed and nondepressed samples.[25]

The striatum

Decreased volumes of the caudate[26] and putamen,[27] which are important structures in the corticostriatal circuit, were observed in depressed samples. This was later replicated in depressed elderly,[28,29] supporting the role of subcortical structures in geriatric depression. Another study found that a decrease in caudate volume predicted psychomotor slowing in older adults with depression.[30] Some studies did not find the above-mentioned differences in basal ganglia volumes; however, this may have been due to differences in sample selection as the patients were younger[31] and free of medical comorbidities; specifically, cardiovascular risk.[32]

The anterior cingulate cortex

Though the entire cingulate cortex was initially thought to be involved with emotion and behavior, the more recent understanding is that the anterior cingulate cortex (ACC) is important in emotion, whereas the posterior part is more important in visuospatial function and memory.[33] The ACC is further subdivided into "affect" and "cognition,"[33] which are implicated in geriatric depression.[34] Some of the functions of the ACC salient to depression include conditioned emotional learning, vocalizations associated with expressing internal states, assessment of motivational content, and assigning emotional valence to stimuli.[33]

In a meta-analysis of several structures involved in depression, the ACC had the largest effect, with depressed individuals having smaller ACC volumes.[10] Though not specific to elderly samples, some studies have demonstrated decreased volumes of the ACC in depressed individuals,[35,36] whereas others failed to do so.[37,38] Another study that limited its sample to the elderly found significant bilateral reductions in gray matter volume in the ACC.[39]

The OFC

The OFC functions as part of a network that includes the hippocampus, amygdala, and basal ganglia. It is involved in integrating sensory experiences and in emotional- and reward-related learning and decision making.[40] In elderly samples, compared with nondepressed subjects, depressed cohorts exhibit smaller OFC volumes.[39,41,42] There have been similar findings in younger adults,[37,43] although negative results have also been reported.[44] The decreased in OFC volume in the depressed is consistent with postmortem findings that show a reduction in the density of pyramidal neurons in this region in the depressed.[45]

In a study that examined the functional implications of the OFC in depressed elderly, decreased left OFC volume was associated with poorer performance on the Benton Visual Retention Test (BVRT).[46] The BVRT measures perception of spatial relations and memory for newly learned material. Depressed elderly with smaller left OFC volumes made more preservative errors and scored lower on the overall test.[46] Further, smaller medial orbitofrontal gyri volume was found to be associated with impairment in both basic and instrumental activities of daily living.[47] Though no causal inferences can be made from either of the above cross-sectional studies, they do expand our current understanding of the mechanisms that underlie cognitive dysfunction and functional impairment in depression.

Voxel-based Morphometry

VBM is a highly automated method with a hypothesis-free approach, not requiring a priori assumptions about the relevance of specific brain regions. VBM consists of the following four steps: (1) spatial normalization that transforms all the subjects' data into the same stereotactic space; (2) partitioning the spatially normalized images into segments such as gray matter, white matter, and cerebrospinal fluid; (3) preprocessing the gray matter segment to make enable further voxel-by-voxel analysis to be comparable to the ROI approach; and (4) comparing the segment of interest such as the gray matter between the groups voxel-by-voxel.[48] VBM is a more recently described method compared with the ROI approach and the literature in geriatric depression using this technique is still in its early stages. Results from recent studies using this technique are encouraging in that the regions that have been identified are by often those that have been identified by previous structural and functional studies. As the literature from VBM is not as voluminous as that from traditional morphometric methods, results about different brain structures are presented together in this section.

In a study of 30 depressed and 47 nondepressed elderly, depressed patients were found to have smaller right hippocampal volumes compared with control subjects. Also, the volume of the hippocampal-entorhinal cortex was inversely associated with the duration since the first episode of depression.[49] In another study, VBM revealed decreases in the volume of the right rostral hippocampus, in the right amygdala, and the medial OFC bilaterally.[50] Additionally, the gray matter volume of both the right and left medial OFC correlated negatively with scores on the geriatric depression scale.[50]

In-patients with late-onset depression were found to have smaller volumes in several regions of gray matter, including the insula and the posterior cingulate region, and white matter, including the subcallosal cingulate cortex, floor of lateral ventricles, parahippocampal region, insula, and the cerebellum.[51] Compared with the depressed who did not attempt suicide, those who attempted suicide had decreased gray matter and white matter volume in the frontal, parietal, and temporal regions, as well as the insula, lentiform nucleus, midbrain, and the cerebellum.[51]

In a study that examined first-episode remitted geriatric depression, patients with remitted depression had smaller volumes of right superior frontal cortex, left postcentral cortex, and right middle temporal gyrus; and larger left cingulate gyrus volume compared with healthy control subjects.[52] In patients with remitted depression, the volume of the left cingulated gyrus correlated negatively with scores on the Rey Auditory Verbal Learning Test and delayed recall[52]—providing further evidence that specific brain regions involved in depression might also be involved in cognitive impairment seen so often in the depressed elderly.

A limitation of the aforementioned studies is their small sample size, which ranged from 34[50] to 67.[49] Though many of the published studies have found significant associations, negative findings have also been reported[53] and larger sample sizes that could clarify these discrepancies are needed. False-positives are an inherent problem in any technique where the number of comparisons is large and the sample size small; as in the case of VBM. However, several statistical methods to control for this have been described.[48,54] Another disadvantage that might be specific to geriatric depression is that this technique does not differentiate between vascular and degenerative causes of differences in regional brain volume. Despite the above limitations, early results are promising and VBM has the potential to identify new structural variations that could expand our current understanding of geriatric depression.

WHITE MATTER PATHOLOGY

White matter hyperintensities (WMH) are thought to be caused by small, silent cerebral infarctions.[55] Such silent cerebral infarctions were observed in 65.9% of patients with early- or presenile-onset depression and 93.7% of those with late-onset depression.[55] Early observations that older individuals with depression have a greater severity of clinically silent ischemic disease that is observable as hyperintense lesions on MRI scans,[56] as well as clinical characteristics such as increased cognitive dysfunction,[57] led to the advent of the "vascular depression hypothesis."[58] WMH can be detected by various structural imaging methods including T2-weighted MRI scans, DTI, and magnetization transfer (MT) imaging.

T2-Weighted MRI Studies

On T2-weighted MRI studies, the hyperintense signals are present in the white matter and can be classified into three major groups: periventricular hyperintensities, deep WMH (DWMH), and subcortical hyperintensities. Older depressed individuals have consistently been found to have more WMH than older healthy controls without depression.[59–63] Further, such lesions are more common in late-onset depression compared with early-onset depression.[56] In a cohort of poststroke patients, those who developed poststroke depression were more likely to have severe DWMH (12.8% vs 1.3%; $P = .009$).[64]

Beyond just diagnosis and classification, WMH have been shown to be important in the course of illness and outcome of depression as subcortical white matter lesions were associated with occurrence, persistence, worsening, and severity of depressive symptoms.[65,66] Additionally, greater progression of white matter lesions was associated with poorer treatment outcomes as depressed elderly who had greater WMH volume did not achieve or sustain remission when compared with depressed elderly who had lower WMH volume.[67] Even in the absence of overt cerebrovascular disease, time to relapse was shorter in those who had severe deep white matter lesions.[68]

WMH have also been shown to predict response to antidepressant treatment. WMH burden predicted Montgomery-Asberg Depression Rating Scale (MADRS) scores over a 12-week course of sertraline. Furthermore, WMH correlated with neuropsychological testing measures that also predicted depression outcome with treatment, and both these variables correlated with the Framingham vascular risk factor scores, supporting the vascular depression hypothesis.[69] In another study, patients with depression who failed to remit after a 12-week controlled trial of escitalopram had greater MRI signal hyperintensity burden compared with those who remitted as well as elderly comparisons but, there was no difference in signal hyperintensity burden between those who remitted and elderly control subjects.[70]

Based on the evidence that vascular depression can confer risk for adverse outcomes and is produced by a pathology that separates it from other forms of depression, it has been argued that "subcortical ischemic depression" be considered as a unique and valid diagnosis corresponding to the "vascular depression" hypothesis.[71] In a more recent study replicated in two independent clinical samples, DWMH was found to be the most accurate marker for classifying depression into vascular versus nonvascular depression.[72]

Diffusion Tensor Imaging

DTI is an MRI-based method that measures the self-diffusion of water, which can be isotropic when it occurs equally in all directions when no barriers are present and anisotropic when the diffusion of water tends to follow along external barriers.[1] White matter tracts in the brain form organized barriers along which water can diffuse, making the flow anisotropic. When such tracts are disrupted, the diffusion is less anisotropic. Fractional anisotropy (FA) is a common measure used to characterize the integrity of the neural circuit. Using measures such as FA and apparent diffusion coefficient, DTI can help further our understanding of white matter pathology in geriatric depression by enabling researchers to locate and quantify the structure and orientation of cerebral white matter tracts.

In one of the earlier studies, regions with hyperintensities in the depressed elderly showed increase apparent diffusion coefficient and decreased FA when compared with normal regions, though there was no significant difference in diffusion characteristics between the depressed and nondepressed.[73] A more recent study showed significantly lower FA in the right superior frontal gyrus white matter of depressed patients.[74] Another study of 106 depressed and 84 nondepressed elderly participants found that depressed patients had significantly lower FA in the white matter lateral to the right ACC, bilateral superior frontal gyri, and the left middle frontal gyrus.[75] Such findings have been replicated in different populations. In a Chinese sample, late-life depression was associated with decreased FA in the frontal (superior and middle frontal gyrus) and temporal (right parahippocampal gyrus) regions.[76]

Diffusion anisotropy was lower in several regions of the brain, including right superior frontal gyrus, left inferior frontal gyrus, left middle temporal gyrus, right inferior parietal lobule, right middle occipital gyrus, left lingual gyrus, right putamen, and right caudate in patients with first-episode remitted geriatric depression.[77] Though most studies have concentrated on DTI imaging of white matter pathology, a recent study used DTI to examine the integrity of normal-appearing white matter and found that depressed elderly had widespread abnormalities in DTI measures in the prefrontal region.[78] These studies strengthen the evidence for the possibility that decreased FA could affect the connectivity of the dorsolateral prefrontal circuit and the anterior cingulate circuit resulting in disconnection of cortical and subcortical structures, thereby resulting in depression. Further, decreased integrity of white matter tracts are also associated with decreased executive function, commonly seen in late-life depression.[79]

Such microstructural abnormalities have also been shown to be associated with the severity of depressive symptoms and the likelihood of remission with treatment. Higher FA values in a region 8 mm below the anterior commissure-posterior commissure line correlated with lower Hamilton Depression Rating Scale scores.[80] In another study, increased FA in the region 15 mm above the anterior commissure-posterior commissure plane was associated with low remission after treatment with citalopram.[81] Similarly, failure to remit with sertraline was associated with increased FA in the superior frontal gyri and anterior cingulate cortices bilaterally.[82] In another study of depression treatment, depressed patients who had decreased FA compared with nondepressed patients showed an increase in frontal FA after electroconvulsive treatment.[83]

Magnetization Transfer MRI

MT-MRI is another MRI-based method used to examine biophysical properties of brain tissue. MT-MRI uses the two types of water molecules present in biological tissues: free water and water bound to molecules. Proton MRI detects signal from mobile protons or free water, which have longer T2 relaxation times. The T2 relaxation times of protons associated with macromolecules are too short to be detected by conventional MRI. However, coupling between the bound and free protons allows the bound protons to influence the spin state of the mobile ones. MT imaging requires two image acquisitions in which the first is similar to an MRI study. The second, which is the MT acquisition, is acquired by first saturating the bound water by an off-resonance radiofrequency pulse, which negates the potential for the bound water to create a signal, which then creates a signal reduction relative to the first image. The difference in signal intensity between the two images is the MT ratio (MTR).[1,84,85]

One of the earliest studies using MTR in late-life depression found that older depressed patients had lower MTRs in the genu and splenium of the corpus callosum, the neostriatum, and the occipital white matter.[84] Of note, all of these differences were in normal-appearing white matter tracts that were free of hyperintense lesions.[84] In a more recent study with a larger sample size of 55 older patients with depression and –24 comparison subjects, depressed patients had lower MTRs in multiple left hemisphere frontostriatal and limbic regions, including white matter lateral to the lentiform nuclei, dorsolateral and dorsomedial prefrontal, dorsal anterior cingulate, subcallosal, periamygdalar, insular, and posterior cingulate regions, complementing previous findings from volumetric and DTI studies.[86]

MRS and Biochemical Correlates of Depression

MRS is another noninvasive imaging method that, unlike all the other techniques described above, characterizes chemical and cellular features in vivo. In the brain, concentrations and mobility of low-molecular-weight chemicals can be measured as spectral peaks that can then be used to identify abnormalities in brain regions that appear normal in MRI.[87] The measurements are usually not absolute and are presented as the ratio of the measure of interest to a standard metabolite such as creatine (Cr).[1]

In a preliminary study of 20 elderly patients with depression and 18 comparison subjects, myo-inositol (MI) to Cr and choline (Cho) to Cr ratios were significantly higher in the frontal white matter in the depressed group.[88] A subsequent study explored the relationship between these metabolites in a voxel in the dorsolateral cortex and cognitive function in the elderly. Among nondepressed subjects, cognition positively correlated with Cho to Cr and MI to Cr ratios, and negatively correlated with phosphocholine to Cr ratio in the four domains of verbal learning, recognition, recall, and hypothesis generation; whereas, depressed patients did not have consistent relationships between the metabolites.[89] Thus, imaging studies have revealed both neuroanatomic as well as biochemical changes in the frontostriatal circuitry that may be associated with cognitive changes in depression.

In a more recent study, patients with late-life major depressive disorder had a significantly lower N-acetyl aspartate (NAA) to Cr ratio in the left frontal white matter, and higher Cho to Cr and MI to Cr ratios in the left basal ganglia when compared with the control subjects.[90] Furthermore, the MI correlated with global cognitive function.[90]

In older patients whose depression responded to treatment, concentrations of total NAA, Cho, and Cr were significantly decreased in the prefrontal cortex; whereas, concentrations of NAA and MI were significantly elevated in the left medial temporal lobe.[91] These investigators concluded that reduced neuronal phospholipid and energy metabolism in the prefrontal cortex persists in clinically improved depression and that the elevated metabolites in the temporal lobe might be associated with glial cell changes in the amygdala.[91]

MRS of the brain before antidepressant treatment of poststroke depression followed by a second MRS 6 months after revealed changes in metabolites in various regions.[92] Before treatment, NAA to Cr ratios in the bilateral hippocampus and thalami were significantly lower in poststroke depression patients than in controls. Cho to Cr ratios were significantly higher in the bilateral hippocampus and left thalamus in poststroke depression patients than in controls. Furthermore, Hamilton Depression Rating Scale scores significantly correlated with the Cho to Cr ratios in the left and right hippocampus. After treatment, patients had significantly higher NAA to Cr ratios in the left hippocampus and bilateral thalami, and significantly lower Cho to Cr ratios in the bilateral hippocampus and left thalamus.[92] This longitudinal study sheds light on some of the biochemical changes that occur in the brain with antidepressant treatment. The authors postulate that these changes might be due to the neurotrophic effects of antidepressants.

SUMMARY

This article has highlighted some of the important findings in geriatric depression from structural imaging. Depression is a complex disease with multiple causes as evidenced by the many structures involved and the different kinds of lesions that are associated with the illness.

Evolution of imaging methods and the refinement of their techniques have enabled the identification and assessment of many potential biomarkers and endophenotypes in depression. The future of imaging research will be multimodal, in which identified structural variations will be used to inform and improve hypotheses for further testing and confirmation by other techniques. In the case of the OFC, an initial neuroanatomic difference of decreased volume among the depressed[42] was studied with cognitive neurological testing, which found that this volumetric difference was associated with decreased performance in tests.[46] Furthermore, lower OFC volumes were associated with functional disability.[47] Thus, findings from imaging studies can be explored using different research methods to interrogate the varied aspects of depression and the many negative outcomes it portends. When consistently replicated, such findings might serve as imaging phenotypes that can identify vulnerability and predict treatment efficacy.[93]

REFERENCES

1. Hoptman MJ, Gunning-Dixon FM, Murphy CF, et al. Structural neuroimaging research methods in geriatric depression. Am J Geriatr Psychiatry 2006;14(10): 812–22.
2. Steffens DC, Byrum CE, McQuoid DR, et al. Hippocampal volume in geriatric depression. Biol Psychiatry 2000;48(4):301–9.
3. Sheline YI. Hippocampal atrophy in major depression: a result of depression-induced neurotoxicity? Mol Psychiatry 1996;1(4):298–9.
4. Lloyd AJ, Ferrier IN, Barber R, et al. Hippocampal volume change in depression: late- and early-onset illness compared. Br J Psychiatry 2004;184:488–95.

5. O'Brien JT, Lloyd A, McKeith I, et al. A longitudinal study of hippocampal volume, cortisol levels, and cognition in older depressed subjects. Am J Psychiatry 2004; 161(11):2081–90.

6. Hickie I, Naismith S, Ward PB, et al. Reduced hippocampal volumes and memory loss in patients with early- and late-onset depression. Br J Psychiatry 2005;186: 197–202.

7. Ballmaier M, Narr KL, Toga AW, et al. Hippocampal morphology and distinguishing late-onset from early-onset elderly depression. Am J Psychiatry 2008;165(2): 229–37.

8. Ashtari M, Greenwald BS, Kramer-Ginsberg E, et al. Hippocampal/amygdala volumes in geriatric depression. Psychol Med 1999;29(3):629–38.

9. Pantel J, Schroder J, Essig M, et al. Quantitative magnetic resonance imaging in geriatric depression and primary degenerative dementia. J Affect Disord 1997; 42(1):69–83.

10. Koolschijn PC, van Haren NE, Lensvelt-Mulders GJ, et al. Brain volume abnormalities in major depressive disorder: a meta-analysis of magnetic resonance imaging studies. Hum Brain Mapp 2009;30(11):3719–35.

11. Videbech P, Ravnkilde B. Hippocampal volume and depression: a meta-analysis of MRI studies. Am J Psychiatry 2004;161(11):1957–66.

12. Campbell S, Marriott M, Nahmias C, et al. Lower hippocampal volume in patients suffering from depression: a meta-analysis. Am J Psychiatry 2004;161(4): 598–607.

13. Sheline YI, Mittler BL, Mintun MA. The hippocampus and depression. Eur Psychiatry 2002;17(Suppl 3):300–5.

14. Frodl TS, Koutsouleris N, Bottlender R, et al. Depression-related variation in brain morphology over 3 years: effects of stress? Arch Gen Psychiatry 2008;65(10): 1156–65.

15. Gould E, McEwen BS, Tanapat P, et al. Neurogenesis in the dentate gyrus of the adult tree shrew is regulated by psychosocial stress and NMDA receptor activation. J Neurosci 1997;17(7):2492–8.

16. Gould E, Tanapat P, McEwen BS, et al. Proliferation of granule cell precursors in the dentate gyrus of adult monkeys is diminished by stress. Proc Natl Acad Sci U S A 1998;95(6):3168–71.

17. Czeh B, Michaelis T, Watanabe T, et al. Stress-induced changes in cerebral metabolites, hippocampal volume, and cell proliferation are prevented by antidepressant treatment with tianeptine. Proc Natl Acad Sci U S A 2001;98(22): 12796–801.

18. Taylor WD, Steffens DC, Payne ME, et al. Influence of serotonin transporter promoter region polymorphisms on hippocampal volumes in late-life depression. Arch Gen Psychiatry 2005;62(5):537–44.

19. Frodl T, Schule C, Schmitt G, et al. Association of the brain-derived neurotrophic factor Val66Met polymorphism with reduced hippocampal volumes in major depression. Arch Gen Psychiatry 2007;64(4):410–6.

20. Benjamin S, McQuoid DR, Potter GG, et al. The brain-derived neurotrophic factor Val66Met polymorphism, hippocampal volume, and cognitive function in geriatric depression. Am J Geriatr Psychiatry 2010;18(4):323–31.

21. Convit A, De Leon MJ, Tarshish C, et al. Specific hippocampal volume reductions in individuals at risk for Alzheimer's disease. Neurobiol Aging 1997;18(2):131–8.

22. Killiany RJ, Moss MB, Albert MS, et al. Temporal lobe regions on magnetic resonance imaging identify patients with early Alzheimer's disease. Arch Neurol 1993; 50(9):949–54.

23. Sheline YI, Barch DM, Donnelly JM, et al. Increased amygdala response to masked emotional faces in depressed subjects resolves with antidepressant treatment: an fMRI study. Biol Psychiatry 2001;50(9):651–8.

24. Frodl T, Meisenzahl EM, Zetzsche T, et al. Larger amygdala volumes in first depressive episode as compared to recurrent major depression and healthy control subjects. Biol Psychiatry 2003;53(4):338–44.

25. Munn MA, Alexopoulos J, Nishino T, et al. Amygdala volume analysis in female twins with major depression. Biol Psychiatry 2007;62(5):415–22.

26. Krishnan KR, McDonald WM, Escalona PR, et al. Magnetic resonance imaging of the caudate nuclei in depression. Preliminary observations. Arch Gen Psychiatry 1992;49(7):553–7.

27. Husain MM, McDonald WM, Doraiswamy PM, et al. A magnetic resonance imaging study of putamen nuclei in major depression. Psychiatry Res 1991;40(2):95–9.

28. Krishnan KR. Neuroanatomic substrates of depression in the elderly. J Geriatr Psychiatry Neurol 1993;6(1):39–58.

29. Parashos IA, Tupler LA, Blitchington T, et al. Magnetic-resonance morphometry in patients with major depression. Psychiatry Res 1998;84(1):7–15.

30. Naismith S, Hickie I, Ward PB, et al. Caudate nucleus volumes and genetic determinants of homocysteine metabolism in the prediction of psychomotor speed in older persons with depression. Am J Psychiatry 2002;159(12):2096–8.

31. Lacerda AL, Nicoletti MA, Brambilla P, et al. Anatomical MRI study of basal ganglia in major depressive disorder. Psychiatry Res 2003;124(3):129–40.

32. Lenze EJ, Sheline YI. Absence of striatal volume differences between depressed subjects with no comorbid medical illness and matched comparison subjects. Am J Psychiatry 1999;156(12):1989–91.

33. Devinsky O, Morrell MJ, Vogt BA. Contributions of anterior cingulate cortex to behaviour. Brain 1995;118(Pt 1):279–306.

34. Alexopoulos GS, Gunning-Dixon FM, Latoussakis V, et al. Anterior cingulate dysfunction in geriatric depression. Int J Geriatr Psychiatry 2008;23(4):347–55.

35. Botteron KN, Raichle ME, Drevets WC, et al. Volumetric reduction in left subgenual prefrontal cortex in early onset depression. Biol Psychiatry 2002;51(4):342–4.

36. Caetano SC, Kaur S, Brambilla P, et al. Smaller cingulate volumes in unipolar depressed patients. Biol Psychiatry 2006;59(8):702–6.

37. Bremner JD, Vythilingam M, Vermetten E, et al. Reduced volume of orbitofrontal cortex in major depression. Biol Psychiatry 2002;51(4):273–9.

38. Brambilla P, Nicoletti MA, Harenski K, et al. Anatomical MRI study of subgenual prefrontal cortex in bipolar and unipolar subjects. Neuropsychopharmacology 2002;27(5):792–9.

39. Ballmaier M, Toga AW, Blanton RE, et al. Anterior cingulate, gyrus rectus, and orbitofrontal abnormalities in elderly depressed patients: an MRI-based parcellation of the prefrontal cortex. Am J Psychiatry 2004;161(1):99–108.

40. Kringelbach ML. The human orbitofrontal cortex: linking reward to hedonic experience. Nat Rev Neurosci 2005;6(9):691–702.

41. Taylor WD, Macfall JR, Payne ME, et al. Orbitofrontal cortex volume in late life depression: influence of hyperintense lesions and genetic polymorphisms. Psychol Med 2007;37(12):1763–73.

42. Lai T, Payne ME, Byrum CE, et al. Reduction of orbital frontal cortex volume in geriatric depression. Biol Psychiatry 2000;48(10):971–5.

43. Lacerda AL, Keshavan MS, Hardan AY, et al. Anatomic evaluation of the orbitofrontal cortex in major depressive disorder. Biol Psychiatry 2004;55(4):353–8.

44. Hastings RS, Parsey RV, Oquendo MA, et al. Volumetric analysis of the prefrontal cortex, amygdala, and hippocampus in major depression. Neuropsychopharmacology 2004;29(5):952–9.
45. Rajkowska G. Postmortem studies in mood disorders indicate altered numbers of neurons and glial cells. Biol Psychiatry 2000;48(8):766–77.
46. Steffens DC, McQuoid DR, Welsh-Bohmer KA, et al. Left orbital frontal cortex volume and performance on the Benton Visual Retention Test in older depressives and controls. Neuropsychopharmacology 2003;28(12):2179–83.
47. Taylor WD, Steffens DC, McQuoid DR, et al. Smaller orbital frontal cortex volumes associated with functional disability in depressed elders. Biol Psychiatry 2003; 53(2):144–9.
48. Ashburner J, Friston KJ. Voxel-based morphometry—the methods. Neuroimage 2000;11(6 Pt 1):805–21.
49. Bell-McGinty S, Butters MA, Meltzer CC, et al. Brain morphometric abnormalities in geriatric depression: long-term neurobiological effects of illness duration. Am J Psychiatry 2002;159(8):1424–7.
50. Egger K, Schocke M, Weiss E, et al. Pattern of brain atrophy in elderly patients with depression revealed by voxel-based morphometry. Psychiatry Res 2008; 164(3):237–44.
51. Hwang JP, Lee TW, Tsai SJ, et al. Cortical and subcortical abnormalities in late-onset depression with history of suicide attempts investigated with MRI and voxel-based morphometry. J Geriatr Psychiatry Neurol 2010;23:171–84.
52. Yuan Y, Zhu W, Zhang Z, et al. Regional gray matter changes are associated with cognitive deficits in remitted geriatric depression: an optimized voxel-based morphometry study. Biol Psychiatry 2008;64(6):541–4.
53. Koolschijn PC, van Haren NE, Schnack HG, et al. Cortical thickness and voxel-based morphometry in depressed elderly. Eur Neuropsychopharmacol 2010; 20(6):398–404.
54. Baudewig J, Dechent P, Merboldt KD, et al. Thresholding in correlation analyses of magnetic resonance functional neuroimaging. Magn Reson Imaging 2003; 21(10):1121–30.
55. Fujikawa T, Yamawaki S, Touhouda Y. Incidence of silent cerebral infarction in patients with major depression. Stroke 1993;24(11):1631–4.
56. Krishnan KR, Hays JC, Blazer DG. MRI-defined vascular depression. Am J Psychiatry 1997;154(4):497–501.
57. Alexopoulos GS, Meyers BS, Young RC, et al. Clinically defined vascular depression. Am J Psychiatry 1997;154(4):562–5.
58. Alexopoulos GS, Meyers BS, Young RC, et al. 'Vascular depression' hypothesis. Arch Gen Psychiatry 1997;54(10):915–22.
59. Coffey CE, Wilkinson WE, Weiner RD, et al. Quantitative cerebral anatomy in depression. A controlled magnetic resonance imaging study. Arch Gen Psychiatry 1993;50(1):7–16.
60. Greenwald BS, Kramer-Ginsberg E, Krishnan RR, et al. MRI signal hyperintensities in geriatric depression. Am J Psychiatry 1996;153(9):1212–5.
61. Krishnan KR, McDonald WM, Doraiswamy PM, et al. Neuroanatomical substrates of depression in the elderly. Eur Arch Psychiatry Clin Neurosci 1993;243(1):41–6.
62. Kumar A, Bilker W, Jin Z, et al. Atrophy and high intensity lesions: complementary neurobiological mechanisms in late-life major depression. Neuropsychopharmacology 2000;22(3):264–74.
63. Taylor WD, MacFall JR, Payne ME, et al. Greater MRI lesion volumes in elderly depressed subjects than in control subjects. Psychiatry Res 2005;139(1):1–7.

64. Tang WK, Chen YK, Lu JY, et al. White matter hyperintensities in post-stroke depression: a case control study. J Neurol Neurosurg Psychiatry 2010;81:1312–5.

65. Steffens DC, Krishnan KR, Crump C, et al. Cerebrovascular disease and evolution of depressive symptoms in the cardiovascular health study. Stroke 2002; 33(6):1636–44.

66. Heiden A, Kettenbach J, Fischer P, et al. White matter hyperintensities and chronicity of depression. J Psychiatr Res 2005;39(3):285–93.

67. Taylor WD, Steffens DC, MacFall JR, et al. White matter hyperintensity progression and late-life depression outcomes. Arch Gen Psychiatry 2003;60(11):1090–6.

68. O'Brien J, Ames D, Chiu E, et al. Severe deep white matter lesions and outcome in elderly patients with major depressive disorder: follow up study. BMJ 1998; 317(7164):982–4.

69. Sheline YI, Pieper CF, Barch DM, et al. Support for the vascular depression hypothesis in late-life depression: results of a 2-site, prospective, antidepressant treatment trial. Arch Gen Psychiatry 2010;67(3):277–85.

70. Gunning-Dixon FM, Walton M, Cheng J, et al. MRI signal hyperintensities and treatment remission of geriatric depression. J Affect Disord 2010;126:395–401.

71. Taylor WD, Steffens DC, Krishnan KR. Psychiatric disease in the twenty-first century: the case for subcortical ischemic depression. Biol Psychiatry 2006; 60(12):1299–303.

72. Sneed JR, Rindskopf D, Steffens DC, et al. The vascular depression subtype: evidence of internal validity. Biol Psychiatry 2008;64(6):491–7.

73. Taylor WD, Payne ME, Krishnan KR, et al. Evidence of white matter tract disruption in MRI hyperintensities. Biol Psychiatry 2001;50(3):179–83.

74. Taylor WD, MacFall JR, Payne ME, et al. Late-life depression and microstructural abnormalities in dorsolateral prefrontal cortex white matter. Am J Psychiatry 2004; 161(7):1293–6.

75. Bae JN, MacFall JR, Krishnan KR, et al. Dorsolateral prefrontal cortex and anterior cingulate cortex white matter alterations in late-life depression. Biol Psychiatry 2006;60(12):1356–63.

76. Yang Q, Huang X, Hong N, et al. White matter microstructural abnormalities in late-life depression. Int Psychogeriatr 2007;19(4):757–66.

77. Yuan Y, Zhang Z, Bai F, et al. White matter integrity of the whole brain is disrupted in first-episode remitted geriatric depression. Neuroreport 2007;18(17):1845–9.

78. Shimony JS, Sheline YI, D'Angelo G, et al. Diffuse microstructural abnormalities of normal-appearing white matter in late life depression: a diffusion tensor imaging study. Biol Psychiatry 2009;66(3):245–52.

79. Murphy CF, Gunning-Dixon FM, Hoptman MJ, et al. White-matter integrity predicts stroop performance in patients with geriatric depression. Biol Psychiatry 2007;61(8):1007–10.

80. Nobuhara K, Okugawa G, Sugimoto T, et al. Frontal white matter anisotropy and symptom severity of late-life depression: a magnetic resonance diffusion tensor imaging study. J Neurol Neurosurg Psychiatry 2006;77(1):120–2.

81. Alexopoulos GS, Kiosses DN, Choi SJ, et al. Frontal white matter microstructure and treatment response of late-life depression: a preliminary study. Am J Psychiatry 2002;159(11):1929–32.

82. Taylor WD, Kuchibhatla M, Payne ME, et al. Frontal white matter anisotropy and antidepressant remission in late-life depression. PLoS One 2008;3(9):e3267.

83. Nobuhara K, Okugawa G, Minami T, et al. Effects of electroconvulsive therapy on frontal white matter in late-life depression: a diffusion tensor imaging study. Neuropsychobiology 2004;50(1):48–53.

84. Kumar A, Gupta RC, Albert Thomas M, et al. Biophysical changes in normal-appearing white matter and subcortical nuclei in late-life major depression detected using magnetization transfer. Psychiatry Res 2004;130(2):131–40.

85. Henkelman RM, Stanisz GJ, Graham SJ. Magnetization transfer in MRI: a review. NMR Biomed 2001;14(2):57–64.

86. Gunning-Dixon FM, Hoptman MJ, Lim KO, et al. Macromolecular white matter abnormalities in geriatric depression: a magnetization transfer imaging study. Am J Geriatr Psychiatry 2008;16:255–62.

87. Dager SR, Corrigan NM, Richards TL, et al. Research applications of magnetic resonance spectroscopy to investigate psychiatric disorders. Top Magn Reson Imaging 2008;19(2):81–96.

88. Kumar A, Thomas A, Lavretsky H, et al. Frontal white matter biochemical abnormalities in late-life major depression detected with proton magnetic resonance spectroscopy. Am J Psychiatry 2002;159(4):630–6.

89. Elderkin-Thompson V, Thomas MA, Binesh N, et al. Brain metabolites and cognitive function among older depressed and healthy individuals using 2D MR spectroscopy. Neuropsychopharmacology 2004;29(12):2251–7.

90. Chen CS, Chiang IC, Li CW, et al. Proton magnetic resonance spectroscopy of late-life major depressive disorder. Psychiatry Res 2009;172(3):210–4.

91. Venkatraman TN, Krishnan RR, Steffens DC, et al. Biochemical abnormalities of the medial temporal lobe and medial prefrontal cortex in late-life depression. Psychiatry Res 2009;172(1):49–54.

92. Huang Y, Chen W, Li Y, et al. Effects of antidepressant treatment on N-acetyl aspartate and choline levels in the hippocampus and thalami of post-stroke depression patients: a study using (1)H magnetic resonance spectroscopy. Psychiatry Res 2010;182(1):48–52.

93. Savitz JB, Drevets WC. Imaging phenotypes of major depressive disorder: genetic correlates. Neuroscience 2009;164(1):300–30.

Immunity, Aging, and Geriatric Depression

Sarah Shizuko Morimoto, PsyD, George S. Alexopoulos, MD*

KEYWORDS

• Immunity • Aging • Depression • Geriatrics

The cause of geriatric depression is not well understood. Attempts to identify causes that contribute to geriatric depression have focused on the role of its comorbid disorders and on the effects of the aging process. Geriatric depression afflicts patients with significant medical comorbidity.[1] When it occurs, depression worsens the outcomes of many medical illnesses and increases mortality. In addition to medical morbidity, geriatric depression is often accompanied by cognitive impairment.[2] Cognitive impairment may improve, but is rarely eliminated, during periods of remission.[3] The persistence of cognitive impairment suggests that geriatric depression occurs in the context of impairment of neural structures associated with cognitive functions. The causes of impairment of these structures are variable and include vascular and neurodegenerative diseases and pronounced aging-related changes. In sum, geriatric depression occurs during broad disruption of bodily and brain functions and, once established, its pathophysiology further contributes to this disruption.

Changes in the immune system mediate disruptive processes of diseases often comorbid with geriatric depression. Inflammation is the central process underlying the sickness behavior accompanying many of the generalized diseases including cancer, organ failure, and infections. Proinflammatory states resulting from immune responses to a variety of pathophysiological events contribute to central nervous system (CNS) abnormalities in neurodegenerative and cerebrovascular diseases. Specifically, inflammatory processes interact with amyloid deposition and lead to pathological changes of Alzheimer disease.[4,5] Similar inflammatory responses contribute to other neurodegenerative diseases.[6] Inflammation is among the initial vascular events leading to cerebral infarction, and it also plays a role in the neuronal destruction following cerebrovascular infarction or embolism.[7] Nonetheless, the role

This work was supported by NIMH grants T32 MH19132, R01 MH079414, and P30 MH085943 to Dr Alexopoulos.

Disclosures: Dr Morimoto, none. Dr Alexopoulos has received grant support by Forest Pharmaceuticals, holds equity of Johnson and Johnson, and has served in the Speakers Bureau of Forest, Astra Zeneca, Lilly, Merck, BMS, and Novartis.

Weill Cornell Institute of Geriatric Psychiatry, 21 Bloomingdale Road, White Plains, NY 10605, USA

* Corresponding author. New York Presbyterian Hospital, 21 Bloomingdale Road, White Plains, NY 10605.

E-mail address: gsalexop@med.cornell.edu

of inflammation in geriatric depression in patients without vascular and neurodegenerative diseases remains unclear.

Stress, a contributor to geriatric depression, leads both to behavioral and to immune changes.[8,9] Moreover, challenge to the immune system is often followed by behavioral changes reminiscent of behavioral responses to stress.[10–12] These findings suggest that immune changes may be at least 1 of the mechanisms by which stress leads to behavioral disorders.

We suggest that geriatric depression is the behavioral syndrome par excellence in which inflammatory processes are likely to play a central causal role. We base this assertion on the several observations. Geriatric depression occurs in the context of medical and neurological illnesses in which inflammatory processes play a significant pathogenetic role. Both aging[13–15] and depression[12] are associated with pronounced and prolonged immune responses. Geriatric depression exacerbates the symptoms of its comorbid medical and neurological disorders,[16] raising the question of whether depression-related inflammatory changes mediate the worsening of their outcomes. Geriatric depression often occurs in persons exposed to chronic adversity (stress), a state that both challenges the immune system and is known to contribute to geriatric depression. This article describes the immune functions of the CNS and summarizes animal and human literature on immune changes that occur during aging and depression.

THE 2 IMMUNE SYSTEMS

Historically, the CNS has been considered an immune-privileged organ, separate from the peripheral immune system, and shielded from the circulatory system by the blood-brain barrier.[17] However, the 2 immune systems interact and engage in mutual maintenance of homeostasis.[15] This communication serves as a sensory pathway through which peripheral immune stimulation informs the brain and influences behavior.[18]

CNS CELLULAR IMMUNE COMPONENT

The CNS immune system is regulated by both macroglial and microglial cells. During insult, injury, or invasion of pathogens, microglial cells are the primary first responders, becoming active before any other brain cells.[19] Microglial cells make up roughly 20% of all glia. However, in an activated state, they may encompass more surface area than astrocytes.[20,21]

Microglia respond to subtle alterations in their environment, and have the ability to differentiate between self/nonself when encountering molecules not present in healthy CNS, such as pathogens, blood clotting factors, intracellular constituents released by necrotic cells, or immunoglobulin-antigen complexes,[22] before pathological changes are detectable.[23] Microglia also respond when neurons are injured as a result of trauma, infection, ischemia, or neurodegeneration. During trauma, microglia become active early in the process via the release of adenosine triphosphate (ATP), neurotransmitters, cytokines, ion changes, or loss of inhibitor molecules.[22] Their ability to respond selectively to molecules related to neurotransmission allows them to monitor their environment continuously. Therefore, the quiescent microglia phase represents a state of constant vigilance to changes in their microenvironment.[19]

Microglia show rapid morphological transformation from resting state to activated state.[19,24] Microglial activation is dictated by the needs of their microenvironment and is stimulus dependent.[15] During the activated phase, microglia proliferate, retract their cellular processes, and increase expression of cell surface molecules. Further activation turns microglia into phagocytes, which are phenotypically and morphologically indistinguishable from macrophages in the periphery. These brain macrophages secrete cytokines, growth factors, oxygen and nitrogen free radicals, neurotransmitters, and proteolytic enzymes.[17,21,24,25] Through the release of these mediators, microglia influence the differentiation and survival of other CNS cells such as neurons, astrocytes, and oligodendrocytes.[17] Activated microglia also produce Trk A, Trk B, and Trk C receptors, and respond to and produce brain-derived neurotrophic factor (BDNF).[26]

Astrocytes, recruited by microglia, are part of the CNS immune response.[27] Once activated, astrocytes metabolize extracellular neurotransmitters, produce extracellular matrix molecules (ECM), and provide neurotrophic support to damaged neurons.[28] Like microglia, astrocytes produce cytokines and chemokines. They also play a role in the synthesis of ECM molecules by microglia. Subsequently, ECM molecules may stimulate production of cytokines and growth factors by microglia that trigger astroglial proliferation.[28]

The activation of microglia can be both neuroprotective and neurotoxic.[19] Microglia facilitate the return to homeostasis after neurophysiological insult by participating in tissue repair after injury, removing cytokines and invading microorganisms, and by secreting wound healing factors. However, excessive or prolonged activation of microglia can be cytotoxic through the release of excitatory amino acids, quinolinic acid, and cytokines.[29]

CNS HUMORAL IMMUNE COMPONENT

Cytokines are a diverse group of polypeptides associated with immune cell function and chemotaxis in both the CNS and the periphery.[6] Virtually all cells in the CNS have been shown to produce and respond to a range of cytokines,[17] although, in normal conditions, cytokine production in the CNS is low to undetectable.[6] Cytokines play a critical role in maintaining homeostasis through the removal of damaged cells and clearing of infections, as well as tissue repair and neuroregeneration. However, depending on the magnitude, length, and timing of their induction, cytokine cascades are capable of exacting severe tissue damage and have been implicated in the pathogenesis of a range of neurodegenerative disorders, stroke, and multiple sclerosis.[6]

PERIPHERY: BRAIN IMMUNE COMMUNICATION

Following exposure to pathogens, the nonspecific immune response begins rapidly with the activation of neutrophils and macrophages in the periphery. These cells engulf and destroy pathological agents and also release cytokines. Cytokines then recruit additional immune cells to the site of infection or injury. They also initiate the peripheral acute-phase response to fight infection and repair the host tissue. The stimulated peripheral immune system may progress to an antigen-specific, adaptive immune response by recruiting T and B lymphocytes. Once the invading pathogen has been neutralized, the peripheral immune system returns to a quiescent state so that it minimizes damage to tissue by the inflammatory response. Communication between the peripheral immune system and the brain initiates immunologic, physiological, and behavioral responses to insult or infection.[30]

The brain receives information from the periphery about the immune status of the organism and, in turn, may change the organism's behavior. Inflammatory cytokines communicate the immune status of the periphery to the CNS through the following mechanisms: (1) active transport; certain cytokines (interleukin [IL]-1β, IL-6, tumor necrosis factor [TNF]α, and IL-1α) cross the blood-brain barrier through a saturable transport system.[31] (2) Crossing at circumventricular organs; cytokines may enter the CNS in the areas of the circumventricular organs where the blood-brain barrier is more permeable or absent. (3) Humoral route; cytokines may bind to receptors within cerebral blood vessels and induce the production of second messengers that then diffuse into the brain and alter neural activity.[32] (4) neural route; peripheral cytokines may directly stimulate vagal and trigeminal afferents fibers, which can carry visceral sensory information to the CNS.[33–35] Activation of the neural pathway sensitizes target brain structures for the production and action of cytokines that may diffuse from the circumventricular organs and the choroid plexus into the brain. The periphery-CNS immune communication is redundant.[30] The afferent neural pathways are quicker and more direct than other forms of transport. However, all forms of communication rely on the production of proinflammatory cytokines by microglial cells in the brain.[29]

AGING, CNS IMMUNITY, AND BEHAVIOR

Aging increases the brain's inflammatory responses. With aging, there is an increase in glia activation, inflammatory mediators, and atrophy.[13–15] Both human and animal studies show that genes related to cellular stress and inflammation are upregulated with age, whereas genes related to synaptic function, growth factors, and trophic support are downregulated.[13,15,36] Neurogenesis also decreases with age, in part because of the effects of cytokines secreted by activated microglia.[37]

A combination of both senescence of microglia and increased secretion of inflammatory proteins may contribute to the proinflammatory shift during aging. Activation of microglia places a burden on the cells' metabolic mechanisms, which can only tolerate high levels of activity for short time periods.[14] Activated microglia are prone to die more often and more quickly than nonactivated microglia.[14] Microglial losses are replenished by mitosis of parenchymal microglia, or by migration of bone marrow progenitor cells. Both processes are enhanced during times of injury or inflammation.[38,39] The mitotic potential of microglia is not reduced, and perhaps is even enhanced in old age.[40] Therefore, increased mitosis, coupled with increased activation, may promote production of senescent microglia.[14]

Dystrophic microglia may increase in the aging brain. These microglia are characterized by abnormalities in cytoplasmic structure such as deramified, atrophic, or fragmented processes.[14] Dystrophic microglia secrete diminished levels of neurotrophic factors and have limited phagocytic function. The combination of diminished neurotrophic factors and downregulated phagocytosis with increased secretion of inflammatory mediators may lead to both neuron loss and inefficient clearance of toxic substances associated with neurodegenerative disease.[15]

Along with immune cellular changes, aging attenuates the ability of the peripheral immune system to initiate an effective immune response[41] and increases the innate immune activity.[11,29] These changes result in increased peripheral immune stimulation and, through periphery-CNS communication, to increased production of inflammatory markers in the CNS.[30,42–44]

In addition to influencing central and peripheral immune responses, aging disrupts communication between the periphery and the CNS. Peripheral immune stimulation in healthy older subjects produces both an increased and discordant CNS inflammatory response compared with younger subjects.[29,30] Increased immune reactivity, combined with exaggerated CNS immune response to stimulus, may leave some older adults in a chronic state of neuroinflammation characterized by continuous production of proinflammatory cytokines.[29,45] Therefore, aging renders microglia hypervigilant and prone to excessive and prolonged release of cytokines when challenged by immune stimuli.[42–44,46,47]

In aged mice, lipopolysaccharide injections caused both exaggerated neuroinflammatory response and prolonged sickness behavior compared with younger adult mice.[48] In these mice, sickness behavior lasted almost twice as long as in younger mice and was associated with a pronounced induction of peripheral and brain idoleamine 2,3-dioxygenase (DOC) and a much higher rate of turnover in brain serotonin.[48] Discordant central inflammatory response to peripheral stimulation can have damaging effects to an organism because of the behavioral effects and neurotoxicity associated with the disproportionate release of proinflammatory cytokines in the brain.[29]

IMMUNE CHANGES IN GERIATRIC DEPRESSION

Limited information exists on the role of the immune system in geriatric depression. Most findings are derived from aging animal experiments, on models of stress and depression, and on sparse clinical studies.

Proinflammatory cytokines exert profound effects on behavior. The set of behaviors occurring after insult or infection has been collectively referred to as sickness behavior.[10,11] Behavioral symptoms include reduced food and water intake, decreased exploration, decreased social interaction, increased somnolence, as well as changes in both mood and cognition.[11,49] In humans, sickness behavior shares many symptoms and signs with major depression. This resemblance led to the suggestion that depression is a behavioral response to proinflammatory changes.[12]

The complexity of sickness behavior suggests that it is mediated by neural systems including structures mediating the depressive syndrome. As an example, IL-1, a proinflammatory cytokine, has receptors in the granule cell layer of the dentate gyrus, the pyramidal cell layer of the hippocampus, the anterior pituitary gland,[50] and the endothelial cells of the brain venules. High densities of IL-1 receptors were found in the preoptic and supraoptic areas of the hypothalamus and the subfornical organ, and lower densities in the paraventricular hypothalamus, cortex, nucleus of the solitary tract, and the ventrolateral medulla.[51] Cytokines do not only affect neurons but also modulate the function of both endothelial and glial cells.[11]

Aging increases inflammatory responses in distinct brain areas. In old rodents, glia cultures and brain sections, including those of areas related to mood processing, had greater increases in IL-6, IL-1β, and TNFα compared with younger animals after challenge with lipopolysaccharide.[45,52] Coronal sections of the cerebral cortex of aged mice spontaneously produce higher levels of IL-6 than do sections from adult animals.[53,54] IL-6 is not only increased in the whole brain of older animals but is concentrated in the hippocampus, cerebral cortex, and cerebellum compared with younger cohorts.[45,53] Taken together, these observations suggest that aging of the brain's inflammatory responses may lead to abnormalities in neural systems related to the development of depressive syndromes.

Geriatric depression is often accompanied by cognitive dysfunction. Although cytokine receptors are spread throughout the CNS, the highest levels of cytokine binding occurs in areas related to both learning and memory, including the hippocampus.[50] Increased levels of IL-1β have been shown to disrupt long-term potentiation (LTP), a cellular mechanism important in the consolidation of memory. In animals, injection of IL-1 β can impair hippocampal-dependent memory performance.[55] In addition, behavioral performance on tests of spatial learning memory can be disrupted by infection or peripheral immune activation and the resultant cytokine upregulation.[56,57]

Exposure to stress not only serves as a precipitating factor of depressive episodes in late-life but also promotes inflammation and influences cognitive functions and behavior. Chronic stress enhances the aging-related proinflammatory state by activating microglia and upregulating the expression of cell surface antigens.[8,9] Earlier exposure to a particular stressor can prime microglia and increase their inflammatory response.[8,58] Mild stress also increases cytokine production and decreases learning and memory functions in aged and adult mice. However, if stressors are repeated for several days, only aged animals continue to show cognitive impairment, whereas adult mice return to baseline performance. Similarly, external stressors increased circulating IL-1β and IL-6 and promoted cognitive impairment in older adults.[49]

The inflammatory response to immune challenge influences neural systems responsible for mood regulation. In humans, typhoid injection produced an inflammatory response of increased circulating IL-6 and development of sad mood. Worsening of mood during inflammatory responses correlated with enhanced activity within the subgenual anterior cingulate cortex (ACC) during processing of emotional stimuli.[59] The subgenual cingulate is a central node of the emotional control system, which often dysfunctions in depression. Inflammation-associated mood change reduces connectivity of the subgenual ACC to amygdala, medial prefrontal cortex, nucleus accumbens, and superior temporal sulcus, and is modulated by peripheral IL-6.[59] In addition, a single nucleotide polymorphism (SNP) of the gene encoding the inflammatory cytokine IL-1β has been associated with both reduced activity of the anterior cingulate and the amygdala in response to emotional stimuli and with nonremission of major depression following antidepressant treatment.[60] These findings raise the question of whether inflammatory processes participate in the mechanisms mediating the development of depressive and cognitive symptoms in late-life, especially during exposure to chronic stress.

Studies of older depressed patients or elders at risk for depression documented abnormalities in inflammatory responses. A recent meta-analysis showed that depressed patients have higher concentrations of IL-6 and TNFα compared with control subjects.[61] Epidemiologic studies found an association of increased IL-6 with depressive symptoms after controlling for likely confounding variables.[62–65] In geriatric depressed patients, peripheral inflammatory markers were correlated with the severity of depressive symptoms overall[66–69] as well as with cognitive symptoms of depression.[70] IL-6 was associated with increased suicide risk, with the highest levels of IL-6 correlating with the most violent suicide attempts.[71] In addition, inflammatory markers predicted depressive symptoms in older adults during 3-year and 6-year follow-ups.[72] Caregiving for an ill relative also increases both depressive symptoms and inflammatory markers in the elderly. In cross-sectional studies, family caregivers of patients with dementia had higher levels of circulating IL-6 than age-matched controls.[73] Other studies have indicated that not only are circulating cytokine levels higher but the response to immune challenge lasts longer in stressed elderly populations. Specifically, elderly caregivers had a prolonged increase in IL-6 of up to 4 weeks following influenza vaccine, whereas there was no IL-6 change in noncaregiving age-matched controls.[74] In addition to depressed mood, increased inflammatory indices are associated with development of cognitive impairment, disability, and mortality in late-life.[47,74–76]

Pharmacological studies provide indirect evidence in support of the inflammation hypothesis of depression. Although definitive studies are lacking, there is early evidence that classic antidepressants may influence inflammatory processes and, conversely, anti-inflammatory agents may have antidepressant action. Animal studies have shown that tricyclic antidepressants reduce proinflammatory, and increase anti-inflammatory, cytokines.[77–79] Some antidepressants ameliorate sickness behavior and reduce production of cytokines in animal models of inflammation.[80] Select antidepressants may reduce serum cytokines,[81–83] although this finding needs to be confirmed. Pretreatment cytokine plasma levels may influence the response to antidepressants.[84,85] Moreover, there is anecdotal evidence that the anti-inflammatory agent minocycline augments the action of some antidepressants in major depression.[86] Similarly, the cyclo-oxygenase-2 inhibitor celecoxib may augment the efficacy of reboxetine and fluoxetine in major depression.[87,88] The anti-inflammatory agent etanercept reduced symptoms of depression in patients with psoriasis.[89]

TRANSGENIC ANIMALS

Several transgenic inflammatory animal models have been developed and can be used to test the relationship of inflammatory responses to depressionlike behavior. This article presents a selective summary of some such models.

The GFAP-IL6 transgenic mouse presents an upregulation of IL-1α/β and TNFα as well as gliosis of both astrocytes and microglia in the cerebellum, brain stem, and subcortical regions.[90] Functional deficits in this mouse include various learning impairments, decreased locomotor and exploratory behavior, reduced long-term potentiation in hippocampal slices, and abnormal hypothalamic-pituitary-adrenal axis responses to immobilization stress. In contrast, IL-6–deficient mice are less sensitive to the behavioral effects of IL-1β or to lipopolysaccharide injected centrally or peripherally. For example, IL-6 knockout mice are resistant to lipopolysaccharide-induced deficits in spatial working memory. These mice still show an increase in plasma TNFα and IL-1β when immune challenged, but do not show the working memory deficits that the knockin mice show. In this sample, working memory performance was associated with reduction in TNFα and IL-1β production in the neuronal cell layer of the hippocampus in the IL-6 knockout mice.[57]

Type 1 IL-1 receptor knockout mice do not respond to the administration of IL-1 but do show behavioral changes in response to lipopolysaccharide injection, perhaps mediated by the proinflammatory cytokine TNFα. This observation indicates that the reduction of expression of one cytokine can be replaced by the actions of a complementary cytokine mediator. However, blockade of IL-1 action through the administration of IL-1 receptor antagonist reduces sickness behavior, part of which is a reduction of social exploration[91] and food intake, suggesting that IL-1 may be a critical mediator of sickness behavior.[11,91]

The knockout mice of the anti-inflammatory cytokine IL-10 respond to lipopolysaccharide injection with exaggerated and prolonged sickness behavior and an increase in CNS proinflammatory cytokines.[11] Aging reduces IL-10 production. Therefore, aging-related reduction of IL-10 may be one of the mechanisms promoting the proinflammatory state of late-life.

SUMMARY

Aging disrupts peripheral and CNS immune responses and influences communication between the periphery and the CNS. Consequently, immune stimulation produces both exaggerated and discordant CNS inflammatory responses in older adults. The net result of these changes is a proinflammatory state characterized by senescence of microglia and increased secretion of inflammatory proteins.

Aging may exacerbate the effects of stress in the CNS, leading to behavioral and cognitive changes similar to those of the depressive syndrome. Chronic stress exacerbates age-related increases in inflammation. Earlier exposure to a particular stressor can prime microglia and increase their inflammatory responses.

Sparse direct information exists on the role of inflammation in geriatric depression. Proinflammatory proteins have profound behavioral effects. Sickness behavior, the behavioral syndrome caused by brain inflammatory processes, resembles the depressive syndrome and often occurs in disorders comorbid with geriatric depression. The complexity of sickness behavior suggests that it is mediated by neural systems distributed throughout brain and includes networks responsible for mood regulation. Animal studies suggest that brain areas related to mood processing have increased inflammatory responses during aging. The connectivity among mood-regulating structures may be modulated by inflammatory responses.

Some inflammatory markers have been found to be increased in geriatric depression and their levels are correlated with the severity of the syndrome. Furthermore, peripheral cytokine levels were associated with suicide risk. In addition to depressed mood, increased inflammatory indices may be associated with development of cognitive impairment, disability, and mortality in late-life. Conditions increasing the risk for depression, such as caregiving, may increase both depressive symptoms and inflammatory markers in the elderly.

The role of inflammation in geriatric depression needs further investigation. The clinical lesson derived from the available information is that depressed older adults should be examined to identify disorders or risk factors with known associations with inflammation. Autoimmune disorders and vascular risk factors such as hyperlipidemia and increased C-reactive protein are examples of such conditions. It is premature to use anti-inflammatory agents in the treatment of the depression syndrome of older adults. However, treatment of comorbid conditions increasing CNS inflammatory responses can have general health benefits and should be part of clinical practice.

Neuroimaging and electrophysiological studies may identify microstructural abnormalities and disturbances in activation and function of neural networks associated with the inflammatory processes accompanying geriatric depression. Transgenic animal models may help to identify candidate anti-inflammatory agents that later may be tested in clinical trials of geriatric depression.

REFERENCES

1. Alexopoulos GS. Depression in the elderly. Lancet 2005;365(9475):1961–70.
2. Lockwood KA, Alexopoulos GS, Van Gorp WG. Executive dysfunction in geriatric depression. Am J Psychiatry 2002;159(7):1119–26.
3. Murphy CF, Alexopoulos GS. Longitudinal association of initiation/perseveration and severity of geriatric depression. Am J Geriatr Psychiatry 2004;12(1):50–6.
4. Bell M, Bryson G, Greig T, et al. Neurocognitive enhancement therapy with work therapy: effects on neuropsychological test performance. Arch Gen Psychiatry 2001;58(8):763–8.
5. Wenk GL. Neuropathologic changes in Alzheimer's disease. J Clin Psychiatry 2003;64(Suppl 9):7–10.
6. Wang J, Asensio VC, Campbell IL. Cytokines and chemokines as mediators of protection and injury in the central nervous system assessed in transgenic mice. Curr Top Microbiol Immunol 2002;265:24–48.
7. Ropper AH, Brown RH. Adams and Victor's principles of neurology. New York: McGraw-Hill; 2005. p. 686–704.
8. Frank MG, Baratta MV, Sprunger DB, et al. Microglia serve as a neuroimmune substrate for stress-induced potentiation of CNS pro-inflammatory cytokine responses. Brain Behav Immun 2007;21(1):47–59.
9. Buchanan JB, Sparkman NL, Chen J, et al. Cognitive and neuroinflammatory consequences of mild repeated stress are exacerbated in aged mice. Psychoneuroendocrinology 2008;33(6):755–65.

10. Hart BL. Biological basis of the behavior of sick animals. Neurosci Biobehav Rev 1988;12(2):123–37.
11. Dantzer R, O'Connor JC, Freund GG, et al. From inflammation to sickness and depression: when the immune system subjugates the brain. Nat Rev Neurosci 2008;9(1):46–56.
12. Nakano Y, Baba H, Maeshima H, et al. Executive dysfunction in medicated, remitted state of major depression. J Affect Disord 2008;111(1):46–51.
13. Lu T, Pan Y, Kao SY, et al. Gene regulation and DNA damage in the ageing human brain. Nature 2004;429(6994):883–91.
14. Streit WJ, Miller KR, Lopes KO, et al. Microglial degeneration in the aging brain– bad news for neurons? Front Biosci 2008;13:3423–38.
15. Lucin KM, Wyss-Coray T. Immune activation in brain aging and neurodegeneration: too much or too little? Neuron 2009;64(1):110–22.
16. Alexopoulos GS, Kelly RE Jr. Research advances in geriatric depression. World Psychiatry 2009;8(3):140–9.
17. Jones TB, Lucin KM, Popovich PG. The immune system of the brain. The hypothalamus-pituitary-adrenal axis. Elsevier; 2008.
18. Blalock JE. The syntax of immune-neuroendocrine communication. Immunol Today 1994;15(11):504–11.
19. Kreutzberg GW. Microglia: a sensor for pathological events in the CNS. Trends Neurosci 1996;19(8):312–8.
20. Lawson LJ, Perry VH, Dri P, et al. Heterogeneity in the distribution and morphology of microglia in the normal adult mouse brain. Neuroscience 1990;39(1):151–70.
21. Banati RB, Graeber MB. Surveillance, intervention and cytotoxicity: is there a protective role of microglia? Dev Neurosci 1994;16(3–4):114–27.
22. Hanisch UK, Kettenmann H. Microglia: active sensor and versatile effector cells in the normal and pathologic brain. Nat Neurosci 2007;10(11):1387–94.
23. Boya J, Carbonell AL, Calvo J, et al. Ultrastructural study on the origin of rat microglia cells. Acta Anat (Basel) 1987;130(4):329–35.
24. Gehrmann J, Banati RB, Kreutzberg GW. Microglia in the immune surveillance of the brain: human microglia constitutively express HLA-DR molecules. J Neuroimmunol 1993;48(2):189–98.
25. Giulian D, Baker TJ, Shih LC, et al. Interleukin 1 of the central nervous system is produced by ameboid microglia. J Exp Med 1986;164(2):594–604.
26. Nakajima K, Kikuchi Y, Ikoma E, et al. Neurotrophins regulate the function of cultured microglia. Glia 1998;24(3):272–89.
27. Blasko I, Stampfer-Kountchev M, Robatscher P, et al. How chronic inflammation can affect the brain and support the development of Alzheimer's disease in old age: the role of microglia and astrocytes. Aging Cell 2004;3(4):169–76.
28. Darlington CL. Astrocytes as targets for neuroprotective drugs. Curr Opin Investig Drugs 2005;6(7):700–3.
29. Dilger RN, Johnson RW. Aging, microglial cell priming, and the discordant central inflammatory response to signals from the peripheral immune system. J Leukoc Biol 2008;84(4):932–9.
30. Godbout JP, Johnson RW. Age and neuroinflammation: a lifetime of psychoneuroimmune consequences. Neurol Clin 2006;24(3):521–38.
31. Banks WA. Cytokine's CVs and the blood-brain barrier. San Diego (CA): Academic Press; 2001.
32. Maier SF, Watkins LR. Immune-to-central nervous system communication and its role in modulating pain and cognition: Implications for cancer and cancer treatment. Brain Behav Immun 2003;17(Suppl 1):S125–31.

33. Maier SF, Goehler LE, Fleshner M, et al. The role of the vagus nerve in cytokine-to-brain communication. Ann N Y Acad Sci 1998;840:289–300.

34. Goehler LE, Gaykema RP, Hansen MK, et al. Vagal immune-to-brain communication: a visceral chemosensory pathway. Auton Neurosci 2000;85(1–3):49–59.

35. Romeo HE, Tio DL, Rahman SU, et al. The glossopharyngeal nerve as a novel pathway in immune-to-brain communication: relevance to neuroimmune surveillance of the oral cavity. J Neuroimmunol 2001;115(1–2):91–100.

36. Lee CK, Weindruch R, Prolla TA. Gene-expression profile of the ageing brain in mice. Nat Genet 2000;25(3):294–7.

37. Carpentier PA, Palmer TD. Immune influence on adult neural stem cell regulation and function. Neuron 2009;64(1):79–92.

38. Graeber MB, Tetzlaff W, Streit WJ, et al. Microglial cells but not astrocytes undergo mitosis following rat facial nerve axotomy. Neurosci Lett 1988;85(3):317–21.

39. Flügel A, Bradl M, Kreutzberg GW, et al. Transformation of donor-derived bone marrow precursors into host microglia during autoimmune CNS inflammation and during the retrograde response to axotomy. J Neurosci Res 2001;66(1):74–82.

40. Conde JR, Streit WJ. Effect of aging on the microglial response to peripheral nerve injury. Neurobiol Aging 2006;27(10):1451–61.

41. Gruver AL, Hudson LL, Sempowski GD. Immunosenescence of ageing. J Pathol 2007;211(2):144–56.

42. Wei J, Xu H, Davies JL, et al. Increase of plasma IL-6 concentration with age in healthy subjects. Life Sci 1992;51(25):1953–6.

43. Ershler WB, Sun WH, Binkley N, et al. Interleukin-6 and aging: blood levels and mononuclear cell production increase with advancing age and in vitro production is modifiable by dietary restriction. Lymphokine Cytokine Res 1993;12(4):225–30.

44. Hager K, Machein U, Krieger S, et al. Interleukin-6 and selected plasma proteins in healthy persons of different ages. Neurobiol Aging 1994;15(6):771–2.

45. Ye SM, Johnson RW. Increased interleukin-6 expression by microglia from brain of aged mice. J Neuroimmunol 1999;93(1–2):139–48.

46. Ershler WB. Interleukin-6: a cytokine for gerontologists. J Am Geriatr Soc 1993;41(2):176–81.

47. Maggio M, Guralnik JM, Longo DL, et al. Interleukin-6 in aging and chronic disease: a magnificent pathway. J Gerontol A Biol Sci Med Sci 2006;61(6):575–84.

48. Godbout JP, Chen J, Abraham J, et al. Exaggerated neuroinflammation and sickness behavior in aged mice following activation of the peripheral innate immune system. FASEB J 2005;19(10):1329–31.

49. Sparkman NL, Johnson RW. Neuroinflammation associated with aging sensitizes the brain to the effects of infection or stress. Neuroimmunomodulation 2008;15(4–6):323–30.

50. Parnet P, Kelley KW, Bluthé RM, et al. Expression and regulation of interleukin-1 receptors in the brain. Role in cytokines-induced sickness behavior. J Neuroimmunol 2002;125(1–2):5–14.

51. Konsman JP, Vigues S, Mackerlova L, et al. Rat brain vascular distribution of interleukin-1 type-1 receptor immunoreactivity: relationship to patterns of inducible cyclooxygenase expression by peripheral inflammatory stimuli. J Comp Neurol 2004;472(1):113–29.

52. Terao A, Apte-Deshpande A, Dousman L, et al. Immune response gene expression increases in the aging murine hippocampus. J Neuroimmunol 2002;132(1–2):99–112.

53. Ye SM, Johnson RW. An age-related decline in interleukin-10 may contribute to the increased expression of interleukin-6 in brain of aged mice. Neuroimmunomodulation 2001;9(4):183–92.
54. Xie Z, Morgan TE, Rozovsky I, et al. Aging and glial responses to lipopolysaccharide in vitro: greater induction of IL-1 and IL-6, but smaller induction of neurotoxicity. Exp Neurol 2003;182(1):135–41.
55. Rachal Pugh C, Fleshner M, Watkins LR, et al. The immune system and memory consolidation: a role for the cytokine IL-1beta. Neurosci Biobehav Rev 2001;25(1):29–41.
56. Barrientos RM, Higgins EA, Biedenkapp JC, et al. Peripheral infection and aging interact to impair hippocampal memory consolidation. Neurobiol Aging 2006; 27(5):723–32.
57. Sparkman NL, Buchanan JB, Heyen JR, et al. Interleukin-6 facilitates lipopolysaccharide-induced disruption in working memory and expression of other proinflammatory cytokines in hippocampal neuronal cell layers. J Neurosci 2006;26(42):10709–16.
58. Johnson JD, O'Connor KA, Deak T, et al. Prior stressor exposure sensitizes LPS-induced cytokine production. Brain Behav Immun 2002;16(4):461–76.
59. Harrison NA, Brydon L, Walker C, et al. Inflammation causes mood changes through alterations in subgenual cingulate activity and mesolimbic connectivity. Biol Psychiatry 2009;66(5):407–14.
60. Baune BT, Dannlowski U, Domschke K, et al. The interleukin 1 beta (IL1B) gene is associated with failure to achieve remission and impaired emotion processing in major depression. Biol Psychiatry 2010;67(6):543–9.
61. Dowlati Y, Herrmann N, Swardfager W, et al. A meta-analysis of cytokines in major depression. Biol Psychiatry 2010;67(5):446–57.
62. Dentino AN, Pieper CF, Rao MK, et al. Association of interleukin-6 and other biologic variables with depression in older people living in the community. J Am Geriatr Soc 1999;47(1):6–11.
63. Penninx BW, Kritchevsky SB, Yaffe K, et al. Inflammatory markers and depressed mood in older persons: results from the Health, Aging and Body Composition study. Biol Psychiatry 2003;54(5):566–72.
64. Tiemeier H, Hofman A, van Tuijl HR, et al. Inflammatory proteins and depression in the elderly. Epidemiology 2003;14(1):103–7.
65. Bremmer MA, Beekman AT, Deeg DJ, et al. Inflammatory markers in late-life depression: results from a population-based study. J Affect Disord 2008; 106(3):249–55.
66. Diniz BS, Teixeira AL, Talib L, et al. Interleukin-1beta serum levels is increased in antidepressant-free elderly depressed patients. Am J Geriatr Psychiatry 2010; 18(2):172–6.
67. Diniz BS, Teixeira AL, Talib LL, et al. Increased soluble TNF receptor 2 in antidepressant-free patients with late-life depression. J Psychiatr Res 2010;44: 917–20.
68. Thomas AJ, Davis S, Morris C, et al. Increase in interleukin-1beta in late-life depression. Am J Psychiatry 2005;162(1):175–7.
69. Grassi-Oliveira R, Brietzke E, Pezzi JC, et al. Increased soluble tumor necrosis factor-alpha receptors in patients with major depressive disorder. Psychiatry Clin Neurosci 2009;63(2):202–8.
70. Gimeno D, Kivimäki M, Brunner EJ, et al. Associations of C-reactive protein and interleukin-6 with cognitive symptoms of depression: 12-year follow-up of the Whitehall II study. Psychol Med 2009;39(3):413–23.

71. Lindqvist D, Janelidze S, Hagell P, et al. Interleukin-6 is elevated in the cerebro-spinal fluid of suicide attempters and related to symptom severity. Biol Psychiatry 2009;66(3):287–92.

72. Milaneschi Y, Corsi AM, Penninx BW, et al. Interleukin-1 receptor antagonist and incident depressive symptoms over 6 years in older persons: the InCHIANTI study. Biol Psychiatry 2009;65(11):973–8.

73. Lutgendorf SK, Garand L, Buckwalter KC, et al. Life stress, mood disturbance, and elevated interleukin-6 in healthy older women. J Gerontol A Biol Sci Med Sci 1999;54(9):M434–9.

74. Harris TB, Ferrucci L, Tracy RP, et al. Associations of elevated interleukin-6 and C-reactive protein levels with mortality in the elderly. Am J Med 1999;106(5):506–12.

75. Ferrucci L, Harris TB, Guralnik JM, et al. Serum IL-6 level and the development of disability in older persons. J Am Geriatr Soc 1999;47(6):639–46.

76. Weaver JD, Huang MH, Albert M, et al. Interleukin-6 and risk of cognitive decline: MacArthur studies of successful aging. Neurology 2002;59(3):371–8.

77. Kubera M, Kenis G, Bosmans E, et al. Effects of serotonin and serotonergic agonists and antagonists on the production of interferon-gamma and inter-leukin-10. Neuropsychopharmacology 2000;23(1):89–98.

78. Kubera M, Kenis G, Bosmans E, et al. Plasma levels of interleukin-6, interleukin-10, and interleukin-1 receptor antagonist in depression: comparison between the acute state and after remission. Pol J Pharmacol 2000;52(3):237–41.

79. Kubera M, Kenis G, Budziszewska B, et al. Lack of a modulatory effect of imip-ramine on glucocorticoid-induced suppression of interferon-gamma and interleukin-10 production in vitro. Pol J Pharmacol 2001;53(3):289–94.

80. Yirmiya R, Tio DL, Taylor AN. Effects of fetal alcohol exposure on fever, sickness behavior, and pituitary-adrenal activation induced by interleukin-1 beta in young adult rats. Brain Behav Immun 1996;10(3):205–20.

81. Maes M, Song C, Lin AH, et al. Negative immunoregulatory effects of antidepres-sants: inhibition of interferon gamma and stimulation of interleukin-10 secretion. Neuropsychopharmacology 1999;20(4):370–9.

82. Lin A, Song C, Kenis G, et al. The in vitro immunosuppressive effects of moclo-bemide in healthy volunteers. J Affect Disord 2000;58(1):69–74.

83. Szuster-Ciesielska A, Tustanowska-Stachura A, Slotwińska M, et al. In vitro immu-noregulatory effects of antidepressants in healthy volunteers. Pol J Pharmacol 2003;55(3):353–62.

84. O'Brien SM, Scully P, Fitzgerald P, et al. Plasma cytokine profiles in depressed patients who fail to respond to selective serotonin reuptake inhibitor therapy. J Psychiatr Res 2007;41(3–4):326–31.

85. Eller T, Vasar V, Shlik J, et al. Pro-inflammatory cytokines and treatment response to escitalopram in major depressive disorder. Prog Neuropsychopharmacol Biol Psychiatry 2008;32(2):445–50.

86. Pae CU, Marks DM, Han C, et al. Does minocycline have antidepressant effect? Biomed Pharmacother 2008;62(5):308–11.

87. Muller N, Schwarz MJ, Dehning S, et al. The cyclooxygenase-2 inhibitor celecoxib has therapeutic effects in major depression: results of a double-blind, randomized, placebo controlled, add-on pilot study to reboxetine. Mol Psychiatry 2006;11(7):680–4.

88. Akhondzadeh S, Jafari S, Raisi F, et al. Clinical trial of adjunctive celecoxib treat-ment in patients with major depression: a double blind and placebo controlled trial. Depress Anxiety 2009;26(7):607–11.

89. Tyring S, Gottlieb A, Papp K, et al. Etanercept and clinical outcomes, fatigue, and depression in psoriasis: double-blind placebo-controlled randomised phase III trial. Lancet 2006;367(9504):29–35.
90. Chiang CS, Stalder A, Samimi A, et al. Reactive gliosis as a consequence of interleukin-6 expression in the brain: studies in transgenic mice. Dev Neurosci 1994;16(3–4):212–21.
91. Konsman JP, Tridon V, Dantzer R. Diffusion and action of intracerebroventricularly injected interleukin-1 in the CNS. Neuroscience 2000;101(4):957–67.

Suicide in Older Adults

Yeates Conwell, MD*, Kimberly Van Orden, PhD, Eric D. Caine, MD

KEYWORDS

• Suicide • Older adult • Aged • Prevention

Suicide at any age is a tragedy for the individual, his or her family and friends, and the communities of which he or she is a part. At a population level, suicide is also a major public health problem, accounting for over 34,500 deaths each year in the United States[1] and an estimated 1 million or more worldwide.[2] The largest number of suicides occurs in younger and middle-aged adults, and suicide deaths in youth and young adults capture the bulk of media attention. This article, however, makes the case that late-life suicide is a cause for great concern that warrants ongoing attention from researchers, health care providers, policy makers, and society at large. Acknowledging the complexity and multidetermined nature of suicidal behavior in older adults, this article provides a framework for its understanding on which to base its prevention. The article reviews the evidence for factors that place older adults at risk for suicide, or protect them from it. Taken individually, however, risk factors offer relatively weak guidance for implementation of successful suicide prevention initiatives because, at the individual level, their ability to predict who will die by suicide is so poor. The authors argue then from a public health perspective for understanding suicide as a developmental process to which risk and protective factors contribute in defining a trajectory to suicide over time. Translation of that developmental perspective into preventive interventions next requires identification of opportunities to intervene, the sites or points of engagement where older adults can best be detected, and interventions made to alter their suicidal trajectories. Finally, the authors introduce the notion that suicide preventive interventions target individuals or groups at different levels of risk at different points on the developmental trajectory toward death by suicide, offering examples of each and recommending their strategic, combined application to create an effective, community level response to the mounting problem of suicide in older adults.

This work was supported in part by Grant Number T32MH20061 from the National Institute of Mental Health.
The authors have nothing to disclose.
Department of Psychiatry, University of Rochester Medical Center, 300 Crittenden Boulevard, Rochester, NY 14642, USA
* Corresponding author.
E-mail address: yeates_conwell@urmc.rochester.edu

Psychiatr Clin N Am 34 (2011) 451–468
doi:10.1016/j.psc.2011.02.002
0193-953X/11/$ – see front matter © 2011 Elsevier Inc. All rights reserved.

psych.theclinics.com

THE EPIDEMIOLOGY OF SUICIDE IN LATER LIFE

In most countries throughout the world that report such statistics to the World Health Organization, suicide rates tend to rise as a function of age for both men and women to a peak in old, old age.[2] There is great variability, however. In Canada, for example, suicide rates peak at midlife for both men and women and decline slightly thereafter. In recent years the United States has exhibited the same pattern for the overall population. **Fig. 1**, however, shows a more complex picture when rates are considered as a function of age, gender, and race. For both black and white women, rates rise through midlife and fall thereafter; black men experience two peaks of risk, one in young adulthood and the second in old age. Most striking is the higher rate at every point in the life course for white men, rising to a peak in the oldest age group of over 45 suicides per 100,000 population per year, over 4 times the nation's overall age-adjusted rate of 11.5 suicides per 100,000 population per year.[1]

There is good news and bad news in trends with regard to aging and suicide over time in the United States, where, as depicted in **Fig. 2**, the overall rate of suicide fell slowly but steadily from 1985 through 2000, after which it has begun to rise again marginally.[1] Reductions in rates among youth, young adults, and those over age 65 largely accounted for the decrease. Indeed, since 1986 rates have dropped among older adults in the United States by over 35%, even as suicide rates have risen by almost 20% over the last 8 years among those ages 35 to 64. While the steady reduction in suicide rates among older adults is encouraging, the recent rise in rates by those in the middle years is a cause for serious concern. Birth cohorts tend to carry with them a characteristic propensity to suicide as they age. The baby boom cohort, those born between 1946 and 1964, has had relatively higher suicide rates at any given age than earlier or subsequent birth cohorts. As well, the leading edge of the baby boom cohort will reach age 65 in 2011, fueling rapid growth over the next 20 years in the total size of the older adult population. Demographers estimate that by the year 2030 over 71 million US citizens will be age 65 or older, or 20% of the US population.[3] Therefore, as the baby boom cohort, a group with historically high rates of suicide, enters older adulthood, the time of greatest risk, in such large numbers, one can anticipate that the rate of suicide in men and women will rise again, resulting in substantial increases in the absolute numbers of senior citizens dying by their own hands.

RISK AND PROTECTIVE FACTORS

To design interventions with the objective of reducing suicide-related morbidity and mortality, one must understand its causes. Establishing causation of a complex, multi-determined, rare and dire outcome such as suicide is a daunting task. However, identification of risk and protective factors can guide prevention efforts. Much of what is known about factors that place older adults at risk for suicide, or protect them from it, has been learned from retrospective analysis of the characteristics, backgrounds, and circumstances of people who kill themselves, an approach known as the psychological autopsy (PA) method.[4] Although subject to recall bias and other limitations inherent to retrospective data collection, the PA approach has advantages as well, including a detailed focus on those who die by suicide. It remains unclear how applicable lessons learned from the study of suicidal ideation and attempts in later life are to the understanding of completed suicide. Longitudinal cohort studies in which sufficient numbers die by suicide to allow meaningful analyses are unfeasible because suicide is a relatively rare event. Furthermore, even in longitudinal studies, the time between a subject's most recent assessment and death, a critical period for

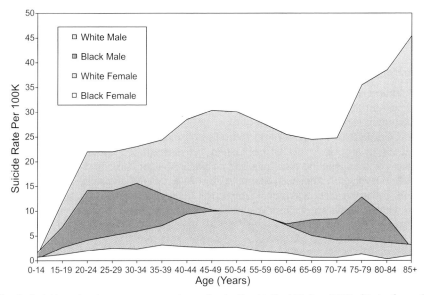

Fig. 1. Suicide rates by age, race, and gender in the United States, 2007. (*Data from* the Centers for Disease Control and Prevention, 2010.)

understanding the more immediate precipitants of suicidal behavior, would require retrospective analysis. Reinforced by studies demonstrating the validity of the PA method,[5,6] various investigators have applied it in case–control studies that provide remarkably consistent findings.[7–21] Results indicate that specific factors in domains of psychiatric illness, social connectedness of the older person with his or her family, friends, and community, physical illness, and functional capacity appear to influence

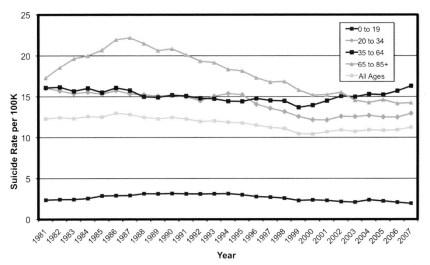

Fig. 2. 1981–2007, US suicide rates per 100,000 population, all races, both sexes. (*Data from* the Centers for Disease Control and Prevention, 2010.)

risk for suicide. They in turn operate against a backdrop of individual's culture, personality, and neurobiological milieu. The authors examine briefly the evidence for each in turn.

Psychiatric Illness

Of all factors examined in PA studies of older adults, psychiatric illness consistently emerges as the most prominent. **Table 1** lists rates of psychiatric and substance use disorders reported in samples of older people who died by suicide in a range of studies. **Table 2** lists results from PA studies that included a control group, allowing calculation of an odds ratio (OR) reflecting the strength of the association between specific axis 1 psychiatric disorders and suicide in the second half of life. The lessons are clear. Psychiatric illness is present in from 71% to 97% of suicides, with affective disorder being the most common. In particular, major depression is most closely associated. Primary psychotic disorders, including schizophrenia, schizoaffective illness, and delusion disorder, as well as anxiety disorders, tend to be present in lower proportions. The prevalence of substance use disorders was highly variable in these studies, reflecting differences in the measures used, the populations examined, and their sociocultural context. Rates of problem drinking, for example differ markedly in the East[9] and West.[21]

As indicated in **Table 2**, the odds of an older adult having any axis 1 diagnosis were between 44 and 113 times higher for suicides than matched controls. The highest ORs were observed for mood disorders, with lower ORs and generally more mixed results in those studies that examined substance abuse and dependence, schizophrenia, and anxiety disorders. The wide variation between studies in the strength of associations observed can also be accounted for by methodological differences, including the choice of control group. For example, Harwood and colleagues[12] compared completed suicides with controls who died of natural causes in hospital, whereas the other listed studies used living community controls. Consequently Harwood and colleagues reported, for example, that the diagnosis of dementia or delirium was significantly less common in suicides than controls, a counterintuitive finding not observed in the other studies and likely explained by high rates of cognitive disorders and confusional states in hospitalized and terminally ill elders. The PA method may be poorly suited to the study of dementia and delirium, the signs and symptoms of which, particularly early in the course of illness when the patient may be at relatively greater risk,[22,23] are less likely to be apparent in community settings to family members and other proxy informants. Other biological[24] and epidemiologic[22] data provide at least preliminary evidence that dementia too is associated with increased risk of suicide in older adults.

Physical Health and Functioning

In addition to psychiatric illness, physical ill health and functional impairments contribute to risk for suicide in later life. Because the base rates of physical illness and disability are so high in this population, however, their usefulness in identifying individual elders who warrant intervention is weak. For instance, record linkage studies have consistently found that individuals with malignancies (other than common skin cancers) are at approximately 2 times greater risk for suicide than those without.[25] Other diverse conditions such as human immunodeficiency virus (HIV)/ acquired immunodeficiency syndrome (AIDS), epilepsy, Huntington disease and multiple sclerosis, renal and peptic ulcer disease, heart and lung diseases, spinal cord injury, and systemic lupus erythematosus also have been found to be associated with increased suicide risk in some studies.[25–27] Relative risks for suicide associated with these conditions are in the range of 1.5 to 4 times higher.

Although the relative risk for suicide associated with any specific condition may be small, as the number of an individual's acute and chronic conditions increases, so does his or her cumulative risk. Juurlink and colleagues[26] linked prescription records of all residents of Ontario, Canada, aged 65 years and older with provincial coroners' reports of suicide in a case–control analysis. They found that patients with 3 physical illnesses had approximately a threefold increase in estimated relative risk for suicide compared with subjects who had no diagnosis, whereas older adults who had 7 or more illnesses had approximately 9 times greater risk for suicide.

Beyond the number of physical illnesses, it is likely that the perceived meaning of those illnesses, their impact on function, pain, and threats to autonomy and personal integrity play pivotal roles as well. For example, in a case-controlled comparison of suicides over age 50 years with living demographically matched controls, the authors' group found in multivariate analyses that the presence of any impairment in instrumental activities in daily living (IADLs) was significantly associated with suicide case status independent of the effects of physical and mental health disorder diagnoses.[21] Elsewhere the authors have noted that elderly suicide decedents commonly communicated a belief to others that they had cancer that on autopsy was unconfirmed. Yet there was no other indication of thought disorder or cognitive impairment.[28] Perceived health status may ultimately prove to have greater salience to late-life suicide and its prevention than objective measures, just as has been observed in association with natural death and all-cause mortality.[29]

Although relatively little research has examined associations between pain and suicide in older adults, several studies suggest that it may be an especially important issue among older men. Juurlink and colleagues,[26] for example, reported that the association between severe pain and suicide was somewhat stronger for men (OR = 9.9) than women (OR = 3.3). Similarly, Sirey and colleagues[30] found a stronger association between suicidal ideation and chronic pain among older adult men receiving home-delivered meals than women, and in their recent analysis of elderly home care recipients, Li and Conwell[31] found that men with severe and uncontrolled pain were at especially high risk for self-injury ideation, whereas no such association was observed in women.

Cognitive deficits in later life have also been linked to suicide. Dombrovski and colleagues,[32] for example, have reported that elderly suicidal depressives performed worse on measures of frontal executive function as well as memory and attention tests than did nonsuicidal elderly depressives. Frontal executive function may be particularly pertinent to suicidal behavior in older adulthood because of its role in effective management of stressful circumstances. Keilp and colleagues[33] found that adult suicide attempters performed poorly on frontal executive tasks relative to controls, a similar observation to one made by King and colleagues[34] in older adult attempters. The cognitive mechanisms underlying relationships between cognitive control, problem solving, and suicidal behavior remain obscure. Dombrovski and colleagues[35] examined more specific components of decision making for their association with suicidal behavior in old age, focusing in particular on reward/punishment-based learning, abnormalities in which have been related in pathology in ventral prefrontal circuits. Their finding of deficits in depressed attempters supports the notion that late-life suicidal behavior is in some instances associated with impaired decision making based on impaired ability to access and use prior experience, which in turn may be related to underlying age-related ventral prefrontal pathology.[36] Other reports support a link between suicidal behavior in older adults and brain pathology. Ahearn

Table 1
Axis 1 diagnoses made by psychological autopsy in studies of late-life suicide

Study	Location	Age	Sample Size (with Gender Distribution if Available)	Major Depression	Other Mood Disorder	Alcohol Use Disorder	Other Drug Use Disorder	Nonaffective Psychosis	Anxiety Disorder	No Diagnosis[a]
								Diagnosis: Percent With		
Barraclough,[7] 1971	West Sussex, UK	≥65	N = 30 (No gender distribution reported)	87		3		0	—	13
Beautrais,[20] 2002	New Zealand	≥55	N = 31 20 (64.5%) ♂ 11 (35.5%) ♀	86		14		—	—	9
Carney et al,[8] 1994	San Diego, California	≥60	N = 49 29 (59.2%) ♂ 20 (40.8%) ♀	54		22		—	—	14
Chiu et al,[9] 2004	Hong Kong	≥60	N = 70 32 (45.7%) ♂ 38 (54.3%) ♀	53 46.9% ♂ 57.9% ♀	26 34.4% ♂ 18.4% ♀	3 6.3% ♂ 0% ♀	—	9 9.4% ♂ 7.9% ♀	1 0% ♂ 1.4% ♀	14 12.5% ♂ 15.8% ♀
Clark,[10] 1991	Chicago	≥65	N = 54	54	11	19	0	0	2	24
Conwell et al,[11] 1996	Monroe County, New York	55–74	N = 36 28 (77.8%) ♂ 8 (22.2%) ♀	47	17	43	3	6	11	8
		75–92	N = 14 9 (64.3%) ♂ 5 (35.7%) ♀	57	21	27	7	0	0	29

Study	Location	Age	N							
Conwell et al,[21] 2009	Monroe and Onondaga Counties, New York	50–64	N = 33; 23 (69.7%) ♂; 10 (30.3%) ♀	49	39	27	18	9	24	3
		65–99	N = 53; 40 (75.5%) ♂; 13 (24.5%) ♀	51	26	9	2	2	9	23
Harwood et al,[12] 2001	Central England	≥60	100	63		5	5	4	—	23
Henriksson et al,[13] 1995	Finland	≥60	43; 34 (54.1%) ♂; 39 (45.9%) ♀	44	21	25	5	5	9	12
McGirr et al,[14] 2008	Quebec, Canada	50–59	N = 88; 71 (80.5%) ♂; 17 (19.5%) ♀	60		45	—	—	15	—
		60–69	N = 31; 25 (80.6%) ♂; 6 (19.4%) ♀	48		24	—	—	24	—
		>70	N = 21; 19 (90.5%) ♂; 2 (9.5%) ♀	46		39	—	—	23	—
Waern et al,[15] 2002	Goteborg, Sweden	≥65	N = 85; 46 (54.1%) ♂; 39 (45.9%) ♀	46	36	27	8		15	5

[a] Includes cases with insufficient data to allow diagnosis. Note: dashes are used to indicate when data were unavailable.

Table 2
Odds ratios for suicide by axis 1 diagnosis in case-control psychological autopsy studies of older adults

	Harwood et al,[12] 2001	Beautrais,[20] 2002	Waern et al,[15] 2002	Chiu et al,[9] 2004	Conwell et al,[21] 2009
Any Axis 1 Diagnosis	—	43.9	113.1	50.0	44.6
Any Mood Disorder	4.0	184.6	63.1	59.2	47.7
Major Depressive Episode	—	—	28.6	36.3	12.2
Substance Use Disorder	ns	4.4	43.1	ns	ns
Anxiety Disorder	—	—	3.6	ns	5.9
Schizophrenic Spectrum	ns	—	10.7	>1	ns
Dementia/Delirium	0.2	—	ns	ns	ns

Comparison groups are as follows: Harwood and colleagues used older adults who died from natural causes; all other studies used living community controls.
Abbreviation: ns, not significant.

and colleagues,[37] for example, reported that elderly depressives with lifetime histories of suicide attempts had significantly more subcortical gray matter hyperintensities on magnetic resonance imaging (MRI) scans than carefully matched depressives with no previous suicide attempt history, supporting the hypothesis that underlying vascular disease may predispose to late-life depressive illness and suicidal behavior.[38]

Social Factors

PA studies clearly and consistently demonstrate a role for social factors in the pathogenesis, and therefore prevention, of suicide in older adults as well. Two broad categories in this domain warrant special note—stressful life events as predisposing factors and social connectedness as a buffer that serves to reduce suicide risk.

It is clear that stressful life events preceding death by suicide tend to be more numerous and severe among suicides than controls. The events most salient to suicide in later life are those associated with aging—threats associated with ill health and functional impairment as noted above, losses through bereavement, or rupture of relationships with family members and other sources of support. Serious relationship and financial problems distinguished older adult suicides and near-fatal suicide attempters from controls in New Zealand,[20] findings replicated by Rubenowitz and colleagues[16] in Sweden. The authors' group also has reported that family discord and employment change distinguished suicides from controls over the age of 50 years even after adjusting for sociodemographic characteristics and mental disorders.[18]

On both theoretical and empirical bases, the construct of social connectedness may be especially important when understanding late-life suicide and its prevention. Indeed, the Centers for Disease Control has identified as a key strategy for preventing suicidal behavior at all ages "the promotion and strengthening of connectedness at personal, family, and community levels."[39] Holt-Lunstad and colleagues,[40] in a recent meta-analytic review of 148 studies to determine the extent to which social relationships influence risk for mortality, found that overall there was a 50% increased likelihood of survival for participants with stronger social relationships. Furthermore, they noted that the influence of social connectedness on risk for death is comparable to or greater than that associated with well-established risk factors such as smoking, obesity, and physical inactivity. The authors excluded studies in which suicide was included as a cause of death; however, other evidence strongly supports this link as well. PA studies have shown that older adult suicides were significantly less likely to have had a confidante,[41] more likely to live alone than their peers in the community,[7] and less likely to participate in community activities,[19] be active in organizations, or have a hobby.[16] Also, Turvey and colleagues[42] found in analyses of data from a prospective cohort study that having a greater number of friends and relatives in whom to confide was associated with significantly reduced suicide risk in older adults.

The Interpersonal Theory of Suicide[43] offers one way of understanding the relationship of social connectedness with suicide. It proposes that there are 2 proximal causes of the desire for suicide—thwarted belongingness and perceived burdensomeness—with a particularly dangerous level of suicidal desire resulting from the simultaneous presence of both factors. In the presence of an acquired capability for suicide (eg, prior experience with pain or well-developed cognitive models of one's death) these painful psychological states may become lethal. The construct of thwarted belongingness stems from the fundamental need for connectedness posited by Baumeister and Leary[44] as the "need to belong," reflected in indices of social isolation that have been empirically linked with late-life suicide such as living alone, loss of spouse, loneliness, and low social support. Perceived burdensomeness is a construct less fully explored in research, but a common theme heard by clinicians who work with older adults whom they perceive to be at risk. The theory proposes that both family discord and functional impairments are associated with late-life suicide, because both factors are likely to engender perceptions of burdensomeness on others. Conversely, connections to other individuals and to his or her community may serve to protect the older person against the development of suicidal desire in the face of stressful life circumstances. However, according to the theory, only connections that contribute to individuals' need to belong—connections that create positive interactions and feelings of being cared about—will be protective. Thus, relationships characterized by perceived burdensomeness, or other forms of interpersonal discord, will not protect against suicide. Spirituality and religiousness have been cited as protective factors against the development of the depression and suicidality,[19,45] a relationship that might also be understood as a function of connectedness at a spiritual or instrumental level (eg, support provided to an isolated elder by their faith community.) As well, differences in suicide risk as a function of gender and race/ethnicity with aging might be understood in part by the stronger ties to supportive others that women and some minority communities have capacity to establish relative to men and white race groups in general.[46] The Interpersonal Theory proposes that risk factors for suicide, including psychiatric illness, elevate risk for suicide by causing or exacerbating thwarted belongingness, perceived burdensomeness and/or acquired capability. Future research should empirically examine this hypothesis.

Other Factors

Risk factors in psychiatric, physical and functional, and social domains operate in complex interactions against a background colored by one's culture, personality traits, and even neurobiological make up. Suicidal elders have been characterized as timid and seclusive,[47] hostile, rigid, and with an independent style.[47,48] Based on standardized measures and case controlled PA methodology, anankastic (obsessional) and anxious traits were shown to significantly distinguish suicides from elder natural death controls in one study,[12] while in another, the Big-Five personality traits of low Openness To Experience (OTE) and high Neuroticism[49] distinguished the groups.[50] Low OTE is associated with muted affective and hedonic responses, a constricted range of interests, and a strong preference for the familiar over the novel. Duberstein[51] hypothesized that older adults low in OTE are at risk for suicide because they are less well equipped socially and psychologically to manage the challenges of aging and less likely to be recognized as being in distress and need of intervention, another manifestation of poor social connectedness.

Numerous reports of associations between suicidal behavior and a range of neurobiological parameters have emerged from studies of mixed age and younger adult samples.[52] They raise the exciting prospect that genetically mediated abnormalities in central nervous system processes predispose individuals to act impulsively and aggressively in the face of dysphoria, hopelessness, and emergent suicidal ideation in the depressed state. Furthermore, they suggest a possibility that age-related changes in these systems may further account for the rise in suicide rates in later life, particularly if these differences were shown to be more pronounced in men than women. However, few studies have examined neurobiological systems in suicidal older adults, because high rates of medication use and medical comorbidity in older adult suicides and attempted suicides complicate interpretation of findings in such studies. Additional research is necessary on the role of neurobiological factors in late-life suicide, just as it is for factors in other domains and, perhaps most importantly, their interaction in determining risk.

DEVELOPMENTAL TRAJECTORIES

Knowledge of factors that increase or decrease risk for suicide in older adults is necessary but not sufficient for the effective design of preventive interventions. It is insufficient because the factors are so inefficient, either individually or in combinations, for predicting outcomes for any individual. The large number of false-positives that resulted from their widespread use would lead to unnecessary, intrusive, and expensive interventions for those who did not need them, while many false-negative results would leave at-risk elders undetected and unprotected. The limitations of risk and protective factors as tools to predict and prevent suicide are related in part to the fact that risk states are dynamic; they wax and wane over short periods of time. Suicide, therefore, is better understood as a developmental process that evolves over longer periods. **Fig. 3** attempts to capture that process and relate it to a public

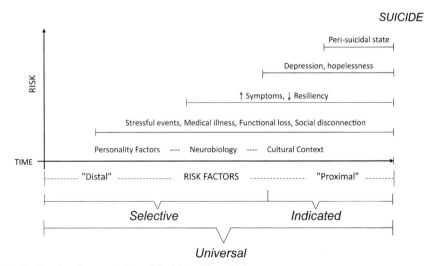

Fig. 3. The developmental model of late-life suicide.

health framework for prevention. The x axis represents the dimension of time. On a foundation of personality characteristics, individual neurobiological factors, and cultural context, each older person encounters stressful events. In the struggle with acute and chronic medical illnesses and functional decline, some become socially disconnected. Relative risk increases among those who are less resilient and develop early symptoms of psychiatric illness. Some become more frankly depressed and hopeless, the most vulnerable of whom enter the perisuicidal state. Risks mount over time with the accumulation of progressively more proximal risk factors or the loss of protective buffers. Those with active ideation and capability of taking their own lives act on their suicidal desire, and many die.

The notion that suicidal processes unfold over time has important implications for prevention. While it connotes a level of complexity that is on one hand daunting, it also indicates opportunities to intervene at multiple points and in many different ways. The authors now turn attention to considering those opportunities for intervention.

APPROACHES TO PREVENTION

A medical model or high-risk approach to suicide prevention would tend to focus on that terminal segment of the developmental process at the right of the diagram in **Fig. 3**, when older adults are at greatest risk. A public health approach would see opportunities for preventive intervention across the entire continuum. Indeed, it would propose that interventions targeting more distal and intermediate factors and stages of the process may result in more lives saved than those restricting focus to higher-risk individuals.[53,54] This premise may apply more directly to older adults than younger age groups, because suicidal behavior in elders is so much more lethal. Studies estimate that as many as 200 young adults attempt suicide for each person who dies by his or her own hand.[55] Among older adults, attempts are far less common, yielding a ratio of perhaps 4 attempts per completed suicide.[56] Whether due to elders' increased isolation and decreased chances of rescue, their greater frailty and hence likelihood of dying as a result of any self-inflicted injury, or the older population's tendency to use more immediately lethal means with greater planning and determination,[57] the implications are clear. Interventions to prevent the development of the suicidal state are especially critical in this age group.

The Institute of Medicine has advocated use of terminology describing preventive interventions at 3 levels: indicated, selective, and universal.[58] **Table 3** provides definitions and examples of each.

Indicated preventive interventions are those that target individuals who have detectable symptoms and other proximal risk factors for suicide. Their objective is typically to diagnose and treat psychiatric disorder to prevent the expression of suicidal behavior. The sites in which indicated preventive interventions are typically mounted include primary care and specialty mental health settings. Because older adults are reluctant to seek care in mental health clinics or providers' offices, however, interventions delivered in primary care are likely to be more effective.[59]

Effective diagnosis and treatment of depression are most often cited as examples of indicated preventive intervention because of the close association between affective illness and suicide in older people. Several lines of evidence reinforce the importance of this approach. In 2009, Stone and colleagues[60] published an analysis of proprietary data submitted to the US Food and Drug Administration (FDA) from 372 double-blind randomized placebo-controlled trials of antidepressants in adults. The analysis was driven by concern that antidepressant administration may in fact exacerbate suicide

Table 3
The language of prevention science applied to suicide in later life[a]

Prevention Approach	Target	Objectives	Examples of Possible Prevention Efforts	Sites to Engage Target
Indicated prevention	Individuals with detectable symptoms or other proximal risk factors for suicide	Treat individuals with precursor signs and symptoms to prevent development of disorder or the expression of suicidal behavior	Train gatekeepers in recognition of depression and suicidality Link outreach and gatekeeper services to comprehensive evaluation and health management services in a continuum of care Implement strategies to provide more accessible, acceptable, and affordable mental health care to elders Increase screening/treatment in primary care settings for elders with depression, anxiety, and substance misuse	Mental health care Primary and specialty medical care Emergency services
Selective prevention	Asymptomatic or presymptomatic individuals or groups with distal risk factors for suicide, or who have a higher-than-average risk of developing mental disorders due to presence of more distal risk factors	Prevent suicide-related morbidity and mortality through addressing specific characteristics that place elders at risk	Promote church-based and community programs to contact and support isolated elders Focus medical and social services on reducing disability and enhancing independent functioning Increase access to home care and rehabilitation services Improve access to pain management and palliative care services	Rehabilitation and long-term care services Pain clinics Pharmacies Home health care Community-based social services Faith communities
Universal prevention	Entire population, not identified based on individual risk	Implement broadly directed initiatives to prevent suicide-related morbidity and mortality through reducing risk and enhancing protective factors	Education of the general public, clergy, the media, and health care providers concerning normal aging, ageism and stigma concerning mental illness, pain and disability management, depression, suicidal behaviors Restrict access to lethal means, such as handguns	Media Legislatures Policy makers

[a] Table developed in collaboration with Kerry Knox, PhD, and Eric D. Caine, MD.

risk among some patients. They found that the relative risk for suicidal ideation or behavior emerging during antidepressant treatment was indeed elevated for participants under age 25, no different than placebo for those aged 25 to 64 years, and significantly reduced for those over age 65 who received antidepressant treatment.

However, affective illness often goes undetected and inadequately treated in primary care settings. Two groups therefore conducted randomized trials in which elderly primary care patients were randomized to receive either care as usual or a collaborative, stepped care intervention in which mental health expertise, physician and patient/family education about depression, use of treatment algorithms, and decision support tools were provided.[61,62] Although there were differences in the details of each intervention (eg, the antidepressants and psychosocial interventions offered), both studies found significantly greater reductions in depressive symptoms and suicidal ideation in depressed older adults who received the experimental interventions.[63,64] Due to sample size limitations, neither trial could assess the effectiveness of the intervention on suicidal behavior, however, and the relatively high proportions of female subjects leave open the question of how effective they would be in reducing attempted and completed suicide among those at greatest risk in later life, men.

Selective preventive interventions target asymptomatic or presymptomatic individuals or groups with more distal risk factors, as depicted in middle and on the left side of **Fig. 3**. They may include, for example, older people with chronic, painful, functionally limiting conditions, or those who have become socially isolated or perceive themselves to be a burden on others. The sites at which one might most effectively and efficiently engage older adults in selective preventive interventions are, therefore, broader than for indicated interventions. They could include, for example, the homes of older people receiving visiting nurse or aide services or home-delivered meals, or in agencies that provide community-based social services. Examples of selective preventive interventions for suicide are rare, although the authors posit that trials designed to prevent incident depression among elders at increased risk for the disorder would achieve the same end. The Telehelp/Telecheck service reported by DeLeo and colleagues[65] represents a rare example of selective prevention in which completed suicide in older adults was the targeted outcome. Based in Padua, Italy, the Telehelp/Telecheck service provided telephone-based outreach, evaluation, and support services to more than 18,000 seniors with a mean age of 80 years. Over 84% were women. During the service's 11 years in operation, there were significantly fewer suicides among its clients than were anticipated in the elder population of that region. Further analyses found the effect was only significant for women, possibly because of the small numbers of men enrolled in the program and/or their resistance to a social outreach intervention of this nature.

Finally, universal preventive interventions target an entire population irrespective of the risk status of any individual or group within it. The sites therefore for universal prevention are ones that allow broad dissemination of public health messages, or via legislative policy forums to effect change in levels of exposure across the population.

Although there are no randomized controlled trials of universal prevention of suicide, ecological studies and natural experiments offer some support for their effectiveness in later life. Hawton and colleagues[66] reported that after legislation was implemented to limit the pack size of paracetamol and salicylates sold over the counter in the United Kingdom, morbidity and mortality from overdose with those medications decreased significantly. Another example in the United States was afforded by passage of the Brady Handgun Violence Prevention Act in 1994. Ludwig and Cooke[67] observed that in the years following implementation of the legislation there was a significantly greater reduction in suicides with a handgun by people over the age of 55 years in those states that newly implemented background checks and waiting periods for gun purchase than in states in which no changes in procedures were necessary.

Because universal, selective, and indicated prevention approaches target the suicidal process at different levels, it is likely that the most effective prevention program for suicide in later life would be one that incorporates elements of each. The best example of a multifaceted prevention program of which the authors are aware is a series of 5 quasi-experimental studies combined in an meta-analysis by Oyama and colleagues.[68] Although the details differed somewhat between studies, each was conducted in a different Japanese rural region with high suicide rates among older people (>160 suicides per 100,000 population). Implemented over 5- to 10-year periods, the interventions included systematic community-wide screening, referral to primary care or mental health care as indicated, and, to varying degrees, public education and socialization programs for seniors. The authors examined changes in the relative risk or incidence risk ratios for suicide in older adults before and after the program's implementation and relative to neighboring reference regions of similar size and character. Overall, risk was significantly reduced in men and women when follow-up was conducted by a psychiatrist, but only in women when follow-up was conducted by general practitioners. Again, older men proved relatively more resistant to the effects of preventive intervention.

SUMMARY

Anticipated rapid increases in the size of the older adult population, fueled by aging of the baby boom cohort that life-long has carried a greater propensity to suicide than earlier or later birth cohorts, require urgent attention and allocation of resources to the development and study of approaches to suicide prevention best tailored to older adults. Informed by knowledge of risk and protective factors, models for how those factors function variably and through complex interactions over time to place vulnerable seniors at risk form the basis for that work.

The importance of depression as a pathogenetic factor in late-life suicide makes its detection and effective treatment of paramount importance. Collaborative care delivered by primary care providers informed by mental health expertise has shown promise as an indicated preventive intervention, although its effect in reducing suicide among elderly men remains to be determined. Results of Oyama's meta-analysis cast additional doubt on whether primary care intervention alone will be sufficient, at least for elderly men, who are by far the highest risk group in the United States. Incorporation of additional selective prevention approaches targeting the older adults in a range of community settings should be further developed and tested as a component of any community's comprehensive late-life suicide prevention plan, with special emphasis on maintaining their connectedness to families, friends, and communities. Finally, consideration must be given to universal preventive approaches such as restricting access to highly lethal means by at-risk elders and changing attitudes and biases that inhibit older adults from accessing effective and affordable mental health care.

REFERENCES

1. Centers for Disease Control and Prevention. WISQARS: web-based injury statistics query and reporting system. Available at: http://www.cdc.gov/ncipc/wisqars/default.htm. Accessed August 15, 2010.

2. World Health Organization—Mental Health. Suicide prevention (SUPRE). Available at: http://www.who.int/mental_health/prevention/suicide/suicideprevent/en/. Accessed August 15, 2010.

3. The Merck Company Foundation. The state of aging and health in America. Available at: http://www.cdc.gov/aging. Accessed March 20, 2011.

4. Hawton K, Appleby L, Platt S, et al. The psychological autopsy approach to studying suicide: a review of methodological issues. J Affect Disord 1998;50: 269–76.

5. Conner KR, Conwell Y, Duberstein PR. The validity of proxy-based data in suicide research: a study of patients 50 years of age and older who attempted suicide. II. Life events, social support, and suicidal behavior. Acta Psychiatr Scand 2001; 104(6):452–7.

6. Conner KR, Duberstein PR, Conwell Y. The validity of proxy-based data in suicide research: a study of patients 50 years of age and older who attempted suicide. I. Psychiatric diagnoses. Acta Psychiatr Scand 2001;104(3):204–9.

7. Barraclough BM. Suicide in the elderly: recent developments in psychogeriatrics. Br J Psychiatry 1971;(Suppl 6):87–97.

8. Carney SS, Rich CL, Burke PA, et al. Suicide over 60: the San Diego study. J Am Geriatr Soc 1994;42(2):174–80.

9. Chiu HF, Yip PS, Chi I, et al. Elderly suicide in Hong Kong—a case-controlled psychological autopsy study. Acta Psychiatr Scand 2004;109(4):299–305.

10. Clark DC. Suicide among the elderly. Final report to the AARP Andrus Foundation. Washington, DC: AARP Andrus Foundation; 1991.

11. Conwell Y, Duberstein PR, Cox C, et al. Relationships of age and axis I diagnoses in victims of completed suicide: a psychological autopsy study. Am J Psychiatry 1996;153(8):1001–8.

12. Harwood D, Hawton K, Hope T, et al. Psychiatric disorder and personality factors associated with suicide in older people: a descriptive and case–control study. Int J Geriatr Psychiatry 2001;16(2):155–65.

13. Henriksson MM, Marttunen MJ, Isometsa ET, et al. Mental disorders in elderly suicide. Int Psychogeriatr 1995;7(2):275–86.

14. McGirr A, Renaud J, Bureau A, et al. Impulsive–aggressive behaviours and completed suicide across the life cycle: a predisposition for younger age of suicide. Psychol Med 2008;38(3):407–17.

15. Waern M, Runeson BS, Allebeck P, et al. Mental disorder in elderly suicides: a case–control study. Am J Psychiatry 2002;159(3):450–5.

16. Rubenowitz E, Waern M, Wilhelmson K, et al. Life events and psychosocial factors in elderly suicides—a case–control study. Psychol Med 2001;31(7): 1193–202.

17. Britton PC, Duberstein PR, Conner KR, et al. Reasons for living, hopelessness, and suicide ideation among depressed adults 50 years or older. Am J Geriatr Psychiatry 2008;16(9):736–41.

18. Duberstein PR, Conwell Y, Conner KR, et al. Suicide at 50 years of age and older: perceived physical illness, family discord and financial strain. Psychol Med 2004; 34(1):137–46.

19. Duberstein PR, Conwell Y, Conner KR, et al. Poor social integration and suicide: fact or artifact? A case–control study. Psychol Med 2004;34(7):1331–7.

20. Beautrais AL. A case–control study of suicide and attempted suicide in older adults. Suicide Life Threat Behav 2002;32(1):1–9.

21. Conwell Y, Duberstein PR, Hirsch JK, et al. Health status and suicide in the second half of life. Int J Geriatr Psychiatry 2009;25(4):371–9.

22. Erlangsen A, Zarit SH, Conwell Y. Hospital-diagnosed dementia and suicide: a longitudinal study using prospective, nationwide register data. Am J Geriatr Psychiatry 2008;16(3):220–8.

23. Haw C, Harwood D, Hawton K. Dementia and suicidal behavior: a review of the literature. Int Psychogeriatr 2009;21(3):440–53.

24. Rubio A, Vestner AL, Stewart JM, et al. Suicide and Alzheimer's pathology in the elderly: a case–control study. Biol Psychiatry 2001;49(2):137–45.

25. Harris EC, Barraclough BM. Suicide as an outcome for medical disorders. Medicine (Baltimore) 1994;73(6):281–96.

26. Juurlink DN, Herrmann N, Szalai JP, et al. Medical illness and the risk of suicide in the elderly. Arch Intern Med 2004;164(11):1179–84.

27. Quan H, Arboleda-Florez J, Fick GH, et al. Association between physical illness and suicide among the elderly. Soc Psychiatry Psychiatr Epidemiol 2002;37(4):190–7.

28. Conwell Y, Caine ED, Olsen K. Suicide and cancer in late life. Hosp Community Psychiatry 1990;41(12):1334–9.

29. Kaplan G, Barell V, Lusky A. Subjective state of health and survival in elderly adults. J Gerontol 1988;43(4):S114–20.

30. Sirey JA, Bruce ML, Carpenter M, et al. Depressive symptoms and suicidal ideation among older adults receiving home delivered meals. Int J Geriatr Psychiatry 2008;23(12):1306–11.

31. Li L, Conwell Y. Pain and self-injury ideation in elderly men and women receiving home care. J Am Geriatr Soc 2010;58(11):2160–5.

32. Dombrovski AY, Butters MA, Reynolds CF 3rd, et al. Cognitive performance in suicidal depressed elderly: preliminary report. Am J Geriatr Psychiatry 2008;16(2):109–15.

33. Keilp JG, Sackeim HA, Brodsky BS, et al. Neuropsychological dysfunction in depressed suicide attempters. Am J Psychiatry 2001;158(5):735–41.

34. King DA, Conwell Y, Cox C, et al. A neuropsychological comparison of depressed suicide attempters and nonattempters. J Neuropsychiatry Clin Neurosci 2000;12(1):64–70.

35. Dombrovski AY, Clark L, Siegle GJ, et al. Reward/punishment reversal learning in older suicide attempters. Am J Psychiatry 2010;167(6):699–707.

36. Arango V, Underwood MD, Mann JJ. Postmortem findings in suicide victims. Implications for in vivo imaging studies. Ann N Y Acad Sci 1997;836:269–87.

37. Ahearn EP, Jamison KR, Steffens DC, et al. MRI correlates of suicide attempt history in unipolar depression. Biol Psychiatry 2001;50:266–70.

38. Alexopoulos GS, Meyers BS, Young RC, et al. Vascular depression hypothesis. Arch Gen Psychiatry 1997;54(10):915–22.

39. Centers for Disease Control and Prevention. Connectedness as a strategic direction for the prevention of suicidal behavior: promoting individual, family, and community connectedness to prevent suicidal behavior. 2006. Available at: http://www.cdc.gov/violenceprevention/pdf/Suicide_Strategic_Direction_Full_Version-a.pdf. Accessed August 20, 2010.

40. Holt-Lunstad J, Smith TB, Layton JB. Social relationships and mortality risk: a meta-analytic review. PLoS Med 2010;7(7):e1000316.

41. Miller M. A psychological autopsy of a geriatric suicide. J Geriatr Psychiatry 1977;10(2):229–42.

42. Turvey CL, Conwell Y, Jones MP, et al. Risk factors for late-life suicide: a prospective, community-based study. Am J Geriatr Psychiatry 2002;10(4):398–406.

43. Van Orden KA, Witte TK, Cukrowicz KC, et al. The interpersonal theory of suicide. Psychol Rev 2010;117(2):575–600.
44. Baumeister RF, Leary MR. The need to belong: desire for interpersonal attachments as a fundamental human motivation. Psychol Bull 1995;117(3):497–529.
45. Dervic K, Oquendo MA, Grunebaum MF, et al. Religious affiliation and suicide attempt. Am J Psychiatry 2004;161(12):2303–8.
46. Goldsmith SK, Pellmar TC, Kleinman AM, Bunney WE. Reducing suicide: a national imperative. Washington, DC: The National Academies Press; 2002.
47. Batchelor IRC, Napier MB. Attempted suicide in old age. BMJ 1953;2:1186–90.
48. Clark DC. Narcissistic crises of aging and suicidal despair. Suicide Life Threat Behav 1993;23(1):21–6.
49. Costa PT, McCrae RR. Revised NEO personality inventory and NEO five factor inventory: professional manual. Odessa (FL): PAR; 1992.
50. Duberstein PR. Openness to experience and completed suicide across the second half of life. Int Psychogeriatr 1995;7(2):183–98.
51. Duberstein PR. Are closed-minded people more open to the idea of killing themselves? Suicide Life Threat Behav 2001;31(1):9–14.
52. Mann JJ, Waternaux C, Haas GL, et al. Toward a clinical model of suicidal behavior in psychiatric patients. Am J Psychiatry 1999;156(2):181–9.
53. Rose G. The strategy of preventive medicine. Oxford (UK): Oxford University Press; 1992.
54. Knox KL, Conwell Y, Caine ED. If suicide is a public health problem, what are we doing to prevent it? Am J Public Health 2004;94(1):37–45.
55. Fremouw WJ, dePerczel M, Ellis TE. Suicide risk: assessment and response guidelines. New York: Pergamon Press; 1990.
56. McIntosh JL, Santos JF, Hubbard RW, et al. Elder suicide: research, theory, and treatment. Washington, DC: American Psychological Association; 1994.
57. Conwell Y, Duberstein PR, Cox C, et al. Age differences in behaviors leading to completed suicide. Am J Geriatr Psychiatry 1998;6(2):122–6.
58. Mrazek PJ, Haggerty RJ. Reducing risks for mental disorders: frontiers for preventive intervention research. Washington, DC: National Academy Press; 1994.
59. Bartels SJ, Coakley EH, Zubritsky C, et al. Improving access to geriatric mental health services: a randomized trial comparing treatment engagement with integrated versus enhanced referral care for depression, anxiety, and at-risk alcohol use. Am J Psychiatry 2004;161(8):1455–62.
60. Stone M, Laughren T, Jones ML, et al. Risk of suicidality in clinical trials of antidepressants in adults: analysis of proprietary data submitted to US Food and Drug Administration. BMJ 2009;339:b2880.
61. Bruce ML, Ten Have T, Reynolds CF III, et al. Reducing suicidal ideation and depressive symptoms in depressed older primary care patients: a randomized controlled trial. JAMA 2004;291(9):1081–91.
62. Unutzer J, Katon W, Callahan CM, et al. Collaborative care management of late-life depression in the primary care setting: a randomized controlled trial. JAMA 2002;288(22):2836–45.
63. Alexopoulos GS, Reynolds CFI, Bruce ML, et al. Reducing suicidal ideation and depression in older primary care patients: 24-month outcomes of the PROSPECT study. Am J Psychiatry 2009;166:882–90.
64. Unutzer J, Tang L, Oishi S, et al. Reducing suicidal ideation in depressed older primary care patients. J Am Geriatr Soc 2006;54(10):1550–6.

65. De Leo D, Dello Buono M, Dwyer J. Suicide among the elderly: the long-term impact of a telephone support and assessment intervention in northern Italy. Br J Psychiatry 2002;181:226–9.

66. Hawton K, Townsend E, Deeks J, et al. Effects of legislation restricting pack sizes of paracetamol and salicylate on self poisoning in the United Kingdom: before and after study. BMJ 2001;322(7296):1203–7.

67. Ludwig J, Cook PJ. Homicide and suicide rates associated with implementation of the Brady Handgun Violence Prevention Act. JAMA 2000;284(5):585–91.

68. Oyama H, Sakashita T, Ono Y, et al. Effect of community-based intervention using depression screening on elderly suicide risk: a meta-analysis of the evidence from Japan. Community Ment Health J 2008;44(5):311–20.

Geriatric Depression in Primary Care

Mijung Park, RN, PhD*, Jürgen Unützer, MD, MPH, MA

KEYWORDS

- Geriatric depression • Primary care • Family caregivers
- Health disparities

Depression is among the leading causes of disability-adjusted life years in the world[1] and a serious public health problem among older adults. General medical settings have been called the de facto mental health care system in the United States,[2] and up to 80% of elderly Americans with depression receive their depression care in primary care.[3] Depression is one of the most common conditions treated in the primary care, and from 1997 to 2002, the proportion of depression visits that took place in the primary care increased from 51% to 64%.[4] Primary care thus presents important opportunities for detecting and treating depressed older adults.

Many older adults prefer to receive their depression treatment in the primary care where providers can address not only mental health problems but also acute and chronic medical conditions that are common in this age group and often comorbid with depression. Primary care providers (PCPs) who provide a continuity of care also have an important opportunity to track depression over time because depression in older adults is often chronic or recurrent. Several research studies over the past 10 years have demonstrated that geriatric depression can be treated effectively when mental health providers effectively partner with their colleagues in the primary care to provide effective consultation and collaborative care.[5] In this article, the authors (1) provide a contextualized overview of, (2) identify trends in, and (3) recommend future directions for the management of geriatric depression in primary care.

EPIDEMIOLOGY OF LATE-LIFE DEPRESSION IN PRIMARY CARE

In community settings, about 5% of adults aged 65 years and more meet research diagnostic criteria for major depression,[6,7] with rates of subsyndromal depression estimated at 8% to 16%.[8] The data from the National Comorbidity Study were used to estimate the projected lifetime risk of major depression to be 23% by age 75 years.[9] Recent epidemiologic data show overall rates of depression to be similar between developed countries (5.5%) and developing countries (5.9%), but rates of depression

Department of Psychiatry and Behavioral Sciences, School of Medicine, University of Washington, 1959 NE Pacific Street, Box 356560, Seattle, WA 98195-6560, USA
* Corresponding author.
E-mail address: parkm5@uw.edu

Psychiatr Clin N Am 34 (2011) 469–487
doi:10.1016/j.psc.2011.02.009
0193-953X/11/$ – see front matter. Published by Elsevier Inc.

psych.theclinics.com

tend to decrease with age in developed countries, whereas rates tend to increase with age in developing countries. Older adults in developed countries were reported to have relatively low average depression rates (2.6%), whereas those in developing countries had an average rate almost 3 times higher (7.5%).[10] The rates of geriatric depression increase to 12% to 30% in institutional settings and up to 50% for residents in long-term care facilities.[11,12] Approximately 5% to 10% of older adults seen in primary care settings have clinically significant depression.[13]

QUALITY OF DEPRESSION TREATMENT IN PRIMARY CARE SETTINGS

Although depression is a common problem in older adults, it is often undetected, undiagnosed, untreated, or undertreated.[14] A recent meta-analysis showed that PCPs detected only 40% to 50% of depression among older adults and that these providers were less successful in detecting depression among older adults than among younger adults.[15] More importantly, only about 1 in 5 older adults with depression receives the effective treatment of depression in primary care.[16] Poor-quality care leads to negative depression outcomes and serious public health problems. In a study of 1198 consecutive suicide attempters in Helsinki, Finland between 1997 and 1998, Suominen and colleagues[17] found that during the 12 months immediately before the attempt, most elderly suicide attempters had a contact with a health care agency. Only 4% of these adults had been diagnosed with a mood disorder before the attempt and only 57% after the attempt. This finding emphasizes the importance of early detection and treatment of late-life depression in primary care.

Barriers to effective late-life depression treatment are at the patient, provider, and system levels.[18,19] Patients may present with somatic rather than emotional complaints, decreasing the likelihood of being diagnosed with depression.[20,21] Patients may also resist a diagnosis of depression and attribute their symptoms to physical causes or to normal aging.[22–24] Patients often have limited knowledge about depression and available treatments. Unique help-seeking patterns among certain population groups, stigma, and poor adherence have been also identified as barriers. Provider barriers include concerns about stigmatizing patients with a psychiatric diagnosis,[25] time pressures,[26,27] inadequate knowledge about diagnostic criteria or treatment options,[28] lack of a psychosocial orientation, and inadequate insight into different cultural presentations of mental disorders.[29] System barriers include productivity pressures; limited mental health coverage; limited availability of mental health specialists, especially for evidence-based psychotherapy[26,30]; lack of systematic approaches for detecting and managing depression[31]; and inadequate continuity of care. Policies that regulate providers' practice contexts and patients' access to evidence-based depression care can also create important barriers to effective treatment.[18]

RISK FACTORS AND PROTECTIVE FACTORS

Risk factors for developing depression after the age 65 years are similar to those in younger individuals and include the female gender, being unmarried, poverty, chronic physical illness, social isolation, and a history or family history of depression.[32] Additional risk factors that are particularly important in older adults include loss and grief, loneliness, and care-taking responsibilities. Other risk factors that increase the likelihood of depression in the medically ill elderly include presence of cognitive impairment, age greater than 75 years, poor social support, active alcohol abuse, and lower educational attainment.[33]

Protective factors include social support and social activities, such as volunteering and physical activity.[34] Religion and spirituality may play an important part in many older adults' lives.[35] These factors may allow older adults to experience life as meaningful despite losses and challenges and, thereby, reduce the risk of depression. It is also possible that the positive effect of religion on mental health is mediated by the social connectedness and the social support derived from taking part in religious and associated social activities.

Loss and Grief

In the United States, 800,000 Americans lose their spouse each year, leaving 11 million widows and 2 million widowers, a total of 7% of the population.[36] The death of a spouse is associated with declining mental and physical health, increased suicide and nonsuicide mortality, and reduced income.[37] A grieving person may also have more somatic symptoms, medical visits, and accidents. Major depression, substance abuse, anxiety disorders, and posttraumatic stress disorder are common within the first year of the spouse's death.[37,38] Specifically, 29% to 58% of widowed person meet criteria for major depression at 1 month, and 25% still meet these criteria at 3 months.[39] Meeting criteria for major depression at 2 months markedly increases the risk of having major depression at 1 year.[40] Although loosing a loved one is an extremely stressful experience for all, evidence suggests that widowhood leads to higher rates of depressive symptoms for men than women.[41,42] With the aging of the population, older adults also experience other important losses, such as losses of children and grand children, which can be even more devastating than the loss of a spouse.

Caregiving Responsibilities

The risk of depression is particularly large for those older adults who are taking care of a significant other with serious medical or cognitive impairments.[43] Studies have shown that the burden from caregiving can compromise immune, cardiovascular, and endocrine functioning and increase the risk for morbidity and mortality.[44,45] A study showed that minor depressive symptoms were common in caregivers of spouses with dementia, but only those who had prior histories of major depression developed major depression.[46]

Medical Illness

Eighty-eight percent of older adults have one or more chronic illnesses, with one-quarter of this group having 4 or more conditions.[47] These chronic conditions significantly impair older adults' health and ability to function.[48] Degenerative arthritis, particularly osteoarthritis, affects 50%, hypertension 40%, hearing loss 30%, urinary incontinence up to 30%, heart disease 30%, diabetes mellitus 15%, and significant impairment of vision up to 15% of population aged 65 years or more.[36] Medical illness is a well-established risk factor for depression. Between 14% and 37% of older medical outpatients suffer from clinically significant depressive syndromes, and as many as 40% of older medical inpatients have been found to have clinically significant depressive symptoms. The associated functional impairment may be a greater risk factor for depression than the physical illness per se.[49,50]

Conversely, comorbid depression has shown a strong association with increased morbidity and mortality, delayed recovery, and negative prognosis among those with medical illness. The rates of comorbid depression are especially high in certain illnesses such as neurologic disorders, endocrine disease (eg, hypothyroidism), myocardial infarction, and cancer. Depression rates of 29% to 36% have been found in stroke,[51] 30% to 50% in Alzheimer disease,[52] and up to 76% in Parkinson disease.[53] A variety of changes on magnetic resonance imaging have been associated with depression,[54] and these findings are consistent with a subtype of late-life and late-onset depression, that is, vascular depression.[55,56]

Several physiologic mechanisms have been proposed to explain the relationship between depression and comorbid physical illness, but this relationship is likely bidirectional and more complex than any single theory can explain. Depression is also associated with poor adherence to treatment, lower physical activity, poor diet, and other health risk behaviors. Such behavioral effects of depression may lead to poor outcomes in chronic medical diseases such as diabetes.[57]

CLINICAL PRESENTATION

With high rates of chronic medical illnesses, biological changes, sociodevelopmental challenges related to aging, and atypical depression symptom presentations, geriatric patients can present substantial diagnostic challenges. The symptoms of late-life depression are often attributed to normal aging, grief, physical illness, or dementia, and providers and patients miss important opportunities to initiate treatment for what is an eminently treatable health problem.[14] In the following section, the authors briefly summarize the clinical presentation of late-life depression in primary care.

Atypical Presentation of Depression

Older adults do not always fit the typical picture of depression, and some may not report feeling sad at all. PCPs should consider such clinical presentations and look for other indicators such as anhedonia, avolition, unexplained physical symptoms, low energy, or fatigue. Depressed patients may attribute symptoms to physical causes or stressful life events or simply reply "I don't know" to questions eliciting their understanding of depressive symptoms. Depressed patients may not participate in physical, speech, or occupational therapy and feel negative or hopeless about the treatments offered. Expressions such as "I just can't do this" or "I can't seem to do anything any more" are common and may be signs of a patient's decreased self-efficacy, motivation, and ability to participate in self-care because of depression. Other common feelings and expressions are "I am not needed," "nobody needs me," or "I feel I am just in everyone's way." Such utterances may indicate a patient's loss of self-worth or sense of loneliness. Among the oldest old, dysphoric mood may be less evident and reliable as an indicator of depression. In this case, the absence of positive effect and anhedonia may be a better indicator.[58,59]

Conversely, life experience and wisdom may protect or buffer older adults from developmental challenges to some degree; this is one potential explanation for lower rates of major depression with increasing age. Depression is less likely if the patient retains a sense of humor, responds warmly to affection from family and caregivers, shows an interest in life and pleasurable activities, looks forward to family visits, readily accepts assistance, actively participates in treatment, and points to reasonable causes for pain.

Overlap Between Chronic Medical Illness and Emotional and Physical Pain

In the medically ill elderly, depressive symptoms may be overlooked because these symptoms are assumed to be caused by concurrent medical illnesses. Many of the symptoms of depression, such as lower energy, fatigue, loss of appetite, and sleep disturbance, are also associated with somatic illnesses. Somatic complaints may suggest presence of depression, especially if they are out of proportion to underlying medical disorders.[22] Only 25% to 30% of primary care patients present with purely affective or cognitive symptoms of depression.[29] Many studies have found an independent and robust relationship between depressive symptoms and chronic physical pain. With older adults, arthritis pain is one the most common correlates of depression.[60–62] The rate of major depression increases in a linear fashion with greater pain severity.[63] Although pain may be an indicator for depression, the authors caution mental health providers that not all pain signifies depression. Older adults often experience pain and suffering from causes such as osteoarthritis along with depression. Although depression treatment may be helpful for such patients,[64] untreated physical pain is a predictor of poor depression treatment response[65] and the most effective treatment includes treatment of depression plus effective pain management.[60]

Minor and Subsyndromal Depression

Most older adults with clinically significant depressive symptoms do not meet standard diagnostic criteria for major depression or dysthymic disorder.[66] Although the prevalence of major depressive illness seems to decrease as one becomes older,[67] the incidence of clinically significant nonmajor forms of depression increases steadily with advancing age and rises steeply among those older than 80 years.[68,69] Patients in this group fall short of meeting diagnostic criteria for major depression because of fewer or limited duration of depression symptoms. Nonetheless, several studies suggest that these patients carry a similar disease burden, including poorer health and social outcomes, functional impairment, and higher health use and treatment costs.[68,70,71] It is important to detect subsyndromal depression because patients with this condition are at a very high risk for subsequent development of major depression, may develop suicidal ideation, and also sustain a fair degree of functional impairment and declined quality of life.[72–74] Unlike major depression, subsyndromal depressive conditions have a relatively small evidence base regarding treatments; existing data suggest that available therapies have modest effects when compared with usual care or placebo.[14,75,76] Targeting interventions for patients with minor and subsyndromal depression may prove useful as both primary and secondary prevention strategies, and clinicians should watch such patients carefully because of the high risk of worsening depression, especially if patients have experienced prior episodes of major depression. Psychosocial treatments may be at least as helpful as medications for older adults with less severe forms of depression,[77] but such treatments are rarely available in busy primary care settings.

TREATMENT MODALITIES FOR MAJOR DEPRESSION AND DYSTHYMIC DISORDER

Although older adults are less likely to access and receive adequate mental health care services than their younger counterparts, late-life depression is treatable with appropriate psychosocial and pharmacologic interventions.[78–80] Evidence shows that depression can be treated in both primary care settings and psychiatric specialty care settings as long as effective treatments are provided. In a recent meta-analysis, Dawson and colleagues[81] found that the remission rate of depression symptoms in interventions in primary care settings range between 50% and 67%, although the studies included did not focus specifically on older adults. Antidepressant medications or psychotherapy are recommended as first-line treatments for depression in older adults,[82] and although millions of prescriptions are written for antidepressant medications in primary care each year, few practices are in a position to offer evidence-based psychotherapies for depression. Physical activity has also been shown to be helpful in late-life depression, and electroconvulsive therapy remains an important and viable treatment option for older adults with psychotic or severe treatment-resistant depression.[83] Several articles by Charles F. Reynolds and Dimitris

N. Kiosses elsewhere in this issue discuss the depression treatment modalities mentioned earlier in detail, and the authors focus on strategies to improve the delivery of efficacious treatments to patients seen in primary care.

DEPRESSION MANAGEMENT STRATEGIES IN PRIMARY CARE
Detection

Geriatric depression in primary care settings is seriously undetected, undiagnosed, and undertreated. Several tools are available to facilitate screening for depression. A single-item screening question is the simplest among all screening tools. A simple question, "Do you often feel sad or depressed?" to which the patient is required to answer either "yes" or "no" was tested in a sample of medically ill patients in the community and had a sensitivity of 69% and a specificity of 90%.[84] The Patient Health Questionnaire (PHQ) 2 asks patient about depressed mood: (1) during the past weeks have you often been bothered by feeling down, depressed, or hopeless? and (2) during the past month have you often been bothered by little interest or pleasure in doing things?[85] This questionnaire is useful in identifying patients at high risk for depression, and it has a sensitivity of 100%, a specificity of 77%, and a positive predictive value of 14% in older adults.[86] Such brief screening tools can be easily administered by office staff or physicians during a primary care visit.

Longer-screening tools are also available: short versions of the Geriatric Depression Scale,[87] the 9-item PHQ (PHQ-9),[88] the 19-item Cornell Scale for Depression in Dementia,[89] the 20-item Center for Epidemiologic Studies Depression Scale,[90] and the Beck Depression Inventory scale.[91] These longer-version tools can also be used to monitor a patient's depression symptoms over the treatment course. Such ongoing symptom tracking is important to evaluate the effectiveness of a treatment. The authors recommend using brief screening tools for the detection and longer-screening tools for the establishment and tracking of treatment progress.

Positive response to these questionnaires should alert the PCP to further evaluate the patient for depression. Not all depressed patients answer positively to these questionnaires, and to address the possibility of false-negatives, clinicians may wish to ask additional questions about depressive symptoms for patients who appear depressed, who have a difficulty engaging in care, or whose functional impairment seems inconsistent with objective medical illness.

Promoting Treatment Engagement and Adherence

Use of health services can be viewed as a complex function of sociodemographic, clinical, and other variables.[92] Variables such as gender, marital status, social class, minority status, education, race and ethnicity play significant roles in rates and patterns of depression care. Other important variables include type of presenting complaints and comorbid medical problems. Prior experiences of patients, family members, and friends with depression treatment in different settings are also important and may be better predictors of treatment engagement and adherence than clinical variables.[92]

Weinberger and colleagues[93] and Sirey and colleagues[94] have studied the challenges with engaging depressed older adults in treatment and have identified several strategies that can be useful in this regard. Once engaged in treatment, it can be challenging for older adults to adhere to an adequate course of pharmacologic or psychosocial treatment of depression. Alexopoulos[95] has proposed several concrete steps to increase treatment adherence among older patients with depression: (1) promote treatment adherence by personalizing depression care, (2) address the constellation of health threats and social constraints that may contribute to poor treatment outcomes, and (3) create comprehensive care algorithms targeting both modifiable predictors and organizational barriers to care.

Family members often play an important role in patients' treatment engagement and adherence. Up to half of depressed older adults fail to take a significant proportion of prescribed antidepressant medication, and recent research indicates that perceived emotional support from family and friends is a critical predictor of adherence.[96] In clinical practice, providers' explicit, expressive, and constant message of commitment to the patients' improvement is an important step to engaging patients and to increasing their adherence to treatment.

Stepped Care

A stepped care approach to treatment first presents patients with relatively simple nonintrusive interventions and proceeds to more intense treatment approaches if patients are not improving as expected. As the first step in a stepped care approach, the patient and supportive family members may be encouraged to try self-directed interventions, such as pleasant events scheduling, physical, or social activities. When these attempts fail to improve depression, more intensive interventions can be offered in the form of guided self-help, which combines a self-help manual with a limited number of brief therapy sessions. More intensive psychosocial or pharmacologic interventions can then be offered at the outpatient level, day treatment, and inpatient level if patients do not improve as expected.

A stepped care model starting with treatments offered in primary care can improve access to care, can alleviate the demand on limited specialty mental health care resources, and may address patients' treatment preferences for less-stigmatized treatments. Bower and Gilbody[97] identified 2 fundamental features for a successful stepped care model: (1) The recommended treatment within a stepped care model should be the least restrictive of those currently available with possible significant health gain. Least restrictive refers to the effect on patients in terms of cost and personal inconvenience. (2) The result of treatment and decision about the treatment provision are monitored systematically, and changes are made if current treatments are not achieving significant health gains. To facilitate such treatment intensification, it is important to use objective measures such as the PHQ-9[88] to monitor depressive symptoms over time.

Collaborative Care

In recent years, collaborative care models have gained significant momentum in the United States, as well as in other countries, such as the United Kingdom, the Netherlands, and Australia. Several interventions have presented a strong evidence for effectiveness with depressed older adults in primary care. Examples include the IMPACT (Improving Mood: Promoting Access to Collaborative Treatment for Late-life Depression)[98] and the PROSPECT (Prevention of Suicide in Primary Care Elderly: Collaborative Trial)[75,99] in the United States and the CADET (Collaborative Depression Trial)[100] in the United Kingdom. Building on a robust evidence base, such collaborative care models are now being widely disseminated in some settings. One such effort is the DIAMOND (Depression Improvement Across Minnesota, Offering a New Direction) program, which uses key components of the IMPACT model and helps practices adapt them to their local context.[101]

The core tenet of collaborative care is that PCPs work closely with their patients and a consulting mental health specialist to treat depression. Patients' clinical outcomes are tracked with structured depression rating scales similar to the way PCPs follow clinical outcomes of other treatments, such as blood pressures in the treatment of hypertension. Treatments are systematically adjusted for patients who do not improve as expected, using evidence-based medication treatments and/or psychotherapies.

A depression care manager (typically a nurse, social worker, or psychologist) working in a primary care practice is responsible for assessing a patient's needs, coordinating an appropriate level of treatment following the stepped care model, supporting a patient's adherence to treatment, and evaluating treatment effectiveness. Such a care management approach ensures close follow-up and contact, supporting streamlined care for the complex multifaceted needs of depressed older adults. This approach also allows providers to incorporate patients' and families' perspectives into depression management (eg, preferences for medication management or evidence-based psychosocial treatments). The care manager works closely with the PCP by educating patients about depression, coaching patients in pleasant events scheduling/behavioral activation, supporting the PCP's antidepressant management, and offering patients a brief course of evidence-based psychotherapy, such as problem-solving treatment in primary care or interpersonal therapy. A consulting psychiatrist consults regularly (usually weekly) on the caseload of patients treated in primary care, focusing on patients who present diagnostic or therapeutic challenges. Such collaborative care programs can double the effectiveness of usual care for depression.[16,18,102]

PRIMARY CARE AS A CONTEXT TO ADDRESS HEALTH DISPARITIES IN GERIATRIC DEPRESSION CARE

Certain population groups are at particularly high risk for poor depression treatment, and the primary care setting is an excellent context to address and reduce such health disparities. These groups include older adults with lower socioeconomic status (SES) or less education, patients from ethnic minority groups, and older men. Older men from ethnic minority groups, for example, are particularly unlikely to receive depression treatment in primary care.[103,104]

There is a strong association between lower SES and less education and higher rates of geriatric depression.[105–109] A growing body of literature also shows that the socioeconomic, physical, and emotional milieus of the area of residence correlates with the rates of geriatric depression. The older adult's level of satisfaction with the neighborhood environment, availability of transportation, and economic character of communities (ie, living in a poor neighborhood) are important determinants of depression among older adults.[110–114] Because of declining health and functioning, older adults may be less adaptable to the environment and more dependent on resources available in their area of residence.[115–117] Older adults with multiple comorbid conditions living in a poor neighborhood may experience difficulties in coordinating clinic visits and actually making it to a clinic because of the lack of transportation. Limited mobility due to declining health, poor public transportation, and a negative neighborhood context (eg, not feeling safe or not feeling connected to neighbors) can increase older adults' feeling of loneliness, further increasing the risk for developing or worsening depression.

Older adults from certain ethnic/racial minority groups have higher rates of depression[118,119] and are less likely to be diagnosed with or treated for depression than their white counterparts.[120,121] These health service disparities in minority populations become increasingly complicated when considering cultural beliefs and practices of health and attitudes to depression care. Culture influences how individuals experience and express depression.[122,123] Minority patients from certain ethnic groups may express their depression more somatically than psychologically.[29,124] Such somatic presentations may reduce the recognition of depression by PCPs or lead to the perception of a patient as difficult.[125] Some minorities may also have less faith in the biological cause of depression, be more skeptical about antidepressant medications, and show stronger preferences for counseling than their white counterparts.[126,127] When pharmaceutical treatment is the only available option, minority patients may be less likely to engage in treatment and more likely to be nonadherent. Our present primary care systems that focus primarily on pharmacologic treatment without considering the unique barriers faced by ethnic and racial minority populations may not be effective in addressing the pattern of disparities observed.[128]

Evidence suggests that collaborative care programs for depression in which care managers support PCPs and offer both pharmacologic and nonpharmacologic treatment options can increase the use of evidence-based depression treatments and improve health outcomes in older minorities and poor older Americans.[129–132] Only minor adaptations were made to meet the cultural needs of the different ethnic groups in published studies of collaborative care, indicating that this approach can address a broad patient population if care managers can adapt the treatment approach to meet the specific needs and preferences of individual patients and families.

Although depression is generally more common in women, such gender differences become less evident in older adults[104] and certain ethnic groups.[133,134] In most settings, depressed men are less likely than their female counterparts to receive recommended care, even though men have the highest risk of committing suicide.[135] The expression of depression symptoms may be particularly challenging for older men who find such help seeking inconsistent with their sense of masculinity, and PCPs may be less likely to ask older men about depression than women.[135] Studies of collaborative care for late-life depression suggest that it may be more challenging to engage men in such programs, but those men who do participate benefit as much from the help offered as do women.[16] The studies also show that widowhood affects men more than women. Thus, close observation is indicated for newly widowed or socially isolated older men who may be at particularly high risk for developing depression.

FAMILY: PARTNERS IN DEPRESSION CARE AND TARGET OF PRIMARY AND SECONDARY PREVENTION

According to a national survey,[44] 44.4 million Americans (21% of people older than 18 years) were providing care to their family members. National data indicate that depressive symptoms in older adults require additional hours of assistance from their family members, with associated costs reaching approximately $9 billion.[136] Family members of depressed older adults experience moderate to high levels of caregiver burden, similar to family caregivers of older adults with Alzheimer disease.[137]

Engaging with and supporting family caregivers of depressed older adults may benefit both patients and family caregivers. Families have a great effect on older adults' health care use, treatment adherence, and depression outcomes, and they can help produce enduring changes in the older person's health behaviors.[138] Among people with depression, social supports are independent predictors of geriatric depression outcomes.[139,140] Older adults with positive family support are less likely to be institutionalized, and the absence of family caregiving is a leading predictor of institutionalization.[44,45] Although positive family support is protective and beneficial to the patient, negative family emotional life, such as hostility and unresolved conflict, are powerful predictors of disease course and mortality in depression.[141–143] Family discord has been identified as a predictor of suicide among older adults.[144]

Caring for an ill family member creates strain and stress to family caregivers and increases morbidity and mortality rates among family caregivers.[145] Caregivers who feel burdened by patients' depressive symptoms may be less able to be supportive regarding the setbacks that patients encounter during treatment, such as treatment side effects and the difficulty of adhering to prescribed treatment.[137,146] By providing support to patients and family members with managing depression and navigating the health care system, it is possible to prevent negative health outcomes in both the patients and their family members. Particularly, family caregivers with a history of major depression along with other risk factors should be considered as targets of secondary prevention. Although the burden of caregiving on the family is apparent across cultures and ethnicities, mental illness may be more burdensome to immigrant and minority families because of social and economic constraints that result from immigration and discrimination[147] and these added stresses may influence and shape their experiences with a mentally ill family member.

Studies have demonstrated the effectiveness of education for older adults and their family members,[148] including a psychoeducational workshop for older adults with recurrent major depression,[149] psychotherapy in primary care,[150] and a behaviorally oriented self-help group led by a nonhealth care professional.[151]

WHERE DO WE GO FROM HERE

Although significant progress in depression treatments has been made in the past decades, much work remains if we want to effectively reach the millions of older adults and their family members who struggle with depression. The authors summarize the opportunities to decrease the public health burden associated with late-life depression in several areas: (1) consumer activation, (2) training of health care providers, and (3) broader system changes.

Consumer Activation

Although much attention has been focused on provider education with the hope of increasing the use of evidence-based treatments, there has been relatively little attention focused on the demand for effective treatments by patients and their family members. Most older adults are not aware of what constitutes evidence-based effective care for depression, and few patients demand such care. Patients who are started on the treatment of depression often receive minimal information about the nature and goals of treatment.[152] In many primary care visits, as little as 1 minute of time is spent in discussing treatment options and plans when patients are started on antidepressant medications.[152] Contrary to the treatments of other health conditions such as hypertension in which a blood pressure measurement is taken at every single contact with the health care system, patients started on depression treatment are rarely systematically followed up and evaluated for treatment response. As a result, partially effective or ineffective treatments are continued for too long or patients drop out of treatment because they give up hope, and millions of Americans remain depressed.

Efforts to improve the management of chronic conditions, such as diabetes, hypertension, or depression, have demonstrated the importance of helping patients become knowledgeable and active collaborators in their own care.[153] Such education efforts are also essential to empower depressed patients and their families to advocate for and participate effectively in treatment. Although direct-to-consumer advertising of antidepressant medication has increased demand for such medications in recent years, careful analysis shows that these advertisements often have limited educational value for increasing effective evidence-based treatments and exclude effective psychosocial treatments.[154] Similar efforts directed at older adults and their family members could include messages that introduce a broader range of effective treatment strategies and empower older adults and their family members to keep asking for changes in treatment until depression is substantially improved, following the stepped care approach outlined earlier.

Training of Health Care Providers

Training in the assessment and management of late-life depression remains an important educational priority for PCPs. Given the strong and consistent support for collaborative care programs in which an interdisciplinary team of primary care and mental health providers effectively collaborate to care for depressed older adults, providers should learn how to practice such effective interdisciplinary team care during their training. The roles of psychiatrists in such teams often vary from traditional outpatient practice or consultation and require training in new skills, such as caseload-focused consultation and support of depression care managers and PCPs in diverse medical settings. Mental health workers trained as psychiatric nurses, social workers, or counselors may need to acquire new skills, such as supporting medication management in primary care, engaging and tracking patients using structured outcome rating scales for depression, and providing evidence-based brief psychosocial treatments such as behavioral activation or problem solving treatment in primary care. Effective collaborative care teams may include members from a broad range of disciplines with varying degrees of training. Provider training in such new skills should be coupled with practice-based support mechanisms, such as electronic health records and patient registries, that can facilitate proactive systematic measurement-based care and effective teamwork.[155]

Broader System Changes

Even with trained providers and active patients and family members, primary care practices often find it challenging to implement evidence-based collaborative care programs that can reach the large numbers of older adults presenting with depression in primary care. Policies that provide financial support for evidence-based collaborative care programs, such as the DIAMOND program in Minnesota,[101] are necessary for medical groups and primary care practices to implement and support such programs. Financial incentives for PCPs to provide evidence-based care management for depression may arise in the context of the movement toward a patient-centered medical home in the United States or through pay-for-performance initiatives, such as a program in the United Kingdom where general practitioners are rewarded financially for performance on the 2 quality indicators for the detection and management of depression.[156]

REFERENCES

1. Murray C, Lopez A. Alternative projections of mortality by cause 1990–2020: Global Burden of Disease Study. Lancet 1997;349:1498–504.
2. Regier DA, Narrow WE, Rae DS, et al. The de facto US mental and addictive disorders service system: epidemiologic catchment area prospective 1-year prevalence rates of disorders and services. Arch Gen Psychiatry 1993;50(2): 85–94.
3. Kessler RC, Birnbaum H, Bromet E, et al. Age differences in major depression: results from the National Comorbidity Survey Replication (NCS-R). Psychol Med 2010;40(2):225–37.

4. Harman JS, Veazie PJ, Lyness JM. Primary care physician office visits for depression by older Americans. J Gen Intern Med 2006;21(9):926–30.

5. Oxman TE, Dietrich AJ, Schulberg HC. Evidence-based models of integrated management of depression in primary care. Psychiatr Clin North Am 2005; 28(4):1061–77.

6. Mojtabai R, Olfson M. Major depression in community-dwelling middle-aged and older adults: prevalence and 2- and 4-year follow-up symptoms. Psychol Med 2004;34(4):623–34.

7. Byers AL, Yaffe K, Covinsky KE, et al. High occurrence of mood and anxiety disorders among older adults: the national comorbidity survey replication. Arch Gen Psychiatry 2010;67(5):489–96.

8. Blazer DG. Depression in late life: review and commentary. Focus 2009;7(1): 118–36.

9. Kessler RC, Berglund P, Demler O, et al. Lifetime prevalence and age-of-onset distributions of DSM-IV disorders in the National Comorbidity Survey Replication. Arch Gen Psychiatry 2005;62(6):593–602.

10. Kessler RC, Birnbaum HG, Shahly V, et al. Age differences in the prevalence and co-morbidity of DSM-IV major depressive episodes: results from the WHO World Mental Health Survey Initiative. Depress Anxiety 2010;27(4):351–64.

11. Teresi J, Abrams R, Holmes D, et al. Prevalence of depression and depression recognition in nursing homes. Soc Psychiatry Psychiatr Epidemiol 2001;36(12): 613–20.

12. Hoover DR, Siegel M, Lucas J, et al. Depression in the first year of stay for elderly long-term nursing home residents in the USA. Int Psychogeriatr 2010; 22:1161–71.

13. Lyness JM, Caine ED, King DA, et al. Psychiatric disorders in older primary care patients. J Gen Intern Med 1999;14(4):249–54.

14. Unutzer J. Diagnosis and treatment of older adults with depression in primary care. Biol Psychiatry 2002;52(3):285–92.

15. Mitchell AJ, Rao S, Vaze A. Do primary care physicians have particular difficulty identifying late-life depression? A meta-analysis stratified by age. Psychother Psychosom 2010;79(5):285–94.

16. Unutzer J, Katon W, Callahan CM, et al. Collaborative care management of late-life depression in the primary care setting: a randomized controlled trial. JAMA 2002;288(22):2836–45.

17. Suominen K, Isometsä E, Lönnqvist J. Elderly suicide attempters with depression are often diagnosed only after the attempt. Int J Geriatr Psychiatry 2004; 19(1):35–40.

18. Unutzer J, Schoenbaum M, Druss BG, et al. Transforming mental health care at the interface with general medicine: report for the presidents commission. Psychiatr Serv 2006;57(1):37–47.

19. Callahan CM. Quality improvement research on late life depression in primary care. Med Care 2001;39(8):772–84.

20. Wittchen H-U, Lieb R, Wunderlich U, et al. Comorbidity in primary care: presentation and consequences. J Clin Psychiatry 1999;60(Suppl 7):29–36.

21. Sheehan B, Banerjee S. Review: somatization in the elderly. Int J Geriatr Psychiatry 1999;14(12):1044–9.

22. Drayer RA, Mulsant BH, Lenze EJ, et al. Somatic symptoms of depression in elderly patients with medical comorbidities. Int J Geriatr Psychiatry 2005; 20(10):973–82.

23. Sarkisian CA, Lee-Henderson MH, Mangione CM. Do depressed older adults who attribute depression to "old age" believe it is important to seek care? J Gen Intern Med 2003;18(12):1001–5.
24. Levkoff SE, Cleary PD, Wetle T, et al. Illness behavior in the aged: implications for clinicians. J Am Geriatr Soc 1988;36(36):622–9.
25. Docherty J. Barriers to the diagnosis of depression in primary care. J Clin Psychiatry 1997;58(Suppl 1):5–10.
26. Hinton L, Franz C, Reddy G, et al. Practice constraints, behavioral problems, and dementia care: primary care physicians' perspectives. J Gen Intern Med 2007;22(11):1487–92.
27. Fiscella K, Epstein RM. So much to do, so little time: care for the socially disadvantaged and the 15-minute visit. Arch Intern Med 2008;168(17):1843–52.
28. Davidson JR, Meltzer-Brody SE. The underrecognition and undertreatment of depression: what is the breadth and depth of the problem? J Clin Psychiatry 1999;60(Suppl 7):4–9.
29. Kirmayer LJ, Young A. Culture and somatization: clinical, epidemiological, and ethnographic perspectives. Psychosom Med 1998;60(4):420–30.
30. Goldman L, Nielsen N, Champion H. Awareness, diagnosis, and treatment of depression. J Gen Intern Med 1999;14(9):569–80.
31. McCall L, Clarke D, Rowle G. A questionnaire to measure general practitioners' attitudes to their role in the management of patients with depression and anxiety. Aust Fam Physician 2002;31:299–303.
32. Vink D, Aartsen MJ, Schoevers RA. Risk factors for anxiety and depression in the elderly: a review. J Affect Disord 2008;106(1–2):29–44.
33. Bruce ML. Psychosocial risk factors for depressive disorders in late life. Biol Psychiatry 2002;52(3):175–84.
34. Hong S-I, Hasche L, Bowland S. Structural relationships between social activities and longitudinal trajectories of depression among older adults. Gerontologist 2009;49(1):1–11.
35. Koenig HG. Religion and depression in older medical inpatients. Am J Geriatr Psychiatry 2007;15(4):282–91.
36. Unutzer J, Katon W, Sullivan M, et al. Treating depressed older adults in primary care: narrowing the gap between efficacy and effectiveness. Milbank Q 1999;77(2):225–56 174.
37. Stroebe M, Schut H, Stroebe W. Health outcomes of bereavement. Lancet 2007;370(9603):1960–73.
38. Zivin K, Christakis NA. The emotional toll of spousal morbidity and mortality. Am J Geriatr Psychiatry 2007;15(9):772–9.
39. Zisook S, Shuchter SR. Depression through the first year after the death of a spouse. Am J Psychiatry 1991;148(10):1346–52.
40. Gilewski MJ, Farberow NL, Gallagher DE, et al. Interaction of depression and bereavement on mental health in the elderly. Psychol Aging 1991;6(1):67–75.
41. Bennett KM, Hughes GM, Smith PT. Psychological response to later life widowhood: coping and the effects of gender. OMEGA 2005;51(1):33–52.
42. van Grootheest DS, Beekman ATF, Broese van Groenou MI, et al. Sex differences in depression after widowhood. Do men suffer more? Soc Psychiatry Psychiatr Epidemiol 1999;34(7):391–8.
43. Vitaliano PP, Young HM, Zhang J. Is caregiving a risk factor for illness? Curr Dir Psychol Sci 2004;13(1):13–6.

44. National Alliance for CAREGIVING/AARP. Caregiving in the US. Washington, DC: National Alliance for CAREGIVING/AARP; 2004.

45. Talley RC, Crews JE. Framing the public health of caregiving. Am J Public Health 2007;97(2):224–8.

46. Russo J, Vitaliano PP, Brewer DD, et al. Psychiatric disorders in spouse caregivers of care recipients with Alzheimer's disease and matched controls: a diathesis-stress model of psychopathology. J Abnorm Psychol 1995; 104(1):197–204.

47. Wolff JL, Starfield B, Anderson G. Prevalence, expenditures, and complications of multiple chronic conditions in the elderly. Arch Intern Med 2002;162(20): 2269–76.

48. Barry LC, Allore HG, Bruce ML, et al. Longitudinal association between depressive symptoms and disability burden among older persons. J Gerontol A Biol Sci Med Sci 2009;64(12):1325–32.

49. Espinoza R, Unutzer J. Diagnosis and management of late-life depression. UpToDate, Waltham, MA, 2005. Available at: http://www.uptodate.com/contents/ diagnosis-and-management-of-late-life-depression?source=search_result& selectedTitle=1%7E8. Accessed July, 2009.

50. Bisschop MI, Kriegsman DMW, Beekman ATF, et al. Chronic diseases and depression: the modifying role of psychosocial resources. Soc Sci Med 2004; 59(4):721–33.

51. Hackett ML, Yapa C, Parag V, et al. Frequency of depression after stroke: a systematic review of observational studies. Stroke 2005;36(6):1330–40.

52. Olin JT, Katz IR, Meyers BS, et al. Provisional diagnostic criteria for depression of Alzheimer disease: rationale and background. Am J Geriatr Psychiatry 2002; 10(2):129–41.

53. Veazey C, Aki SO, Cook KF, et al. Prevalence and treatment of depression in Parkinson's disease. J Neuropsychiatry Clin Neurosci 2005;17(3):310–23.

54. Videbech P, Ravnkilde B. Hippocampal volume and depression: a meta-analysis of MRI studies. Am J Psychiatry 2004;161(11):1957–66.

55. Alexopoulos GS, Meyers BS, Young RC, et al. 'Vascular depression' hypothesis. Arch Gen Psychiatry 1997;54(10):915–22.

56. Baldwin RC. Is vascular depression a distinct sub-type of depressive disorder? A review of causal evidence. Int J Geriatr Psychiatry 2005;20(1):1–11.

57. Lin EH, Katon W, Von Korff M, et al. Relationship of depression and diabetes self-care, medication adherence, and preventive care. Diabetes Care 2004; 27(9):2154–60.

58. Blazer DG. Psychiatry and the oldest old. Am J Psychiatry 2000;157(12): 1915–24.

59. Evans DL, Charney DS, Lewis L, et al. Mood disorders in the medically ill: scientific review and recommendations. Biol Psychiatry 2005;58(3):175–89.

60. Unützer J, Hantke M, Powers D, et al. Care management for depression and osteoarthritis pain in older primary care patients: a pilot study. Int J Geriatr Psychiatry 2008;23(11):1166–71.

61. Bair MJ, Robinson RL, Katon W, et al. Depression and pain comorbidity: a literature review. Arch Intern Med 2003;163(20):2433–45.

62. Turner JA, Ersek M, Kemp C. Self-efficacy for managing pain is associated with disability, depression, and pain coping among retirement community residents with chronic pain. J Pain 2005;6(7):471–9.

63. Carroll LJ, Cassidy JD, Côté P. Depression as a risk factor for onset of an episode of troublesome neck and low back pain. Pain 2004;107(1–2):134–9.

64. Lin EH, Katon W, Von Korff M, et al. Effect of improving depression care on pain and functional outcomes among older adults with arthritis: a randomized controlled trial. JAMA 2003;290(18):2428–9.

65. Thielke SM, Fan MY, Sullivan M, et al. Pain limits the effectiveness of collaborative care for depression. Am J Geriatr Psychiatry 2007;15(8):699–707.

66. Lyness JM, Kim J, Tang W, et al. The clinical significance of subsyndromal depression in older primary care patients. Am J Geriatr Psychiatry 2007;15(3): 214–23. 210.1097/1001.JGP.0000235763.0000250230.0000235783.

67. Mulsant BH, Alexopoulos GS, Reynolds CF III, et al. Pharmacological treatment of depression in older primary care patients: the PROSPECT Algorithm. Focus 2004;2:253–9. Available at: http://focus.psychiatryonline.org/cgi/content/abstract/2/2/253. Accessed April 1, 2004.

68. Lavretsky H, Kumar A. Clinically significant non-major depression: old concepts, new insights. Am J Geriatr Psychiatry 2002;10(3):239–55.

69. Tannock C, Katona C. Minor depression in the aged. Concepts, prevalence and optimal management. Drugs Aging 1995;6(4):278–92.

70. Judd LL, Akiskal HS. The clinical and public health relevance of current research on subthreshold depressive symptoms to elderly patients. Am J Geriatr Psychiatry 2002;10(3):233–8.

71. Lyness J, King D, Cox C, et al. The importance of subsyndromal depression in older primary care patients: prevalence and associated functional disability. J Am Geriatr Soc 1999;47(6):647–52.

72. Remick RA. Diagnosis and management of depression in primary care: a clinical update and review. CMAJ 2002;167(11):1253–60.

73. Lyness JM, Yu Q, Tang W, et al. Risks for depression onset in primary care elderly patients: potential targets for preventive interventions. Am J Psychiatry 2009;166(12):1375–83.

74. Grabovich AB, Lu NP, Tang WP, et al. Outcomes of subsyndromal depression in older primary care patients. Am J Geriatr Psychiatry 2010;18(3):227–35.

75. Bruce ML, Ten Have TR, Reynolds CF III, et al. Reducing suicidal ideation and depressive symptoms in depressed older primary care patients: a randomized controlled trial. JAMA 2004;291(9):1081–91.

76. Oxman TE, Sengupta A. Treatment of minor depression. Am J Geriatr Psychiatry 2002;10(3):256–64.

77. Pinquart M, Duberstein PR, Lyness JM. Treatments for later-life depressive conditions: a meta-analytic comparison of pharmacotherapy and psychotherapy. Am J Psychiatry 2006;163(9):1493–501.

78. Pirraglia PA, Rosen AB, Hermann RC, et al. Cost-utility analysis studies of depression management: a systematic review. Am J Psychiatry 2004;161:2155–62.

79. Mottram PG, Wilson K, Strobl JJ. Antidepressants for depressed elderly. Cochrane Database Syst Rev 2006;1:CD003491.

80. Fournier JC, DeRubeis RJ, Hollon SD, et al. Antidepressant drug effects and depression severity: a patient-level meta-analysis. JAMA 2010;303(1):47–53.

81. Dawson M, Michalak E, Waraich P, et al. Is remission of depressive symptoms in primary care a realistic goal? A meta-analysis. BMC Fam Pract 2004;5:19.

82. Unützer J. Late-life depression. N Engl J Med 2007;357(22):2269–76.

83. Unutzer J. Clinical practice. Late-life depression. N Engl J Med 2007;357(22): 2269–76.

84. Watkins CL, Lightbody CE, Sutton CJ, et al. Evaluation of a single-item screening tool for depression after stroke: a cohort study. Clin Rehabil 2007; 21(9):846–52.

85. Kroenke K, Spitzer RL, Williams JB. The Patient Health Questionnaire-2: validity of a two-item depression screener. Med Care 2003;41(11):1284–92.
86. Li C, Friedman B, Conwell Y, et al. Validity of the Patient Health Questionnaire 2 (PHQ-2) in identifying major depression in older people. J Am Geriatr Soc 2007;55(4):596–602.
87. Yesavage JA, Sheikh JI. Geriatric Depression Scale (GDS)—recent evidence and development of a shorter violence. Clin Gerontol 1986;5(1):165–73.
88. Löwe B, Unützer J, Callahan CM, et al. Monitoring depression treatment outcomes with the patient health questionnaire-9. Med Care 2004;42(12):1194–201.
89. Alexopoulos GS, Abrams RC, Young RC, et al. Cornell scale for depression in dementia. Biol Psychiatry 1988;23(3):271–84.
90. Radloff LS, Teri L. Use of the center for epidemiological studies-depression scale with older adults. Clin Gerontol 1986;5(1):119–36.
91. Beck AT, Steer RA, Carbin MG. Psychometric properties of the Beck Depression Inventory: twenty-five years of evaluation. Clin Psychol Rev 1988;8(1):77–100.
92. de Figueiredo J, Boerstler H, Doros G. Recent treatment history vs clinical characteristics in the prediction of use of outpatient psychiatric services. Soc Psychiatry Psychiatr Epidemiol 2006;41(2):130–9.
93. Weinberger MI, Mateo C, Sirey JA. Perceived barriers to mental health care and goal setting among depressed, community-dwelling older adults. Patient Prefer Adherence 2009;3:145–9.
94. Sirey JA, Bruce ML, Alexopoulos GS. The treatment initiation program: an intervention to improve depression outcomes in older adults. Am J Psychiatry 2005;162(1):184–6.
95. Alexopoulos GS. Personalizing the care of geriatric depression. Am J Psychiatry 2008;165(7):790–2.
96. Voils CI, Steffens DC, Flint EP, et al. Social support and locus of control as predictors of adherence to antidepressant medication in an elderly population. Am J Geriatr Psychiatry 2005;13(2):157–65.
97. Bower P, Gilbody S. Stepped care in psychological therapies: access, effectiveness and efficiency: narrative literature review. Br J Psychiatr 2005;186(1):11–7.
98. Unutzer J, Katon WJ, Fan MY, et al. Long-term cost effects of collaborative care for late-life depression. Am J Manag Care 2008;14(2):95–100.
99. Alexopoulos GS, Reynolds CF III, Bruce ML, et al. Reducing suicidal ideation and depression in older primary care patients: 24-month outcomes of the PROSPECT study. Am J Psychiatry 2009;166(8):882–90.
100. Richards D, Hughes-Morley A, Hayes R, et al. Collaborative Depression Trial (CADET): multi-centre randomised controlled trial of collaborative care for depression—study protocol. BMC Health Serv Res 2009;9(1):188.
101. Korsen N, Pietruszewski P. Translating evidence to practice: two stories from the field. J Clin Psychol Med Settings 2009;16(1):47–57.
102. Gilbody S, Bower P, Fletcher J, et al. Collaborative care for depression: a cumulative meta-analysis and review of longer-term outcomes. Arch Intern Med 2006;166(21):2314–21.
103. Unutzer J, Katon W, Callahan CM, et al. Depression treatment in a sample of 1801 depressed older adults in primary care. J Am Geriatr Soc 2003;51(4):505–14.
104. Klap R, Unroe KT, Unutzer J. Caring for mental illness in the United States: a focus on older adults. Am J Geriatr Psychiatry 2003;11(5):517–24.

105. Breeze E, Fletcher A, Leon D, et al. Do socioeconomic disadvantages persist into old age? Self-reported morbidity in a 29-year follow-up of the Whitehall Study. Am J Public Health 2001;91(2):277–83.

106. Menec VH, Shooshtari S, Nowicki S, et al. Does the relationship between neighborhood socioeconomic status and health outcomes persist into very old age? A population-based study. J Aging Health 2010;22(1):27–47.

107. Rostad B, Deeg D, Schei B. Socioeconomic inequalities in health in older women. Eur J Ageing 2009;6(1):39–47.

108. Miech RA, Shanahan MJ. Socioeconomic status and depression over the life course. J Health Soc Behav 2000;41(2):162–76.

109. Yong-Hong L, Yi-Zhou X, Qing-Xiu L, et al. Education and risk for late life depression: a meta-analysis of published literature. Int J Psychiatr Med 2010;40(1):109–24.

110. Ladin K, Daniels N, Kawachi I. Exploring the relationship between absolute and relative position and late-life depression: evidence from 10 European Countries. Gerontologist 2010;50(1):48–59.

111. Weich S, Twigg L, Lewis G, et al. Geographical variation in rates of common mental disorders in Britain: prospective cohort study. Br J Psychiatr 2005;187(1):29–34.

112. Berke EM, Gottlieb LM, Moudon AV, et al. Protective association between neighborhood walkability and depression in older men. J Am Geriatr Soc 2007;55(4):526–33.

113. La Gory M, Fitpatrick K. The effects of environmental context on elderly depression. J Aging Health 1992;4(4):459–79.

114. Muramatsu N. County-level income inequality and depression among older Americans. Health Serv Res 2003;38(6p2):1863–84.

115. Cagney KA, Browning CR, Wen M. Racial disparities in self-rated health at older ages: what difference does the neighborhood make? J Gerontol B Psychol Sci Soc Sci 2005;60(4):S181–90.

116. Robert SA. Socioeconomic position and health: the independent contribution of community socioeconomic context. Annu Rev Sociol 1999;25(1):489–516.

117. Thompson EE, Krause N. Living alone and neighborhood characteristics as predictors of social support in late life. J Gerontol B Psychol Sci Soc Sci 1998;53B(6):S354–64.

118. Kuo BCH, Chong V, Joseph J. Depression and its psychosocial correlates among older Asian immigrants in North America. J Aging Health 2008;20(6):615–52.

119. Simpson S, Krishnan L, Kunik M, et al. Racial disparities in diagnosis and treatment of depression: a literature review. Psychiatr Q 2007;78(1):3–14.

120. Strothers HS, Rust G, Minor P, et al. Disparities in antidepressant treatment in Medicaid elderly diagnosed with depression. J Am Geriatr Soc 2005;53(3):456–61.

121. Crystal S, Sambamoorthi U, Walkup JT, et al. Diagnosis and treatment of depression in the elderly Medicare population: predictors, disparities, and trends. J Am Geriatr Soc 2003;51(12):1718–28.

122. Kleinman A. Patients and healers in the context of culture: an exploration of the borderland between anthropology, medicine, and psychiatry. Los Angeles (CA). Berkeley (CA): University of California Press; 1981.

123. Kleinman A. Culture and depression. N Engl J Med 2004;351(10):951–3.

124. Pang KY. Symptom expression and somatization among elderly Korean immigrants. Journal of Clinical Geropsychology 2000;6(3):199–212.

125. Jackson JL, Kroenke K. Difficult patient encounters in the ambulatory clinic: clinical predictors and outcomes. Arch Intern Med 1999;159(10):1069–75.

126. Cooper LA, Gonzales JJ, Gallo JJ, et al. The Acceptability of treatment for depression among African-American, Hispanic, and white primary care patients. Med Care 2003;41(4):479–89.

127. Givens JL, Houston TK, Van Voorhees BW, et al. Ethnicity and preferences for depression treatment. Gen Hosp Psychiatr 2007;29(3):182–91.

128. Alegria M, Chatterji P, Wells K, et al. Disparity in depression treatment among racial and ethnic minority populations in the United States. Psychiatr Serv 2008;59(11):1264–72.

129. Ayalon L, Arean PA, Linkins K, et al. Integration of mental health services into primary care overcomes ethnic disparities in access to mental health services between black and white elderly. Am J Geriatr Psychiatry 2007; 15(10):906–12.

130. Arean PA, Ayalon L, Hunkeler E, et al. Improving depression care for older, minority patients in primary care. Med Care 2005;43(4):381–90.

131. Miranda J, Azocar F, Organista KC, et al. Treatment of depression among impoverished primary care patients from ethnic minority groups. Psychiatr Serv 2003;54(2):219–25.

132. Miranda J, Duan N, Sherbourne C, et al. Improving care for minorities: can quality improvement interventions improve care and outcomes for depressed minorities? Results of a randomized, controlled trial. Health Serv Res 2003; 38(2):613–30.

133. Levav I, Kohn R, Golding J, et al. Vulnerability of Jews to affective disorders. Am J Psychiatry 1997;154(7):941–7.

134. Takeuchi DT, Chung RC, Lin KM, et al. Lifetime and twelve-month prevalence rates of major depressive episodes and dysthymia among Chinese Americans in Los Angeles. Am J Psychiatry 1998;155(10):1407–14.

135. Hinton L, Zweifach M, Oishi S, et al. Gender disparities in the treatment of late-life depression: qualitative and quantitative findings from the IMPACT trial. Am J Geriatr Psychiatry 2006;14(10):884–92.

136. Langa KM, Valenstein MA, Fendrick AM, et al. Extent and cost of informal caregiving for older Americans with symptoms of depression. Am J Psychiatry 2004; 161(5):857–63.

137. van Wijngaarden B, Schene AH, Koeter MW. Family caregiving in depression: impact on caregivers' daily life, distress, and help seeking. J Affect Disord 2004;81(3):211–22.

138. Institute of Medicine. Health and behavior: the interplay of biological, behavioral, and social influence. Washington, DC: The national Academied Press; 2001.

139. Martire LM, Schulz R. Involving family in psychosocial interventions for chronic illness. Curr Dir Psychol Sci 2007;16(2):90–4.

140. Lee MS, Crittenden KS, Yu E. Social support and depression among elderly Korean immigrants in the United States. Int J Aging Hum Dev 1996;42(4): 313–27.

141. Hooley JM, Orley J, Teasdale JD. Levels of expressed emotion and relapse in depressed patients. Br J Psychiatry 1986;148:642–7.

142. Koenigsberg HW, Klausner E, Pelino D, et al. Expressed emotion and glucose control in insulin-dependent diabetes mellitus. Am J Psychiatry 1993;150(7): 1114–5.

143. Kim EY, Miklowitz DJ. Expressed emotion as a predictor of outcome among bipolar patients undergoing family therapy. J Affect Disord 2004;82(3):343–52.

144. Rubenowitz E, Waern M, Wilhelmsom K, et al. Life events and psychosocial factors in elderly suicides control study. Psychol Med 2001;31(7):1193–202.

145. Pearlin LI, Aneshensel CS. Caregiving: the unexpected career. Soc Justice Res 2006;7(4):373–90.
146. Perlick DA, Rosenheck RA, Clarkin JF, et al. Impact of family burden and affective response on clinical outcome among patients with bipolar disorder. Psychiatr Serv 2004;55(9):1029–35.
147. Chun KM, Organista B, Martin G, editors. Acculturation: advances in theory, measurement, and applied research. Washington, DC: American Psychological Association; 2003.
148. Schulz R, Martire LM, Klinger JN. Evidence-based caregiver interventions in geriatric psychiatry. Psychiatr Clin North Am 2005;28(4):1007–38.
149. Sherrill J, Frank E, Geary M, et al. Psychoeducational workshops for elderly patients with recurrent major depression and their families. Psychiatr Serv 1997;48(1):76–81.
150. Areán P, Hegel M, Reynolds C. Treating depression in older medical patients with psychotherapy. Journal of Clinical Geropsychology 2001;7(2):93–104.
151. Floyd M, Scogin F, McKendree-Smith NL, et al. Cognitive therapy for depression. Behav Modif 2004;28(2):297–318.
152. Tai-Seale M, McGuire T, Colenda C, et al. Two-minute mental health care for elderly patients: inside primary care visits. J Am Geriatr Soc 2007;55(12): 1903–11.
153. Sorensen S, Pinquart M, Duberstein P. How effective are interventions with caregivers? An updated meta-analysis. Gerontologist 2002;42(3):356–72.
154. Frosch DL, Krueger PM, Hornik RC, et al. Creating demand for prescription drugs: a content analysis of television direct-to-consumer advertising. Ann Fam Med 2007;5(1):6–13.
155. Unutzer J, Choi Y, Cook IA, et al. Clinical computing: a web-based data management system to improve care for depression in a multicenter clinical trial. Psychiatr Serv 2002;53(6):671–8.
156. Lester H, Howe A. Depression in primary care: three key challenges. Postgrad Med J 2008;84:545–8.

Designing Personalized Treatment Engagement Interventions for Depressed Older Adults

Patrick J. Raue, PhD*, Jo Anne Sirey, PhD

KEYWORDS

- Depression • Geriatric • Treatment engagement
- Adherence • Community settings

Major depression affects 0.7% to 1.4% of community-dwelling older adults,[1,2] with higher rates seen in settings in which medical illness, functional disability, and pain are more common. Thus, 6% to 9% of primary care patients,[3,4] 12% of elderly people receiving home-delivered meals,[5] and 14% of elderly home health care patients suffer from major depression.[6]

When treating older depressed adults, clinicians strive to provide appropriate pharmacological and psychotherapeutic interventions to alleviate suffering and promote recovery. In recent years, primary care-based collaborative care interventions have improved depression outcomes as compared with usual care.[7–11] Interventions that are delivered in community and home-based settings have also demonstrated improvement in depressive symptoms.[12–15]

Despite the benefits of such treatment, we are frequently faced with the dual challenges of underutilization of mental health services by older adults and nonadherence to offered interventions. Many conceptual models highlight the importance of an individual's self-identification of distressing symptoms and subsequent decisions on whether and where to seek care (ie, "help-seeking pathways").[16–21] This article focuses on an individual's degree of engagement in depression treatment after a community

This work was supported by Grant Nos. R01 MH084872; R01 MH087562; R01 MH079265; P30 MH085943 from the National Institute of Mental Health.
The authors have nothing to disclose.
Department of Psychiatry, Weill Cornell Medical College, 21 Bloomingdale Road, White Plains, NY 10605, USA
* Corresponding author.
E-mail address: praue@med.cornell.edu

Psychiatr Clin N Am 34 (2011) 489–500
doi:10.1016/j.psc.2011.02.011
0193-953X/11/$ – see front matter © 2011 Elsevier Inc. All rights reserved.

case worker or health care professional has identified depression. The authors define treatment engagement broadly as a process beginning with identification of depression in community settings; moving to a referral for mental health evaluation; making decisions on treatment and acceptance of treatment recommendations; and early adherence and participation in care. The authors focus in particular on older adults encountered in community settings, which include any non–mental health specialty setting such as aging services, primary care, and home health care. These settings are those in which older adults are commonly served, and where untapped opportunities exist for identifying and treating depression.

Barriers and facilitators of engaging in mental health services exist on multiple levels (eg, societal, agency, provider, individual). This article focuses on individual-level factors. In particular, psychosocial factors such as negative attitudes and beliefs about mental illness, and interactional factors such as lack of involvement in medical decision making can undermine older adults' acceptance of mental health interventions. These factors may also play a role in adherence to interventions, and ultimately in depression outcomes. Thus, in light of the evidence base for the care of depressed older adults, the authors describe the need for, and benefits of engaging older adults in treatment using interventions that: (1) target psychological barriers such as stigma and other negative beliefs about depression and its treatment; and (2) increase individuals' involvement in the treatment decision-making process. Personalized treatment engagement interventions designed by the authors' group for a variety of community settings are then presented, including: (1) the Open Door intervention, which targets identification and referral of depressed community-dwelling older adults to mental health service providers; (2) a Shared Decision-Making approach for primary care patients, which targets treatment selection[22]; and (3) the Treatment Initiation Program (TIP), which targets patient adherence to pharmacological depression treatment recommendations by primary care physicians.[23]

PERSONALIZED RESEARCH: A FOCUS ON THE INDIVIDUAL

As outlined in *The Road Ahead: Research Partnership to Transform Services*[24] equitable access is fundamental to fair mental health care service delivery. Elders are less likely than younger adults to use mental health services,[25] and African American adults and elderly have the lowest rates of mental health service use, even when education and income level are accounted for.[26] In addition, when elders do engage in care they are less likely to use specialty mental health facilities,[26,27] thus reducing the number of venues where care may be obtained. There are many barriers to engaging older adults in mental health care. Barriers can emerge from individual (eg, attitudes, mobility), interactional (eg, involvement with health care professionals), systemic (eg, availability of mental health care, lack of parity), and societal factors (eg, ageism, stigma). By targeting the individual and his or her interaction with community workers and health care professionals, as done in this article, clinicians are in a position to implement interventions targeting specific person-by-person factors that affect engagement in care.

In an overview of National Institute of Mental Health (NIMH) priorities, there is a renewed interest in the individual perspective and the impact of psychosocial factors. The clinical vision offered by NIMH[28] outlines the 4 "Ps" of medical research: prediction, preemption, personalization, and participation. To personalize research is to highlight "individual biologic, environment, and social factors" and develop interventions that are targeted to the needs of the individual. This new emphasis may pave the way for greater attention to personal and psychological perspectives on mental illness. When we consider older persons' use of mental health services and treatments, we can view their personal choices as driven in part by social-psychological factors that either hinder or facilitate quality care.

MODELS RELEVANT TO MENTAL HEALTH TREATMENT ENGAGEMENT AND CARE

Several conceptual models identify factors relevant to help-seeking in general, and to treatment engagement in particular. As already mentioned, the focus is on treatment engagement after a community case worker or health care professional has identified depression. The authors define treatment engagement broadly from initial identification of need and referral for mental health evaluation through early adherence and participation in care. The Anderson Behavioral Model of Health Service Use proposes that need, enabling factors, and predisposing factors affect use of services.[29,30] In short, need reflects both perceived and evaluated symptoms. In community settings, a community worker or health care professional may identify the need and refer older adults for further evaluation or treatment, which may take place in either health or mental health settings. Enabling factors include family and community resources. Predisposing factors are demographic characteristics and health beliefs such as attitudes toward health services. Later updates to the Andersen model include provider and organizational-level factors[31] and illustrate multidimensional domains that influence use of services.

Seeking or accepting a recommendation for care is a health behavior that emerges out of an often "non-conscious cost benefit analysis."[32] It is only when older adults are asked about the reasons for their choices and about their personal experiences that their attitudes and beliefs become clear. To accept a recommendation or referral and participate in mental health treatment reflects a balance of predisposing factors, enabling factors, and perceived need for care. Clinicians are generally aware of tangible barriers older adults face due to transportation, lack of mental health parity in insurance costs, and the impact of medical illnesses. But often these factors obscure attitudes toward depression and concerns about treatment that may be equal determinants. Attitudes and beliefs may exacerbate tangible barriers (eg, transportation, cost), making treatment inaccessible. In addition, for older adults with depression, low energy and resignation resulting from depressive symptoms, cognitive deficits, and associated disabilities all compound psychosocial barriers to treatment engagement.[33]

There are several alternative models to the Andersen model that explain individual-level health behavior change, each relevant to different aspects of the treatment engagement process. The Health Belief model[34,35] emphasizes individual perceptions including benefits and barriers. Social Learning Theory[36] emphasizes the importance of self-efficacy. Beliefs are primary according to the Theory of Reasoned Action,[37] including normative beliefs such as social stigma. Other conceptual models take into account interpersonal interactions between individuals and health care providers. For example, Interdependence Theory posits that health behavior change most effectively takes place in the context of relationships characterized by trust, respect, and shared power and decision making.[38–40] The Network Episode model frames care-seeking as a dynamic process where contacts with mental health and lay providers affect an individual's engagement in care over time.[41]

EMPIRICAL FINDINGS RELATED TO TREATMENT ENGAGEMENT
Perceived Illness Severity, Stigma, and Treatment Preferences

The authors' work with community-dwelling older adults from a variety of settings has documented several barriers and facilitators of care, including perceived depression severity, stigma, and preferences for specific types of treatment. Among clients of senior services, the authors found that half of elders diagnosed with depression do not perceive themselves as suffering from an emotional illness.[5] Moreover, research from other groups has documented an association between perceived illness severity and treatment adherence.[42,43] The authors have also documented a high degree of concern by aging service clients about the social costs of being stigmatized for seeking depression treatment. Even for those elders who do initiate care, perceived stigma is a barrier to both participation in treatment and antidepressant medication adherence.[44] Among adult and elderly primary care patients, the authors have found strength of treatment preferences for antidepressant medication or psychotherapy to be associated with treatment initiation and ongoing adherence.[45] A wide array of depression treatment preferences among elderly home health care patients has been documented, with roughly half preferring active treatments as their first choice (eg, antidepressant medication or psychotherapy) and half preferring inactive or complementary approaches (eg, religious activities, do nothing).[46] Patients with current or prior mental health treatment, white or Hispanic patients, those with greater functional impairment, and those with less personal stigma were more likely to prefer an active treatment approach.

Influence of Sociocultural Factors on Treatment Engagement

Race, ethnicity, and cultural factors may play a significant role in the treatment engagement process. For example, barriers to using mental health care may reflect cultural assumptions about need and mental health care.[47] Attributions of depression to difficult life circumstances versus medical causes influence help-seeking and reactions to treatment recommendations.[48–51] Concerns about stigma, fear of involuntary hospitalization, and reluctance to divulge personal information are common among minority elders.[52,53] Religious and spiritual beliefs may contribute to this reluctance and to delays in help-seeking.[54]

Based on resilience theory, resistance to seeking care among minority seniors may reflect effective coping mechanisms and adaptations to surviving poverty, racism, and discrimination into later years that now have become obstacles to health care.[55,56] Preferences for self-reliance, use of home remedies, and care avoidance due to mistrust of health care professionals may be powerful remnants from earlier health care abuses.[55–57] In these cases, the predisposing factors that once served to protect the individual have now become barriers to care.

INTEGRATED MODEL OF THE TREATMENT ENGAGEMENT PROCESS

In conceptualizing the impact of both psychosocial and interactional factors on the treatment engagement process, the authors have integrated aspects of the Andersen, Health Belief, and Interdependence Models (**Fig. 1**). Their model begins at the point where depression is identified. In some cases, older adults recognize the need for treatment and self-refer to health or mental health services. In other instances, a community worker or health care professional identifies depression and introduces the need for further evaluation or treatment. Referral for further evaluation to determine treatment need represents one opportunity for behavioral intervention, given low rates of follow-through by older adults on such referrals (see section on Open Door intervention). Interventions targeting the referral process are appropriate for settings in which mental health care is not available on site but must be pursued elsewhere.

Another opportunity for intervention is the treatment decision-making process between an individual and a health care professional (see section on shared decision making). This process involves some sort of interaction that can range from a simple

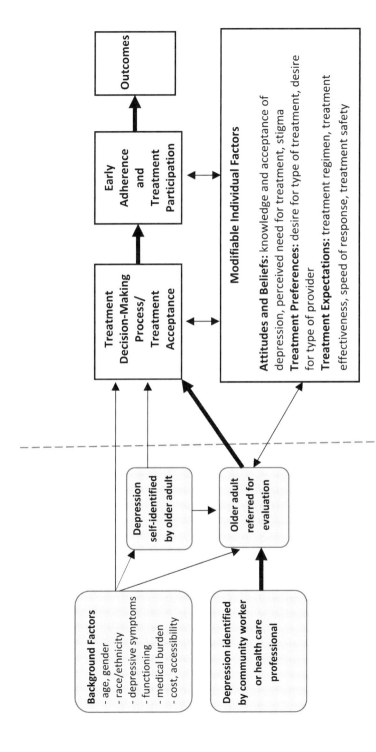

Fig. 1. Treatment engagement process.

treatment recommendation at the most basic end, to education about the effectiveness, side effects, and cost of a treatment approach (or approaches), to a truly mutual collaboration that results in a treatment decision that is tailored to the unique needs and background of the older adult. Interventions targeting treatment decision making are appropriate for settings in which mental health care may or may not be available on site.

Yet another avenue for intervention in the treatment engagement process may focus on early adherence and participation in treatment. These types of interventions address an individual's attitudes and beliefs about depression treatment after treatment recommendations have been given or treatment decisions have been made (see section on Treatment Initiation Program).

Numerous a priori individual and environmental background factors (eg, demographics, clinical status, medical and functional status, personality, cost, accessibility), health care professional factors, and modifiable individual factors affect how older adults respond to a referral for evaluation and how they participate in the treatment decision-making process and ongoing treatment. Interventions that address these areas may help older adults generate more positive and realistic attitudes, beliefs, and expectations about depression treatment, develop more informed treatment preferences, and participate more actively in their care.

TREATMENT ENGAGEMENT INTERVENTIONS

Many collaborative care interventions for depressed individuals attempt to encourage patient involvement in treatment decisions and subsequent treatment adherence. Very few targeted interventions, however, have been developed and tested regarding the treatment engagement process. The PRISM-E study,[58] while not specifically focused on individual attitudes or beliefs, examined organizational changes to primary care in comparison to enhancing the referral process. Colocation of mental health specialists in primary care resulted in improved access to care for older adults, in comparison with "enhanced referral" to specialty services that addressed tangible barriers such as transportation and payment. In another study, a single session of psychoeducation to address stigma in Black adults referred for mental health treatment was found to reduce stigma among those with higher perceived treatment need or greater uncertainty about treatment.[59] Other studies have found shared decision-making interventions for depressed adults to increase their involvement and satisfaction with the treatment decision-making process.[60–64]

The following sections describe 3 personalized treatment engagement interventions designed specifically by the authors for depressed community-dwelling older adults. Each intervention targets potential barriers at different junctures in the treatment engagement process, with the goal of improving treatment adherence and depression outcomes.

The Open Door Intervention

The Open Door study is an NIMH-funded randomized controlled trial of a brief psychosocial intervention focused on the early part of the engagement model: the point at which depression is identified by a community worker who provides aging services. The intervention involves identification of both psychological and tangible barriers to care by a study clinician, who then collaboratively addresses these barriers with the depressed older adult. Its format is two 30-minute face-to-face sessions with one telephone follow-up. Using psychoeducation and problem-solving techniques combined with the inquiry style of motivational interviewing, the goal is to help the depressed older adult engage in a decision analysis about seeking care and to support use of mental health services.

Common barriers that need to be addressed with older depressed adults who receive aging services include a perception that depression is a natural part of aging, or that it is symptomatic of comorbid medical conditions. Older adults often do not readily identify these "symptoms" as abnormal. Instead, many depressed older persons struggle to get moving, take care of themselves and their families, and manage their day-to-day affairs. These persons do not perceive themselves as suffering from a mental illness. From their perspectives the difficulties they encounter are part of life, and therefore cannot be ameliorated by engaging in mental health care.

In a pilot study, the Open Door intervention was offered to all older adults who scored 10 or higher on the PHQ-9 and participated in a home-delivered meal program in Westchester County, New York. Of 32 eligible participants over a 7-month period, the authors found that 3 older adults were already receiving treatment. The study clinician coached these individuals to discuss their continued distress with their existing clinician. Of the remaining 29, 20 (62%) accepted a mental health referral and scheduled a first appointment to be seen by a clinician in the community. Nine (38%) refused a referral. This successful referral rate was notably higher than a historical control rate of 22% (n = 18/171 over a 7-month period). The current NIMH-funded study will allow a fully powered randomized trial to be conducted on the impact of this intervention, in comparison with a control condition where mental health referrals are offered through case management services, on attendance at mental health treatment centers and decrease in depressive symptoms.

Shared Decision Making for Elderly Depressed Primary Care Patients

The authors are currently evaluating a shared decision-making intervention in an NIMH-funded study among older depressed, low-income patients in an inner-city New York hospital.[22] This brief intervention is also focused on an early stage of their engagement model: the point at which a primary care physician has identified depression and introduced the need for some kind of treatment. Developed from the patient-centered view of health care delivery[65] and in reaction to the traditional paternalistic approach in medicine,[66] shared decision making emphasizes a collaborative process, and involves an exchange of information on the pros and cons of different treatment options; exploration of patient expectations and preferences; and formulation of a mutually agreed-upon treatment decision.[66] Decision aid materials are commonly used as part of this process, and aim to clarify personal values and lead to more informed treatment preferences. These interventions attempt to counteract typical symptoms of helplessness, hopelessness, and lack of motivation by increasing patient involvement in their care. This challenge can be compounded in older adults who experience greater medical burden and cognitive impairment, and who have unique sets of psychological and tangible barriers to care.

The shared decision-making intervention is delivered by a nurse within the primary care setting. The intervention consists of one 30- to 40-minute face-to-face meeting between the nurse and older depressed primary care patient, followed by two weekly 10- to 15-minute telephone follow-ups. The intervention is targeted to English-speaking and also to Spanish-speaking patients, in whom barriers to treatment engagement may be even more pronounced. The nurse elicits the patient's treatment experiences, values, preferences, and concerns regarding a variety of treatment approaches including antidepressant medication and psychotherapy. The nurse then uses decision aid materials to educate the patient about each treatment's effectiveness, speed of onset, side effects, and costs, and to clarify the patient's values.

A one-page form presents treatment information in easily understood language, with treatment options presented in column format so patients can compare their relevant characteristics. Education handouts regarding late-life depression for patients and family members are provided for review at home. Telephone follow-ups allow the nurse and patient to review treatment decisions and the patient's ability to implement and adhere to them. The current study will evaluate the impact of this intervention, in comparison with usual care, on patient adherence to antidepressant medication or psychotherapy and on reduction in depressive symptoms.

Treatment Initiation Program in Primary Care

The Treatment Initiation Program in Primary Care (TIP-PC) is a brief intervention focused on a later stage in the authors' engagement model: early adherence among older adults prescribed antidepressant medication by their primary care physicians. TIP-PC targets several psychological barriers that can interfere with antidepressant adherence, including stigma, self-efficacy, resignation about antidepressant limitations, fears about antidepressants, and attribution of depressive symptoms to other causes that would make treatment unnecessary. An understanding is incorporated that while older adults may face many tangible barriers (eg, transportation, medication copayments, and mobility), it is often their attitudes and beliefs that contribute to these barriers seeming insurmountable.

The TIP-PC intervention format is 3 30-minute individual meetings with the patient during the first 6 weeks of pharmacotherapy, followed by 2 follow-up telephone calls at 8 and 10 weeks. The intervention involves: (1) reviewing symptoms and assessing barriers to antidepressant recommendations; (2) assistance in defining personal goals regarding adherence; (3) providing psychoeducation; (4) collaborating to address barriers to adherence; (5) creating an adherence strategy; and (6) facilitating and empowering older adults to speak directly with their physician about treatment concerns.

The authors have conducted a randomized controlled pilot study of TIP-PC among 70 elderly primary care patients in New York City.[23] Subjects were assigned to receive either the TIP-PC intervention or usual care. Analyses indicated that TIP-PC participants had higher rates of antidepressant adherence than usual care participants at 6-, 12-, and 24-week follow-up points. At 12 weeks the majority (82%) of TIP-PC participants were adherent to prescribed antidepressant medication at the 80% level or above, when compared with only 43% of usual care participants. Neither age, gender, nor baseline depression severity modified the impact of TIP-PC. TIP-PC participants also showed a greater decrease in depressive symptoms than usual care participants over the 24-week follow-up period. In collaboration with the University of Michigan (Principal Investigator: Kales), the authors are currently conducting a larger-scale collaborative NIMH-funded study using a similar design.

SUMMARY AND FUTURE DIRECTIONS

Three personalized interventions aimed at identifying and addressing barriers to the treatment engagement of depressed older adults in community settings are described herein. The authors' conceptual model highlights the different junctures at which such interventions may be implemented, ranging from the point at which a referral is provided for further evaluation, to the treatment decision-making process, to early treatment adherence following a specific treatment recommendation. Addressing barriers early in the process can maximize treatment engagement, while ongoing attention to new challenges and barriers can reinforce earlier intervention efforts. If these interventions are found to be useful, the next step will be to disseminate them more widely to other community settings.

Beyond the specific interventions described, there are several promising research agendas regarding treatment engagement. While much of the authors' research is conducted among diverse low-income older adults, there is a need to address the needs of a variety of older adult populations in which barriers to treatment engagement may be unique. For example, sociodemographic and cultural factors may affect the extent to which patients respond to and benefit from interventions. In addition, the authors have investigated discrete interventions focused on very specific junctures of the engagement process. In certain service settings, combined aspects of these interventions may also prove fruitful. For example, addressing treatment barriers and engaging in shared decision making are certainly compatible processes. These interventions may also be blended into other psychotherapeutic, pharmacological, and collaborative care interventions to facilitate engagement. Key issues to investigate when combining such interventions are: the feasibility of their implementation depending on service setting; their effectiveness relative to a single discrete intervention; and their cost. Lastly, as the evidence base builds for the effectiveness of these types of person-centered interventions in improving treatment engagement and clinical outcomes, efforts should turn to designing multifaceted interventions that incorporate organizational issues. For example, adaptations of interventions to specific community agencies are necessary when attempting to maximize their uptake and sustainability.[67] Future research is needed to document factors that facilitate successful adoption and integration of such engagement interventions in community settings that serve older persons.

REFERENCES

1. Henderson AS, Jorm AF, MacKinnon A, et al. The prevalence of depressive disorders and the distribution of depressive symptoms in later life: a survey using Draft ICD-10 and DSM-III-R. Psychol Med 1993;23:719–29.
2. Regier DA, Farmer ME, Rae DS, et al. One-month prevalence of mental disorders in the United States and sociodemographic characteristics: the Epidemiologic Catchment Area study. Acta Psychiatr Scand 1993;88:35–47.
3. Lyness JM, Caine ED, King DA, et al. Psychiatric disorders in older primary care patients. J Gen Intern Med 1999;14:249–54.
4. Schulberg HC, Mulsant B, Schulz R, et al. Characteristics and course of major depression in older primary care patients. Int J Psychiatry Med 1998;28:421–36.
5. Sirey JA, Bruce ML, Carpenter M, et al. Depressive symptoms and suicidal ideation among older adults receiving home delivered meals. Int J Geriatr Psychiatry 2008;23:1306–11.
6. Bruce ML, McAvay GJ, Raue PJ, et al. Major depression in elderly home health care patients. Am J Psychiatry 2002;159:1367–74.
7. Bruce ML, Ten Have TR, Reynolds CF 3rd, et al. Reducing suicidal ideation and depressive symptoms in depressed older primary care patients: a randomized controlled trial. JAMA 2004;291:1081–91.
8. Dietrich AJ, Oxman TE, Williams JW Jr, et al. Re-engineering systems for the treatment of depression in primary care: cluster randomised controlled trial. BMJ 2004;329:602.
9. Gilbody S, Bower P, Fletcher J, et al. Collaborative care for depression: a cumulative meta-analysis and review of longer-term outcomes. Arch Intern Med 2006; 166:2314–21.

10. Hunkeler EM, Katon W, Tang L, et al. Long term outcomes from the IMPACT randomised trial for depressed elderly patients in primary care. BMJ 2006;332: 259–63.

11. Unutzer J, Katon W, Callahan CM, et al. Collaborative care management of late-life depression in the primary care setting: a randomized controlled trial. JAMA 2002;288:2836–45.

12. Banerjee S, Shamash K, Macdonald AJ, et al. Randomised controlled trial of effect of intervention by psychogeriatric team on depression in frail elderly people at home. BMJ 1996;313:1058–61.

13. Ciechanowski P, Wagner E, Schmaling K, et al. Community-integrated home-based depression treatment in older adults: a randomized controlled trial. JAMA 2004;291:1569–77.

14. Gellis ZD, McGinty J, Horowitz A, et al. Problem-solving therapy for late-life depression in home care: a randomized field trial. Am J Geriatr Psychiatry 2007;15:968–78.

15. Rabins PV, Black BS, Roca R, et al. Effectiveness of a nurse-based outreach program for identifying and treating psychiatric illness in the elderly. JAMA 2000;283:2802–9.

16. Rogler LH, Cortes DE. Help-seeking pathways: a unifying concept in mental health care. Am J Psychiatry 1993;150:554–61.

17. Mechanic D. Sociocultural and social-psychological factors affecting personal responses to psychological disorder. J Health Soc Behav 1975;16:393–404.

18. Mechanic D. Removing barriers to care among persons with psychiatric symptoms. Health Aff (Millwood) 2002;21:137–47.

19. Briones DF, Heller PL, Chalfant HP, et al. Socioeconomic status, ethnicity, psychological distress, and readiness to utilize a mental health facility. Am J Psychiatry 1990;147:1333–40.

20. Goldberg D, Huxley P. Mental illness in the community. The pathway to psychiatric care. New York: Tavistock; 1980.

21. Greenley JR, Mechanic D, Cleary PD. Seeking help for psychologic problems. A replication and extension. Med Care 1987;25:1113–28.

22. Raue PJ, Schulberg HC, Lewis-Fernandez R, et al. Shared decision-making in the primary care treatment of late-life major depression: a needed new intervention? Int J Geriatr Psychiatry 2010;25:1101–11.

23. Sirey JA, Bruce ML, Kales HC. Improving antidepressant adherence and depression outcomes in primary care: the treatment initiation and participation (TIP) program. Am J Geriatr Psychiatry 2010;18:554–62.

24. National Advisory Mental Health Council, 2006. Available at: http://www.nimh.nih.gov/about/advisoryboards-and-groups/namhc/reports/road-ahead.pdf. Accessed March 14, 2011.

25. Bartels SJ, Drake RE. Evidence-based geriatric psychiatry: an overview. Psychiatr Clin North Am 2005;28:763–84.

26. Swartz MS, Wagner HR, Swanson JW, et al. Administrative update: utilization of services. I. Comparing use of public and private mental health services: the enduring barriers of race and age. Community Ment Health J 1998;34:133–44.

27. Sirey JA, Meyers BS, Bruce ML, et al. Predictors of antidepressant prescription and early use among depressed outpatients. Am J Psychiatry 1999;156:690–6.

28. National Institute of Mental Health. The National Institute of Mental Health Strategic Plan. (NIH Publication 08-6368). Bethesda (MD): National Institute of Mental Health; 2008. Available at: http://www.nimh.nih.gov/about/strategic-planning-reports/index.shtml. Accessed March 14, 2011.

29. Andersen R. Behavioral model of families' use of health services. Research Series No. 25. Chicago: Center for Health Administration Studies, University of Chicago; 1968.

30. Andersen RM. Revisiting the behavioral model and access to medical care: does it matter? J Health Soc Behav 1995;36:1–10.

31. Andersen RM. National health surveys and the behavioral model of health services use. Med Care 2008;46:647–53.

32. Glanz K, Rimer B, Lewis F, editors. Health behavior and health education: theory, research and practice. 3rd edition. San Francisco (CA): Jossey-Bass; 2002. p. 45–66.

33. Kiosses DN, Alexopoulos GS. IADL functions, cognitive deficits, and severity of depression: a preliminary study. Am J Geriatr Psychiatry 2005;13:244–9.

34. Becker M. The health belief model and personal health behavior. Health Education Monographs 1974;2:326–473.

35. Janz NK, Becker MH. The health belief model: a decade later. Health Educ Q 1984;11:1–47.

36. Bandura A. Social foundations of thought and action: a social cognitive theory. Englewood Cliffs (NJ): Prentice Hall; 1986.

37. Ajzen I, Fisbein M. Understanding attitudes and social behavior. Englewood Cliffs (NJ): Prentice Hall; 1980.

38. Kelley H, Thibaut J. Interpersonal relation: a theory of interdependence. New York: Wiley; 1978.

39. Lewis M, DeVeliis B, Sleath B. Social influence and interpersonal communication in health behavior. In: Glanz K, Rimer B, Lewis F, editors. Health behavior and health education. San Francisco (CA): Jossey-Bass; 2002. p. 240–64.

40. Rusbult C, Van Lange P. Interdependence processes. In: Higgins E, Kruglanski A, editors. Social psychology: handbook of basic principles. New York: Guilford Press; 1996. p. 564–695.

41. Pescosolido BA, Boyer CA, Lubell KM. The social dynamics of responding to mental health problems. In: Aneshensel CS, Phelan JC, editors. Handbook of the sociology of mental health. New York: Kluwer Academic/Plenum Publishers; 1998. p. 441–60.

42. Aikens JE, Nease DE Jr, Nau DP, et al. Adherence to maintenance-phase antidepressant medication as a function of patient beliefs about medication. Ann Fam Med 2005;3:23–30.

43. DiMatteo MR, Haskard KB, Williams SL. Health beliefs, disease severity, and patient adherence: a meta-analysis. Med Care 2007;45:521–8.

44. Sirey JA, Bruce ML, Alexopoulos GS, et al. Stigma as a barrier to recovery: perceived stigma and patient-rated severity of illness as predictors of antidepressant drug adherence. Psychiatr Serv 2001;52:1615–20.

45. Raue PJ, Schulberg HC, Heo M, et al. Patients' depression treatment preferences and initiation, adherence, and outcome: a randomized primary care study. Psychiatr Serv 2009;60:337–43.

46. Raue PJ, Weinberger MI, Sirey JA, et al. Depression treatment preferences in home healthcare. Psychiatr Serv, in press.

47. Alegria M, Canino G, Rios R, et al. Mental health care for Latinos: inequalities in use of specialty mental health services among Latinos, African Americans, and non-Latino Whites. Psychiatr Serv 2002;53:1547–55.

48. Alverson HS, Drake RE, Carpenter-Song EA, et al. Ethnocultural variations in mental illness discourse: some implications for building therapeutic alliances. Psychiatr Serv 2007;58:1541–6.

49. Cabassa LJ, Hansen MC, Palinkas LA, et al. Azucar y nervios: explanatory models and treatment experiences of Hispanics with diabetes and depression. Soc Sci Med 2008;66:2413–24.

50. Guarnaccia PJ, Lewis-Fernandez R, Marano MR. Toward a Puerto Rican popular nosology: nervios and ataque de nervios. Cult Med Psychiatry 2003;27:339–66.

51. Lewis-Fernandez R, Das AK, Alfonso C, et al. Depression in US Hispanics: diagnostic and management considerations in family practice. J Am Board Fam Pract 2005;18:282–96.

52. Alvidrez J, Arean PA, Stewart AL. Psychoeducation to increase psychotherapy entry for older African Americans. Am J Geriatr Psychiatry 2005;13:554–61.

53. Cooper-Patrick L, Gallo JJ, Gonzales JJ, et al. Race, gender, and partnership in the patient-physician relationship. JAMA 1999;282:583–9.

54. Conrad MM, Pacquiao DF. Manifestation, attribution, and coping with depression among Asian Indians from the perspectives of health care practitioners. J Transcult Nurs 2005;16:32–40.

55. Franklin A, Oscar S, Guishard M, et al. Factors contributing to colon cancer beliefs and screening practices for African Americans. Paper presented at the American Psychological Association Annual Meeting. Washington, DC, August 18, 2005.

56. Franklin A, Oscar S, Guishard M, et al. Resilience theory in studying African Americans beliefs and practices toward colon cancer screening. Paper presented at the American Psychological Association Annual Meeting. Washington, DC, August 18, 2005.

57. Figaro MK, Russo PW, Allegrante JP. Preferences for arthritis care among urban African Americans: "I don't want to be cut". Health Psychol 2004;23:324–9.

58. Bartels SJ, Coakley EH, Zubritsky C, et al. Improving access to geriatric mental health services: a randomized trial comparing treatment engagement with integrated versus enhanced referral care for depression, anxiety, and at-risk alcohol use. Am J Psychiatry 2004;161:1455–62.

59. Alvidrez J, Snowden LR, Rao SM, et al. Psychoeducation to address stigma in black adults referred for mental health treatment: a randomized pilot study. Community Ment Health J 2009;45:127–36.

60. Adams JR, Drake RE. Shared decision-making and evidence-based practice. Community Ment Health J 2006;42:87–105.

61. Loh A, Simon D, Wills CE, et al. The effects of a shared decision-making intervention in primary care of depression: a cluster-randomized controlled trial. Patient Educ Couns 2007;67:324–32.

62. Schauer C, Everett A, del Vecchio P, et al. Promoting the value and practice of shared decision-making in mental health care. Psychiatr Rehabil J 2007;31:54–61.

63. Wills C, Franklin M, Holmes-Rovner M. Feasibility and outcomes testing of a patient-centered depression support intervention for depression in people with diabetes. Paper presented at the 4th International Shared Decision Making Conference. Freiburg (Germany), May 30, 2007.

64. Wills CE, Holmes-Rovner M. Integrating decision making and mental health interventions research: research directions. Clin Psychol (New York) 2006;13:9–25.

65. Levenstein JH, McCracken EC, McWhinney IR, et al. The patient-centered clinical method. 1. A model for the doctor-patient interaction in family medicine. Fam Pract 1986;3:24–30.

66. Charles C, Gafni A, Whelan T. Decision-making in the physician-patient encounter: revisiting the shared treatment decision-making model. Soc Sci Med 1999;49:651–61.

67. Alexopoulos GS, Bruce ML. A model for intervention research in late-life depression. Int J Geriatr Psychiatry 2009;24:1325–34.

Index

Note: Page numbers of article titles are in **boldface** type.

Psychiatr Clin N Am 34 (2011) 501–509
doi:10.1016/S0193-953X(11)00039-6
0193-953X/11/$ – see front matter © 2011 Elsevier Inc. All rights reserved.

psych.theclinics.com